Pharmaceutical Chemistry II

Dr. H.P.Tipnis
M.Sc (Tech), M.S., Ph.D (USA)
Former Principal, Bombay College of Pharmacy, Mumbai
Currently : Corporate Advisor, Medicine Shoppe, Mumbai

Dr. A.S.Dhake
Ph.D (Tech.)
Principal, L.B.Rao Institution of Pharmaceutical Education & Research,
Khambhat, Dist.Anand, Gujarat

CAREER
Publications

Pharmaceutical Chemistry II

First Edition : July 2007
First Edition Reprint : September 2009

ISBN : 978-81-88739-51-6

Published by :
Nishad Deshmukh
Career Publications

Reg. Office :
432/B, Deshmukh Bunglow,
Vakil Wadi, Nashik - 422 001.
Maharashtra, India.

Communication Address :
First Floor, Kaveri Smruti,
Ashok Stambh, Nashik - 422 001
Maharashtra, India.
Ph.: (0253) 2311210, 2310421, 2311422, 2576175.
E-mail : publications@careerandyou.com
Visit us : www.careerandyou.com

Pune Office :
First Floor, Gokhale Building,
Tilak Road, Pune - 411 030
Maharashtra, India.
Ph. : (020) 24497602
careerpune@careerandyou.com

Typesetting :
Career Publications

Printer :
Replica Printers
Nashik

Price : Rs. 140/-

Production Y/E/ Pharmaceutical Chemistry - II

(Dhake Sir)

Dedicated to the memory of

Late Prof. E.C. Jorgensen

Professor of Pharmaceutical Chemistry
School of Pharmacy,
University of California,
San Francisco, U.S.A.

"He not only taught me the basics of Pharmaceutical Chemistry, but also how to teach this complex subject; which inspired me to become a teacher of this subject."

Dr. H.P.Tipnis

OUR EARLIER PUBLICATIONS

For B. Pharm

1) Career in Pharmacy : Thoughts & Views : Mr. Milind Wagh
2) Inorganic Pharmaceutical Chemistry (Theory) : Dr. Tipnis & Dr. Dhake
3) Inorganic Pharmaceutical Chemistry (Practical) : Mr. Belsare & Dr. Dhake
4) Anatomy Physiology and Health Education : Mr. Rahul Phate
5) Modern Dispensing Pharmacy : Dr. Pawar & Dr. Gaud
6) Experimental Pharmaceutical Organic Chemistry - A Benchtop Manual : K.S. Jain, P.B. Miniyar & T.S. Chitre
7) Practical Physical Pharmacy : H.N. More & A.A. Hajare
8) Pharmaceutical Microbiology -Experiments and Techniques : Dr. C. R. Kokare
9) Biostatistics : Dr. Sai Subramanian
10) Pathophysiology for Pharmacy : Dr. Prakash Ghadi
11) Introduction to Clinical Biochemistry : Dr. (Mrs.) Dandekar
12) Pharmaceutical Analysis - I (Practical) : Mrs. Sheorey & Ms. Honrao
13) Pharmacology for Pharmacy : Dr. Vivek Bele
14) Pharmacognosy & Phytochemistry Part - I : Dr. Vinod Rangari
15) Pharmacognosy & Phytochemistry Part -II : Dr. Vinod Rangari
16) Principles & Applications of Biopharmaceutics and Pharmacokinetics : Dr. Tipnis & Dr. Amrita Bajaj
17) Business Accounting : Dr. Mahesh Kulkarni
18) Managerial Economics : Prof. Geet, Prof. Morajkar & Mr. Wagh
19) Industrial Psychology and Sociology : Mr. Milind Wagh
20) A Handbook of Experiments in Pre-clinical Pharmacology : Sanjay Kasture
21) Introduction to Pharmaceutics : Dr. A.P. Pawar
22) Pharmaceutical Analysis - III As per RGTU (Bhopal) : N.P. Sengar, R. Agrawal, A. Singh

For D. Pharm

1) Human Anatomy & Physiology : Mr. Rahul Phate
2) Text Book of Biochemistry & Clinical Pathology : Mr. Umekar, Mr. Lohiya, Mr. Kotagale
3) Theory and Practice Pharmaceutics - I : Dr. A.P. Pawar
4) Theory and Practice Pharmaceutics - II : Dr. A.P. Pawar
5) Pharmaceutical Chemistry II : Dr. A.S. Dhake
6) Handbook for Community Pharmacists (Exclusively for Chemists and Druggists) : Dr. A.P. Pawar

Reference Books ....

1) Clinical Pharmacy : Dr.H.P. Tipnis & Dr. Amrita Bajaj
2) Hospital Pharmacy : Dr. Tipnis & Dr. Amrita Bajaj

For GATE Study ....

1) GATE : A Companion (for pharmacy) : Mrs.N.N.Inamdar
2) Pharmacy GATE Solved Question Papers (1988-2006) : Mrs.N.N.Inamdar
3) Career GATE Postal Test Series : For details write to us

Foreign Titles

1) Lexi-com's Pharmacogenomics Handbook : Cavallari, Ellingrod & Kolesar

Preface

This text book of Pharmaceutical Chemistry - Part II, is written for Diploma in Pharmacy (D.Pharm.) students, who will be entering the Second year of their course. The book is written according to the syllabus of the Education Regulations 1991, as notified by the Pharmacy Council of India.

Part II of the pharmaceutical chemistry course of D.Pharm. consists of chemistry of drugs and their therapeutic usage. The book is therefore written to cover the basic part of chemistry of drugs of each class, their therapeutic uses and doses. Structures are also given wherever required and as indicated in the syllabus. Although chemistry of drugs is a very vast subject and volumes have been written, this book contains only the information on selected drugs which are commonly used. The pharmacological classification of drugs is the basis of the chapters, since it is logical that drugs be identified by their therapeutic use, rather than their chemical class. But within the class of similar pharmacological action, drugs are further sub-classified according to their chemical groups, which make it easy to relate the active part of the drug molecule to its therapeutic action. Synthesis of drugs is not included in this book, as it does not form a part of the syllabus.

The authors are thankful to Career Publications, Nashik, for bringing out the book in an attractive form and at the proper time to make it available to students and teachers. We are grateful to the staff and students of the Bombay College of Pharmacy, Bombay, N.D.M.V. P. Samaj's College of Pharmacy, Nashik and L.B.Rao Institute of Pharmaceutical Education and Research, Khambhat for the encouragement given by them in preparing the manuscript. We are open to criticism and suggestions for any further improvement of this book.

Dr. H.P.Tipnis
Dr. A.S.Dhake

Syllabus

(Education Regulation - 1991)

1. Introduction to the nomenclature of organic chemical systems with particular reference to heterocyclic system containing up to 3 rings.
2. The chemistry of following pharmaceutical organic compounds, covering their nomenclature, chemical structure, uses and the important physical and chemical properties [chemical structure of only those compounds marked with asterisk (*)].

   The stability and storage conditions and the different type of pharmaceutical formulations of these drugs and their popular brand names.

- **Antiseptics and Disinfectants** - Proflavine*, benzalkonium chloride, cetrimide, chlorocresol*, chloroxylenol, formaldehyde solution, hexachlorophene, liquified phenol, nitrofurantoin.
- **Sulphonamides** - Sulphadiazine, sulphaguanidine*, phthalylsulphathiazole, succinylsulphathiazole, sulphadimethoxine, sulphamethoxypyridazine, sulphamethoxazole, cotrimoxazole, sulfacetamide*.
- **Antileprotic Drugs** - Clofazimine, thiambutosine, dapsone*, solapsone.
- **Anti-tubercular Drugs** - Isoniazid*, PAS*, streptomycin, rifampicin, ethambutol*, thiacetazone, ethionamide, cycloserine, pyrazinamide*.
- **Antiamoebic and Anthelmintic Drugs** - Emetine, metronidazole*, halogenated hydroxyquinolines, diloxanide furoate, paramomycin, piperazine*, mebendazole, D.E.C*.
- **Antibiotics** - Benzyl penicillin*, phenoxy methyl penicillin*, benzathine penicillin, ampicillin*, cloxacillin, carbenicillin, gentamicin, neomycin, erythromycin, tetracycline, cephalexin, cephaloridine, cephalothin, griseofulvin, chloramphenicol.
- **Antifungal agents** - Undecylenic acid, tolnaftate, nystatin, amphotericin, hamycin.
- **Antimalarial Drugs** - Chloroquine*, amodiaquine, primaquine, proguanil, pyrimethamine*, quinine, trimethoprim.
- **Tranquilisers** - Chlorpromazine*, prochlorperazine, trifluoperazine, thiothixene, haloperidol*, triperidol, oxypertine, chlordiazepoxide, diazepam*, lorazepam, meprobamate.
- **Hypnotics** - Phenobarbital*, butobarbital, cyclobarbital, nitrazepam, glutethimide*, methyprylone, paraldehyde, triclofos sodium.
- **General Anesthetics** - Halothane*, cyclopropane*, diethyl ether*, methohexital sodium, thiopental sodium, trichloroethyelene.
- **Antidepressant Drugs** - Amitriptyline, nortriptyline, imipramine*, phenelzine, tranylcypromine.
- **Analeptics** - Theophylline, caffeine*, coramine*, dextroamphetamine.
- **Adrenergic Drugs** - Adrenaline*, noradrenaline, isoprenaline*, phenylephrine, salbutamol, terbutaline, ephedrine*, pseudoephedrine.
- **Adrenergic Antagonists** - Tolazoline, propranolol*, practolol.
- **Cholinergic Drugs** - Neostigmine*, pyridostigmine, pralidoxime, pilocarpine, physostigmine*.

- **Cholinergic Antagonists** - Atropine*, hyoscine, homatropine, propantheline*, benztropine, tropicamide, biperiden*.
- **Diuretic Drugs** - Furosemide*, chlorothiazide, hydrochlorothaizide, benzthiazide, urea*, mannitol*, ethacrynic Acid.
- **Cardiovascular Drugs** - Ethyl nitrite*, glyceryl trinitrate, alpha methyl dopa, guanethidine, clofibrate, quinidine.
- **Hypoglycemic Agents** - Insulin, chlorpropamide*, tolbutamide, glibenclamide, phenformin*, metformin.
- **Coagulants and Anti-Coagulants** - Heparin, thrombin, menadione*, bishydroxycoumarin, warfarin sodium.
- **Local Anaesthetics** - Lignocaine*, procaine,*, benzocaine.
- **Histamine and Anti-histaminic Agents** - Histamine, diphenhydramine*, promethazine, cyproheptadine, mepyramine, pheniramine, chlorpheniramine*.
- **Analgesics and Antipyretics** - Morphine, pethidine*, codeine, methadone, aspirin*, paracetamol*, analgin, dextropropoxyphene, pentazocine.
- **Non-steroidal anti-inflammatory Agents** - Indomethacin*, phenylbutazone*, oxyphenbutazone, ibuprofen.
- **Thyroxine and Antithyroids** - Thyroxine*, methimazole, methylthiouracil, propylthiouracil.
- **Diagnostic Agents** - Iopanoic acid, propyliodone, sulphobromophthalein sodium indigotindisulphonate, Indigo carmine, Evans blue, Congo red, fluorescein sodium.
  *Anticonvulsants, cardiac glycosides, antiarrhythmic antihypertensives & vitamins.
- **Steroidal Drugs** - Betamethasone, cortisone, hydrocortisone, prednisolone, progesterone, testosterone, estradiol, nandrolone.
- **Anti-neoplastic Drugs** - Actinomycins, azathioprine, busulphan, chlorambucil, cisplatin cyclophosphamide, daunorubicin hydrochloride, fluorouracil, mercaptopurine, methotrexate, mitomycin.

Contents

① Nomenclature of Organic Compounds

"*Chemical Abstracts*" Index nomenclature is the generally accepted standard for chemical nomenclature.

Functions

It is customary to use the term "function" to mean, any atom, group, or arrangement which causes a compound to behave in some characteristic way. Functions are denoted by prefixes or suffixes (e.g., hydroxy and ol for alcohols) according to circumstances.

When a molecule contains more than one kind of functions, then the principal or chief function is expressed in the end of the name and the other functions are denoted by prefixes (as aminobenzoic acid). There are, however, few exceptions to this rule such as ethanolamine.

Order of precedence of functions

The order used by "*Chemical Abstracts*" (C.A.) in descending order is, onium compounds, acids, acid halides, amides, imides, phenols, thiols, amines, oxyamines ($RONH_2$), imines, ethers, sulfides, sulfoxides and sulfones.

Determination of Principal Compound

The largest size structural unit within the compound in question (or longest aliphatic chain) is usually taken for naming the principal or parent compound from which it is derived. This rule is modified, however, by the principle of "treating like things alike". For example, $C_6H_5CH_3$ is called either toluene or methylbenzene rather than phenylmethane. However, $C_6H_5CH_2C_6H_5$ is called diphenylmethane rather than α-phenyltoluene.

Formation of Names of Radicals

Aliphatic hydrocarbons

(1) **Univalent radicals** from alkanes are named by replacing the ending -ane of the hydrocarbon by the ending -yl. eg. methyl, ethyl etc.

(2) **Univalent radicals** from alkenes have endings of -enyl, -ynyl, -dienyl, etc. eg. CH_2=CH- ethenyl (or vinyl), CH_3CH=$CHCH_2$- 2-butenyl.

(3) **Bi or trivalent radicals** from alkanes through removal of the hydrogens from one C atom, the ending -ane is replaced by -ylene or -ylidene. eg. $-CH_2$ methylene, CH_3CH ethylidene.

(4) **Bivalent radicals** formed by removing a H atom from each of two terminal C atoms are named as ethylene, trimethylene, tetramethylene, etc.

(5) **Radicals derived from acids** by removal of -OH are named by changing the ending carboxylic to carbonyl or the ending -oic is changed to -oyl.eg. $C_{12}H_{25}CO$- Tridecanoyl or dodecane-carbonyl.

Aromatic hydrocarbons

Univalent radicals formed by removal of one H atom from the ring are generally named by changing the -ene to -yl. However, the radicals C_6H_5- and $C_6H_5CH_2$ - are named phenyl and benzyl, respectively.

Heterocyclic compounds

Radicals formed by the removal of the H atom from the ring are named changing the ending to -yl. In cases where this would cause ambiguity, only the final e is changed to -yl. eg. pyridine-pyridyl, indole-indolyl, pyrroline-pyrrolinyl, triazole-triazolyl.

Mixed compounds

Radicals formed by removal of a H atom from a side chain of a cylic compound are regarded as substituted aliphatic radicals. eg. $C_6H_5CH_2CH_2CH_2$- 3-phenylpropyl.

Radicals not provided for in the above rules are named by compounding two or more approved names, as dimethylamino $(CH_3)_2N$-.

Numbering

Aliphatic compounds

The "fundamental chain" is numbered from end to end with arabic figures in such a way that the lowest numbers are given in order of preference, first, to the principal function, then to double bonds, then triple bonds, then for point of attachment (of side chains), then for substituents.eg. - $CH_3CH_2CH_2CH(CH_2CH_2Br)CH_2OH$, is named as 2-(2 bromoethyl)-1-pentanol.

The use of primes ('), seconds ("), and indices (as, [2]) are reserved for cases where they are more necessary, as, when trivial names are used in aliphatic acids the carbon atom of the -COOH group is numbered 1. Acid derivatives, like butyryl chloride or propionamide are numbered correspondingly.

Ring compounds

For designating benzene derivatives the conventional abbreviations o-, m-, and p- are used when they cause no ambiguity, otherwise the numbers 1 to 6 are preferred.

The numbering of ring systems conform to the IUPAC 1957 rules, with the exceptions as follows - acridine, anthracene, carbazole, cyclopentano-phenanthrene, phenanthrene, purine and 9H-purine, xanthene and thioxanthene.

Mixed compounds

Where conjunctive names are used, such as, naphthalenepropionic acid, Greek letters are usually used for the side chain. In such cases, the C atom next to the -COOH group is labeled α. With compounds such as butyrophenone, numbers are used for the aliphatic portion and primed numbers for the ring. ($CH_3CH_2CH_2COC_6H_5$, butyrophenone).

'Extra hydrogen' containing compounds

Numbers followed by H are used to indicate the position of hydrogen necessary for the existance of the compound, thus 2H-1, 3-oxazine denotes an oxazine in which there is a CH_2 group instead of CH at position 2 (O at position 1, N at 3), and 3(4H)- quinolone is equivalent to 3, 4-dihydro-3-oxoquinoline.

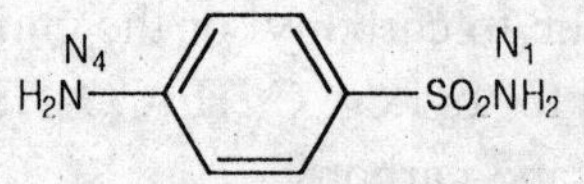

Sulfanilamide

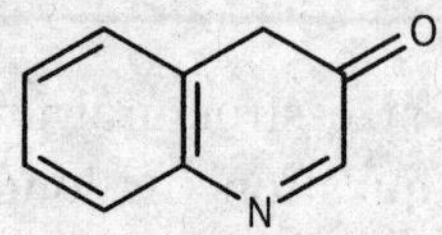

3 (4H) - Quinolone

Naming Heterocyclic Systems

Where common names are lacking, systematic names are formed, the hetero atoms being denoted by the prefixes oxa-, thio-, aza-, and the size of the ring is indicated by characteristic syllables.

Syllable endings indicating heterocyclic ring sizes

3-membered rings end in -ir; 4-membered rings end in -et;

5-membered rings end in -ole; 6-membered rings end in -ine;

7-membered rings end in -ep; 8-membered rings end in -oc.

Naming the parent or principal structure

Preference is given to the largest nitrogenous sytem present; if none is present, then the largest hetero system of any kind is preferred.

Naming hetero systems having side chains

The name of the hetero system is frequently given preference, with the various derivatives, side chains, etc. being indicated by prefixes.

Order of precedence of hetero atoms

The order used is the same for numbering and for combining prefixes in naming. The order is O, S, (Se, Te), N, P, (As, Sb, ...) etc.

Numbering heterocyclic compounds

Numbering starts so as to give first the preferred hetero atom, followed by the other hetero atoms, in order, as low numbers as possible. Example, 5-membered ring compound containing O and N as hetero atoms is an oxazole, ox (oxygen no. 1), az (nitrogen no. 3), the ending -ole indicates the 5-membered ring.

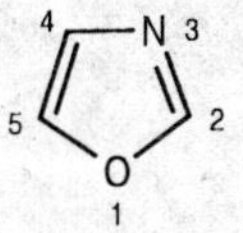

Naming of The Various Classes of Principal or Parent Compounds

Acid anhydrides

Acid anhydrides are designated according to the names of the corresponding acids. eg. acetic anhydride, benzoic anhydride.

Acid halides

Acid halides are named by combining the name of the halogen with the name of the acid radical as acetyl chloride, benzoyl chloride, succinyl chloride.

Acids

A choice is permitted between two systems of nomenclature.

1) **Geneva System** - Wherein the aliphatic acids are regarded as being derived from hydrocarbons of the same number of C atoms.
2) **Carboxylic Nomenclature** - Wherein the acids are regarded as derived from the hydrocarbons by substitution of COOH for a hydrogen atom.

Note : Common or trivial names may also be used.

Examples of nomenclature of acids are,

$CH_3CH_2CH_2COOH$ Butanoic acid
4 3 2 1

$CH_3CH_2CH_2COOH$ 1-propanecarboxylic acid
3 2 1

$CH_3CH_2CH_2COOH$ α butyric acid
γ β α

Notice the numbering and lettering used with the different systems.

The common names and structures of a number of the more commonly used (in pharmaceutical chemistry) acids are,

$CH_2=CHCOOH$	Acrylic acid
$CH_2=C(CH_3)COOH$	Methacrylic acid
$CH_3CH=CHCOOH$	Crotonic acid

$CH_2CH{=}CHCOOH$ Hydrosorbic acid
C_2H_5 (attached to the first C)

C_6H_5COOH Benzoic acid (Benzenecarboxylic acid).

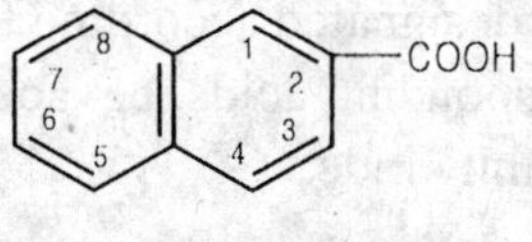

2-Napthoic Acid
(2-Napthalenecarboxylic acid)

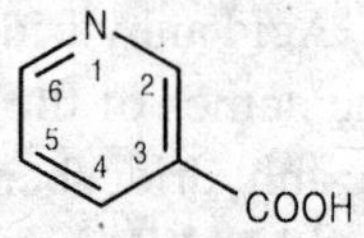

Nicotonic Acid
(3-Pyridinecarboxylic acid)

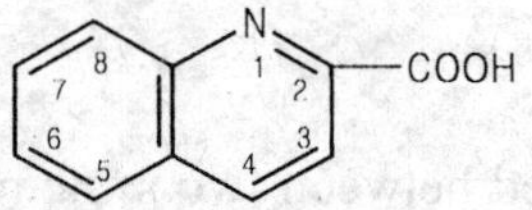

Quinaldic acid
(2-Quinolinecarboxylic acid)

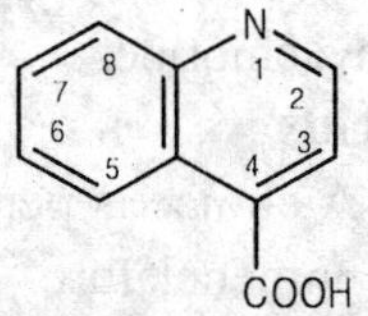

Cinchoninic Acid
(4-Quinolinecarboxylic acid)

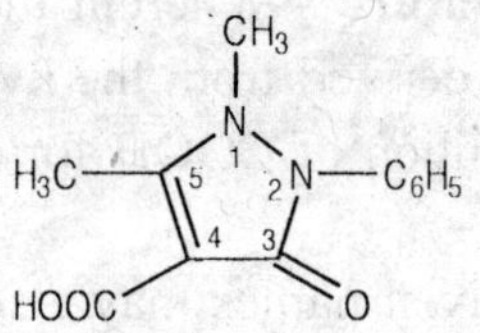

Antipyric acid
(2,3-dihydro-1,5-dimethyl -3-oxo-2-phenyl-4-pyrazole carboxylic acid)

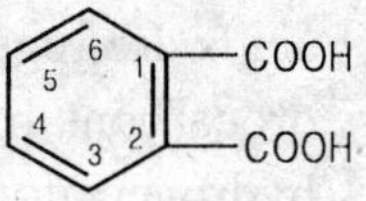

Phthalic acid
(1,2-benzenedicarboxylic acid)

In the naming of compounds having mixed functions, remember that the acid function is preceded only by the onium function so that most compounds containing acid function are given names based on that functional group with the other groups expressed as prefixes.

Amic and Anilic acids

When one carboxyl group of a dicarboxylic acid, having a common or trivial name, has become a carboxamide group, the resulting acid is named as an amic acid. eg. Malonamic acid H_2NOCCH_2COOH, Phthalamic acid p-$H_2NOCC_6H_4COOH$.

N-phenyl or substituted N-phenyl derivatives of such acids are named as anilic acids. Thus $C_6H_5NHOCCH_2CH_2COOH$, succinanilic acid.

However, a mono or diamide of a tricarboxyilc acid is not named in the above manner, but rather as a carbamyl derivative of the acid name of the compound when only the remaining COOH groups are considered. Thus $HOOCCH_2CH_2C(CH_3)(CONH_2)COOH$, is named α-methyl-α-carbamyl-glutaric acid.

Phenols

When no common name exists and the hydroxyl is the chief function, the name is formed by appending -ol to the name of the parent substance. In numbering, the -OH group is given the lowest possible number.

Amides

Amides are named like acids, with the word amide being added to the HC name, or if the carboxylic nomenclature is used, the name ending of carbonamide is used. Common names of acids may be used in naming amides by dropping the "ic acid" or "oic acid" and substituting the name amide to the root of the name.eg. acetamide, propionamide, valeramide, etc.

N-monoaryl derivatives are named as anilides, anisidides, phenetidides, toluidides, etc.

Amides in which the amide N atom is a part of a heterocyclic ring and the acyl group is a side chain, as with morpholides, piperidides, and N-acyl derivatives of other nitrogen heterocycles, are named as acyl derivatives of the ring.

eg.

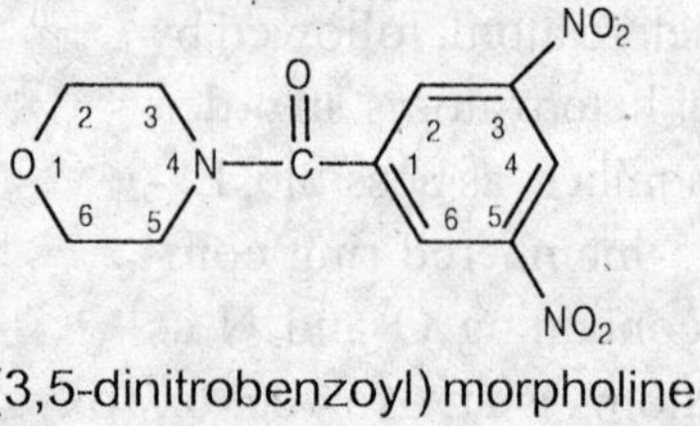

4(3,5-dinitrobenzoyl) morpholine

Carboxamide names take precedence over sulfonamide names, except for sulfanilamide and its derivatives. The radical $RNHSO_2$ is named by combining the name of the radical R with sulfamyl.

eg.

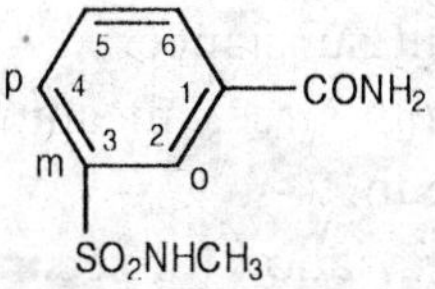

m-Methylsulfamylbenzamide

Amidines

Amidines are named by adding "amidine" to the name of the corresponding CH. If carboxyl is considered as a substituent the ending "carbonamidine" is used.

eg.

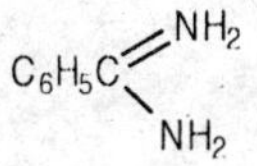

Benzamidine

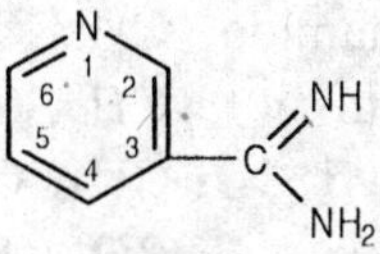

Nicotinamidine

Amines

Amines are named using either a common name or the HC name to which the suffix "amine" is added.

eg.

$C_6H_5NH_2$

Aniline

$H_2NCH_2CH_2NH_2$

Ethylenediamine

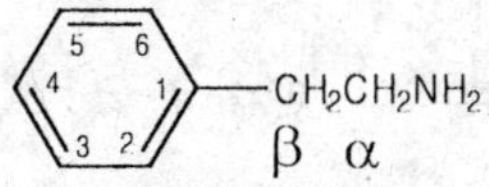

β-Phenythylamine

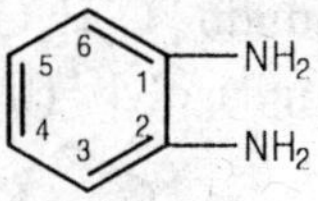

o-Phenylenediamine

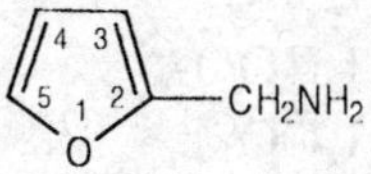

Furfurylamine

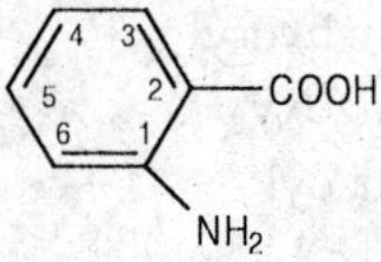

Anthranilic Acid

Note : This name as well as the common or trivial names for the ortho, meta, and para aminobenzene sulfonic acids, namely orthanilic acid, metanilic acid, and sulfanilic acid respectively, should not be confused with the mono-N-phenyl amides of dicarboxylic acids that are named as anilic acids.

Imides

Imides are compounds of a bivalent acid radical and an NH group or a substituted NH group, and thus are derivatives of ring systems. Common names or names derived from carboxylic names are used.

Names from carboxylic names are formed by changing "dicarboxylic acid" to "dicarboximide". Some names are

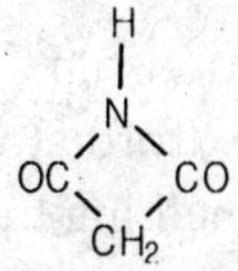

Malonimide

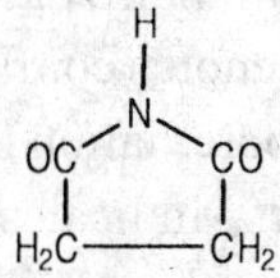

Succinimide (2,5-pyrrolidine-dione)

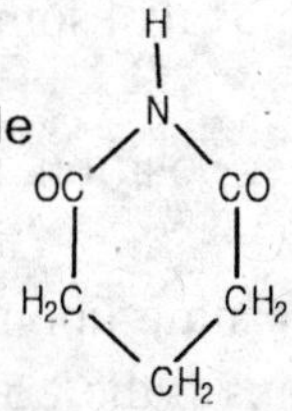

Glutarimide (2,6-piperidine-dione)

Onium compounds

Compounds containing an organic cation including compounds with the suffixes -onium, -olium, -inium, -ylium, -enium.

For aliphatic and cyclic compounds containing pentavalent nitrogen the ending -ine is changed to -onium or -inium, respectively. For those ending in -ole, the ending is changed to -olium. eg. pyridine-pyridinium, imidazole-imidazolium, amine-ammonium.

Ureides

Ureides are acyl derivatives of urea and are named as such; unless they are cyclic ureides when they may have names of their own as barbituric acid.

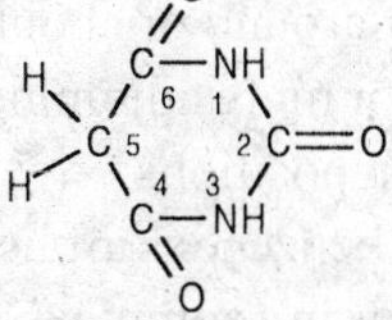

Barbituric acid (Malonylurea)

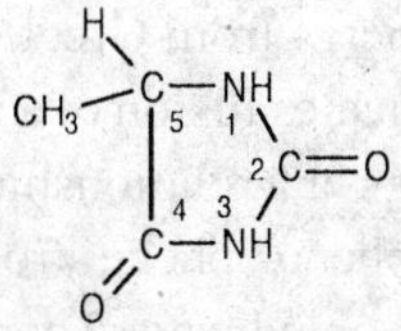

5-methylhydantoin

Miscellaneous Chemical Prefixes

allo - indicating close relationship, often the more stable of 2 geometric isomers.

amphi - from Greek meaning 'on both sides', indicating certain isomer.

apo - denoting formation from another compound.

bisnor - indicating removal of 2 carbon atoms with their H atoms.

D - denotes configurational relationship.

d - abbreviation for dextro-or dextrorotatory.

de,des - indicates removal of something from the molecule.

endo - indicates inner position, as in a ring, not side chain.

epi - from Greek meaning upon, on, to, denotes certain relationships as the 1,5 positions in naphthalene or a bridge connection 9, 10-epidioxy- (9, 10 per oxide)

gem - two groups attached to the same atom.

i - abbreviation for inactive or iso-

L - denotes configurational relationship.

l - abbreviation for levorotatory.

meso - from Greek meaning middle or intermediate.

n - abbreviation for normal.

neo - meaning new as a newer compound related in some way to an older one.

nor - from normal, indicates parent compound from which the compound is derived by removal of 1 or more C atoms with their H atoms.

per - meaning complete or extreme, denotes the highest oxidation state.

peri - from Greek meaning around or about, indicates fusion of a ring to 2 or more adjoining rings or a relationship between positions.

pheno-, phene - from phene, benzene as in phenyl, or indicates 2 benzene rings in a complex.

pro - from Greek meaning before, denotes an antecedent substance.

proto - from Greek meaning false indicates resemblance to.

sec - abbreviation for secondary.

syn - same as cis-meaning on same side.

t - abbreviation for tertiary.

v-, vic- abbreviation for vicinal.

Organic Groups And Radicals

acetamido CH_3CONH-
acetoxy CH_3COO-
acetyl CH_3CO-
alkoxy RO- ('R' is any alkyl radical)
allyl $CH_2=CHCH_2-$
amido $-CONH_2$ (properly, in acid groups only)
amino H_2N-
aniline C_6H_5NH-
azido/triazo $-N=N^+=N^-$
azino $=NN=$
azo $-N=N-$ (as connective)
azoxy $-N(O)N-$
benzamido C_6H_5CONH-
benzimidazolyl (from benzimidazole)

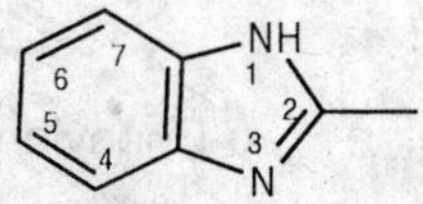

benzhydryl $(C_6H_5)_2CH-$
benzoxy C_6H_5COO-
benzoyl C_6H_5CO-
benzyl $C_6H_5CH_2-$
benzyloxy $C_6H_5CH_2O-$
carbamido/ureido $H_2NCONH-$
carbamoyl H_2NCO-
carbethoxy/ethoxycarbonyl $-C_2H_5OCO-$
carbonyl $C=O$
carboxy HOOC
cetyl/hexadecyl $-C_{16}H_3$
cinnamoyl $C_6H_5CH=CHCO-$
cinnamyl $C_6H_5CH=CHCH_2-$

crotyl - 2 - butenyl $CH_3CH=CH$
cysteinyl $HSCH_2CH(NH_2)CO-$
cystyl $-OCCH(NH_2)CH_2SSCH_2CH$
diazo -N=N
diazonium $N^+=N:$
dimethylamino $(CH_3)_2N-$
dimethylbenzoyl $(CH_3)_2C_6H_3CO$
diphenylmethyl $(C_6H_5)_2CH-$
diphenylmethylene $(C_6H_5)_2CH-$
epidoxy -CO- (to different atoms already united in some other way)
epithio -S- (as epidioxy above)
epoxy -O- (as epidioxy)
ethoxy C_2H_5O-
ethoxycarbonyl C_2H_5OOC-
ethoxyphenyl $C_2H_5OC_6H_4-$
ethylamino C_2H_5NH-
ethylene $-CH_2CH_2-$
ethylenedioxy $-OCH_2CH_2O-$
ethylidene $CH_3CH=$
ethynyl HC≡C
fluorenyl (9 shown)

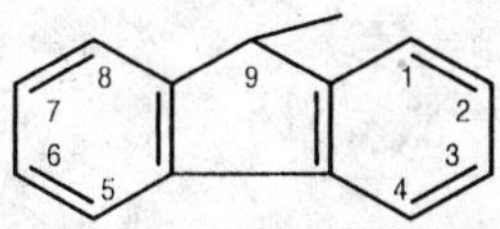

formamido OHCNH-
formyl OHC-
furfuryl

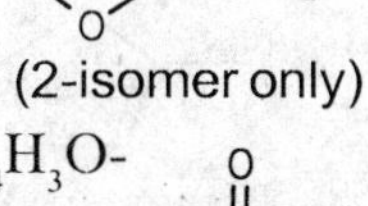

(2-isomer only)

furyl - (two isomers) C_4H_3O-
furoyl - (3-shown)

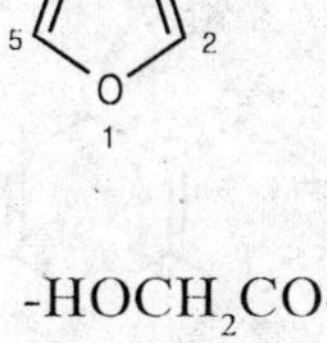

3-furylmethyl
glycolyl/glycololyl $-HOCH_2CO-$
glycyl H_2NCH_2CO-
glyoxalinyl or glyoxalyl/imidazolyl
glyoxylyl/glyoxyloyl -OHCCO-
guanidino - $H_2NC(=NH)NH-$
guanyl/amidino
hydrazi (to the same atom)
hydrazino H_2NNH-
hydrazo -NHNH-
hydroperoxy
hydroxy/hydroxyl -OH
hydroxymethyl $HOCH_2-$
hydroxyamino HONH

(-idene added to any radical usually means a double bond at point of attachment)

imidazolidinyl/imidazolydyl(5-shown)

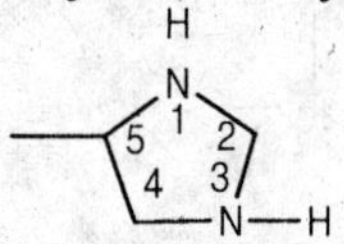

imidazolinyl (2 shown)

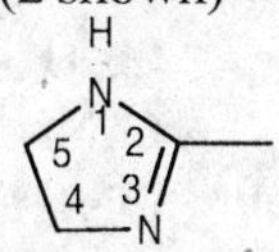

imidazolyl (2 shown)

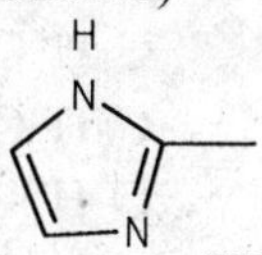

imino HN=
indanyl (C_9H_9-) (1-shown)

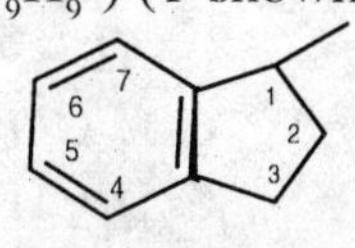

indenyl (C_9H_7-) (1-shown)

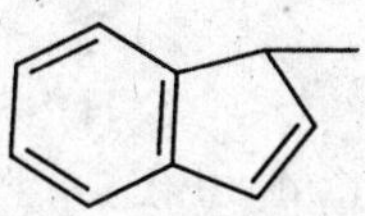

indolinyl (C_8H_8N-) (2-shown)

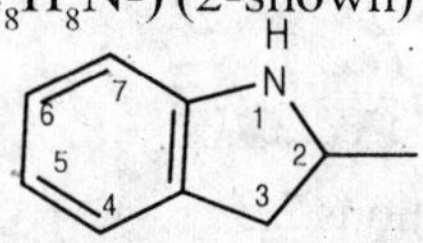

indolyl/indyl (C_8H_6N-) (2-shown)

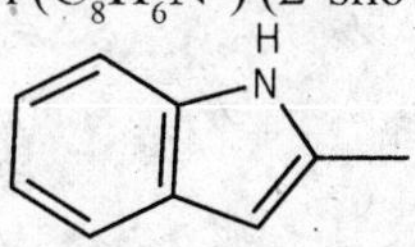

mercapto HS- (used only when unsubstituted)
mercuri -Hg-
methyllyl/2-methylallyl $CH_2{=}C(CH_3)CH_2$-
methene/methylene CH_2
methoxybenzoyl/anisoyl
(o,m or p-$CH_3OC_6H_4CO$-)
methylenedioxy -OCH_2O-
morpholino (4 position only)

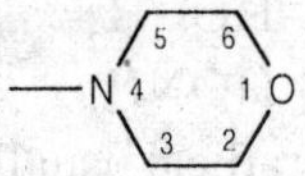

morpholinyl (position 2 or 3)

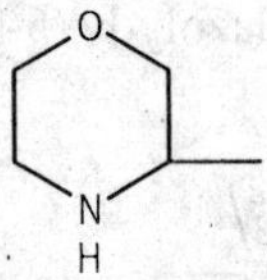

napthal/naphthylmethylene ($C_{10}H_7CH{=}$)
naphthyl $C_{10}H_7$-
nitro O_2N-
nitrosamino ONNH-
nitroso ON-
phenacyl $C_6H_5COCH_2$-
phenethyl $C_6H_5CH_2CH_2$-
phenyl C_6H_5-
phenylacetyl $C_6H_5CH_2CO$-
phenylcarbamoyl C_6H_5NHC0-
phenylene -C_6H_4-
α-phenylphenacyl C_6H_5COCH-
3-phenylpropyl $C_6H_5CH_2CH_2CH_2$-
phenylsulfamyl/phenulsulfamoyl
$C_6H_5NHSO_2$-
phenylsulfonyl $C_6H_5S_2$-
piperidino (1 position only)

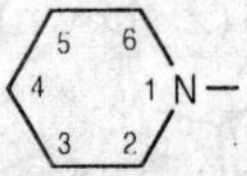

piperidyl (positions 2,3 or 4)

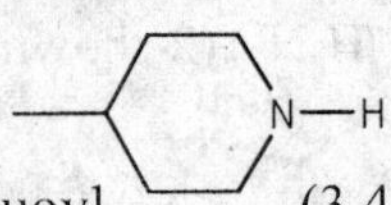

Protocatechuoyl (3,4-$(HO)_2$ C_6H_3CO-

salicyl o-$HOC_6H_4CH_2$-
salicyloyl o-HOC_6H_4CO-
styrene/phenylethylene
sulfamyl/sulfamoyl H_2NSO_2-
sulfanilamido p-$H_2NC_6H_4SO_2NH$-
sulfanilyl p-$H_2NC_6H_4SO_2$-
sulfhydryl/mercapto -SH
sulfino (HO)OS-
sulfo $(HO)O_2S$-
sulfonamido SO_2NH
sulfonyl/sulfuryl -SO_2
sulfinyl/thionyl -SO-
thio -S-
thenyl ($C_4H_3SCH_2$-) (3-shown)

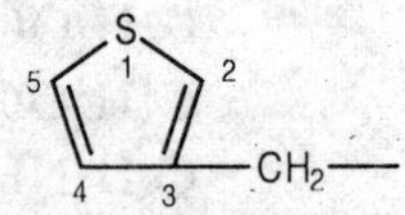

thienyl (C_4H_3S-) (2-shown)

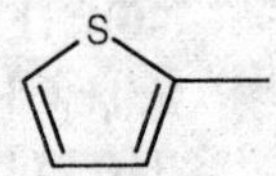

thiazinyl (C_4H_4NS-) (2H-1, 4 thiazin-6-yl shown)

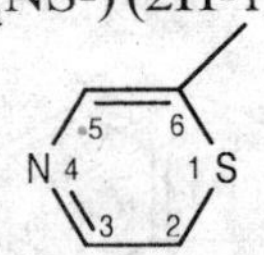

thiazolinyl (C_3H_4NS-) (4H-2-thiazolinyl-shown)

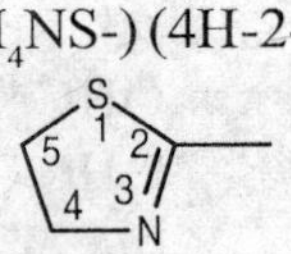

thiazolyl (5-shown)

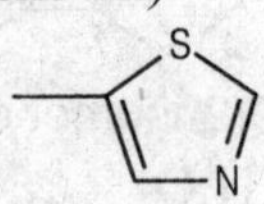

vinyl $CH_2{=}CH$-
xanthenyl/xanthyl ($C_{13}H_9O$-) (9-shown)

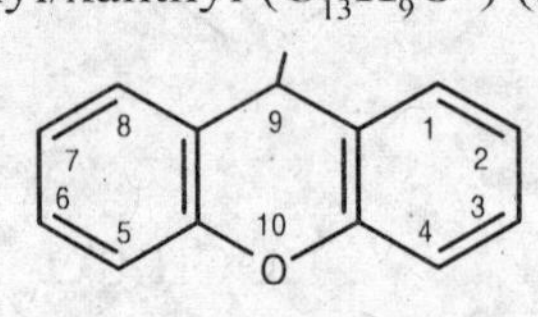

Organic Ring Systems

Nomenclature of heterocyclic compounds

Five membered rings with one hetero atom

Structures of the 3 parent ring systems containing 5 atoms are

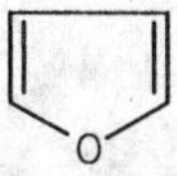
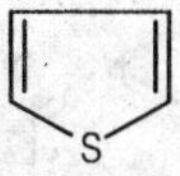
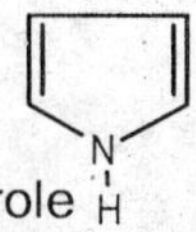

Furan Thiophene Pyrrole

The location of substitutents of these heterocyclic compounds is indicated by either Greek letters or number, eg.

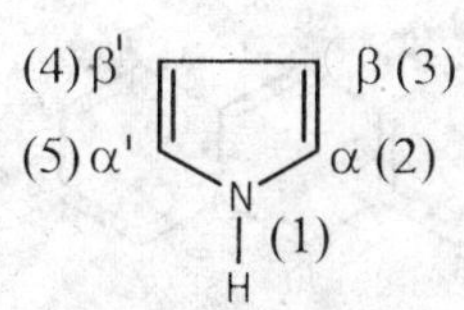

Pyrrole

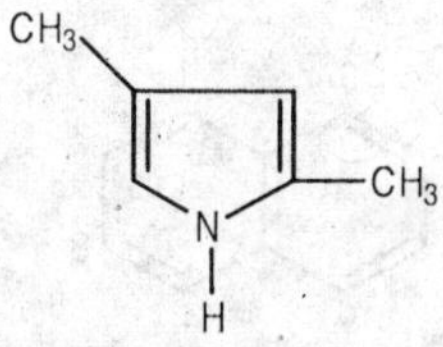

2,4 dimethyl pyrrole or α, β' dimethyl pyrrole

The positions 2,5 and 3,4 are identical in, monosubstituted derivatives.

Reduction products are named as follows:

Dihydro compounds, add suffix -ine to the name of parent compound, thus I becomes pyrroline. Tetrahydro compounds, add suffix -idine, thus II becomes pyrrolidine.

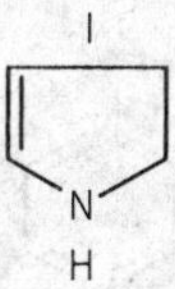

Pyroline

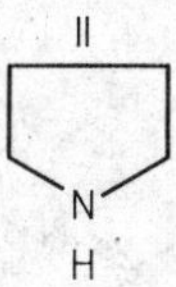

Pyrrolidine

These ring systems may be condensed in the ortho position with benzene ring to form.

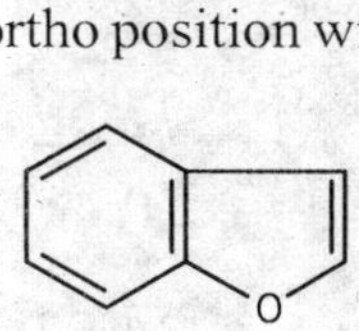

Benzofuran or Coumarone

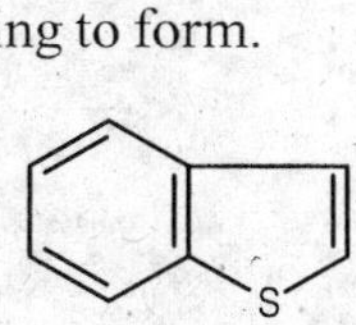

Benzothiophene

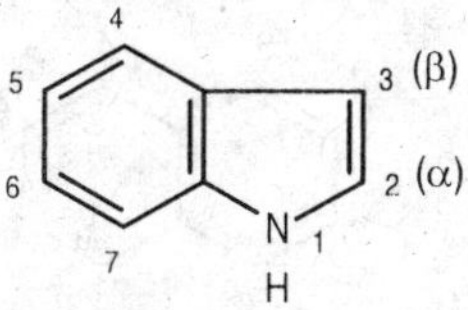

Benzopyrrole or Indole

In combining the prefixes, oxa- for oxygen, thia- for sulfur, and aza- for nitrogen, the same order of precedence is observed as is.used in numbering positions in a ring, i.es. oxygen, sulfur, nitrogen. The numbering starting with the preferred kind of hetero atom, as 1 thus giving hetero atoms, numbers as low as possible.

Five membered rings with 2 hetero atoms

Compounds belonging to this class that have an aromatic character and always contain one or more nitrogen atoms in the ring. They are known as azoles Example are,

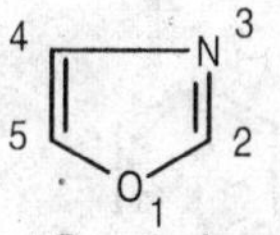
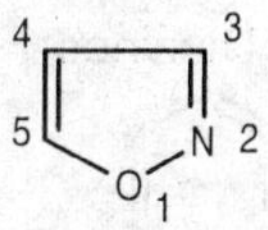
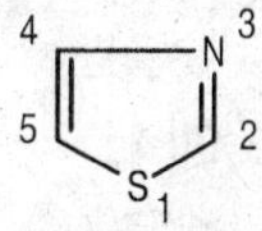

Oxazole Iso-oxazole Thiazole

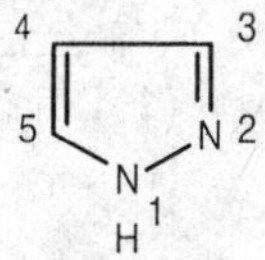
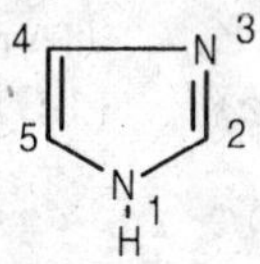

Pyrazole Imidazole

Six-membered rings with one hetero atom

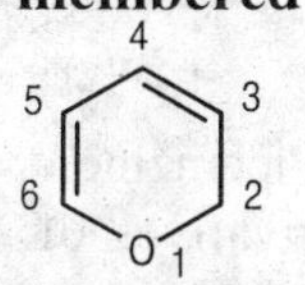
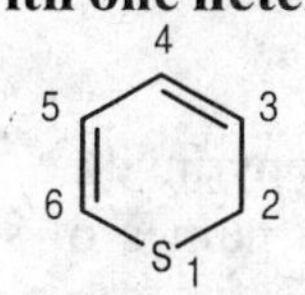

Pyran Thiopyran

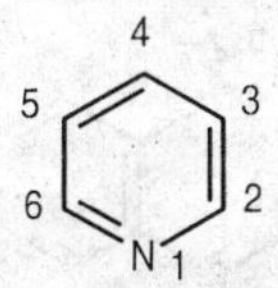
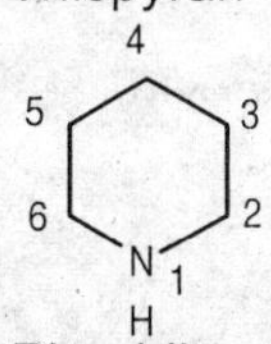

Pyridine Piperidine

The fully reduced pyridine ring is called piperidine. The condensed ring system consisting of a benzene ring fused on a pyran ring, produces benzopyran, while a benzene ring fused on a pyridine ring produces one of 2 common structures.

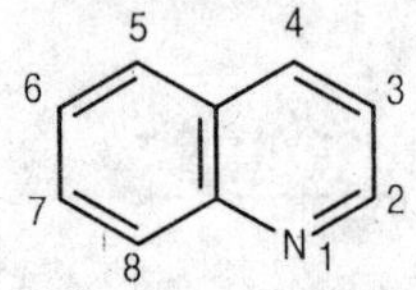

Quinoline

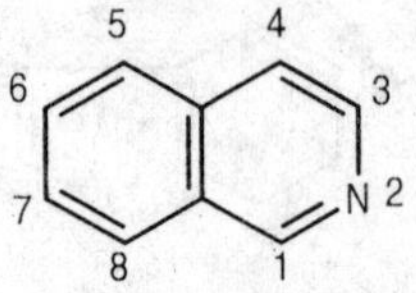

Isoquinoline

Two benzene rings fused onto a pyridine ring produce a di-benzopyridine structure commonly called acridine. Dibenzopyran is commonly called xanthene and is numbered like acridine.

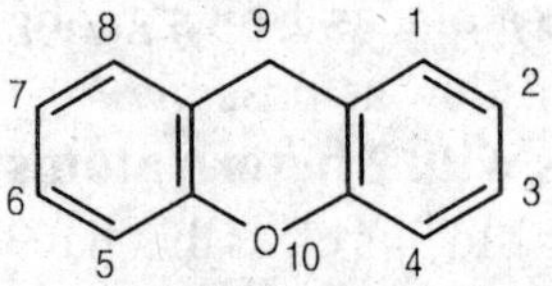

Xanthene

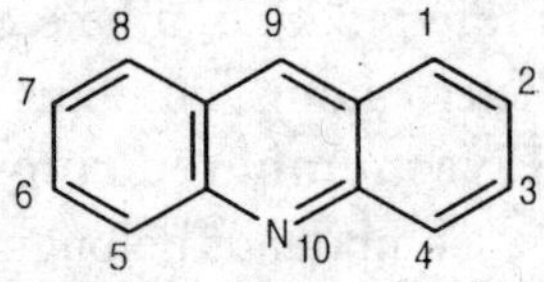

Acridine

Six-membered rings containing two nitrogen atoms

The Diazines

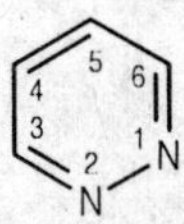

Pyridazine (1,2 diazine)

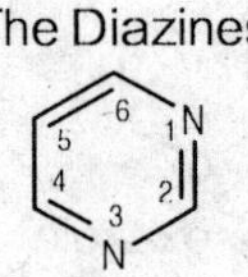

Pyrimidine (1,3 diazine)

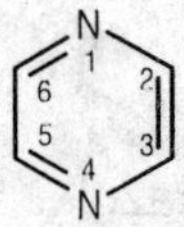

Pyrazine (1,4 diazine)

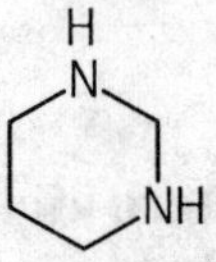

Perhydropyrimidine

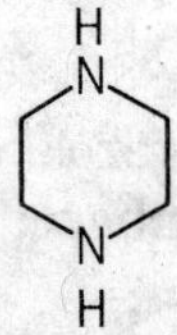

Piperazine

Common names of some derivatives of six-membered rings with two or more hetero atoms.

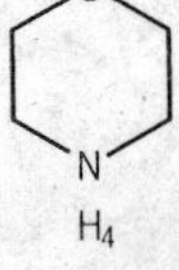

Morpholine

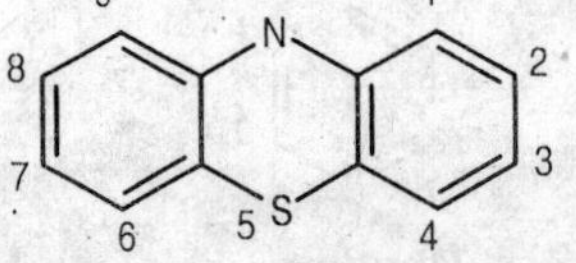

Phenothiazine

(Note the different numbering of these compounds)

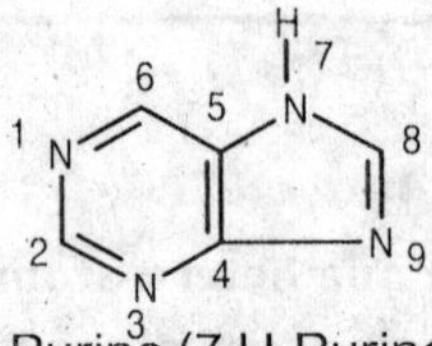

Purine (7 H-Purine)

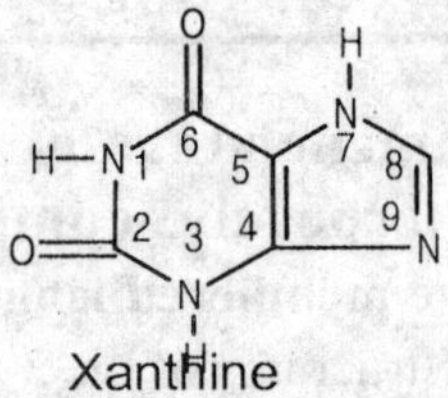

Xanthine

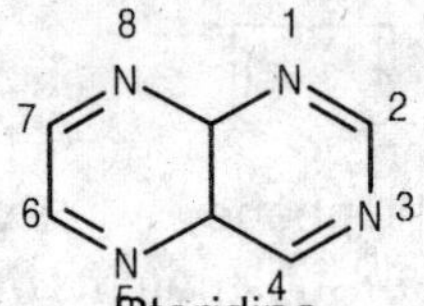

Pteridine

Other common aromatic ring systems

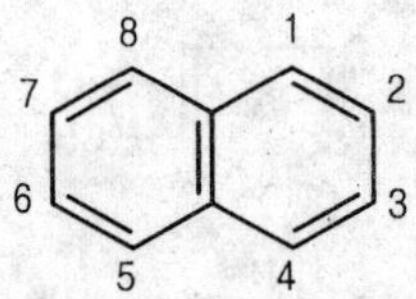

Naphthalene

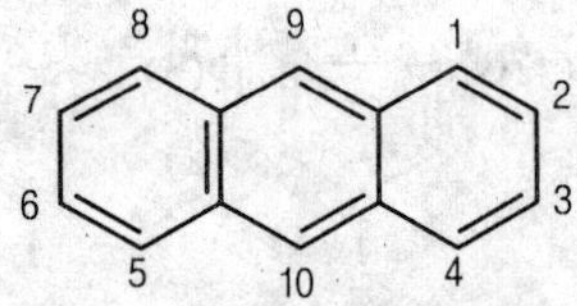

Anthracene

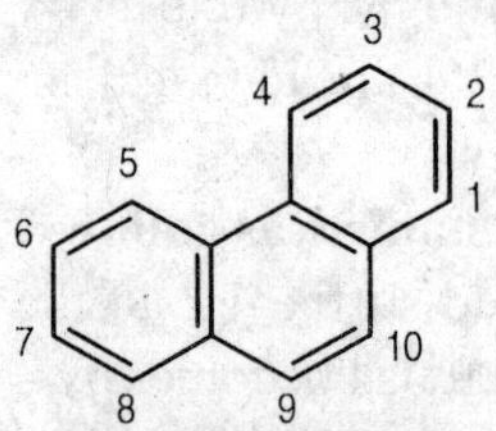

Phenanthrene

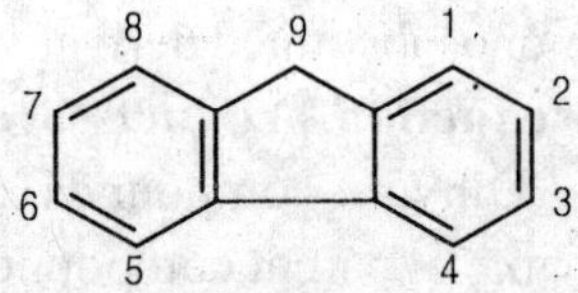

Fluorene

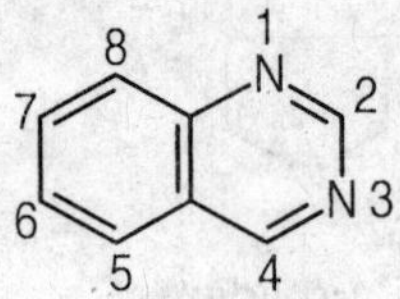

Quinazoline

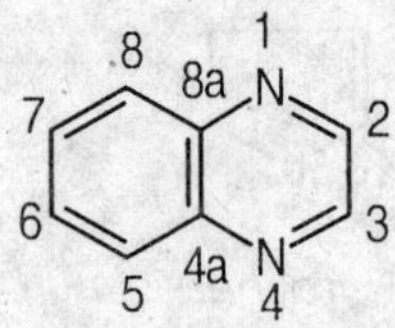

Quinoxaline

Exercise

Q1. Write the structures of the following and name one drug from each group.
1) Aziridine, 2) Imidazole, 3) Indole, 4) Isoxazole, 5) Piperazine, 6) Piperidine, 7) Pyrazole, 8) Pyrimidine, 9) Pyrrolidine, 10) Thiazole (Kachchh Univ. 06)

Q2. What are heterocyclic compounds? Write the structure of Indole, Pyrazine and Phenothiazine. (Karnataka Univ.)

Q3. Give structure and method of numbering of - a) Phenothiazine, b) Barbituric acid, c) Quinoline, d) Thiadiazole, e) Xanthine, f) 4-Imidazoline, g) Pyridazine, h) Furan, i) Acridine, j) Pyridine, k) Pyrazolidine, l) Imidazole, m) Purine, n) Pyrazine, o) Pyrimidine, p) Indole, q) Xanthine, r) Isoxazole, s) Benzimidazole, t) Dibenzoazepine, u) Pyrazole, v) Phenol, w) Thiazole, x) Pyrrole, y) Phthalazine, z) Pyrazoline, (Summer 03, Winter 04, Summer 06, Winter 06, May-June 04).

Q4. Write the formulae of the following - i) Allyl, ii) Acetylthio, iii) Ethoxycarboxyl, iv) Guanidino, v) Vinyl & vi) Glycyl. (Nov 06)

2 Antiseptics and Disinfectants

Antiseptics and disinfectants are local anti-infective agents. While both antiseptics and disinfectants are used with the purpose of destroying harmful microorganisms, antiseptics are applied to living tissues while disinfectants are applied to inanimate objects. Disinfectants are bactericidal and rapidly produce an irreversibly lethal effect. Antiseptics have a bacteriostatic effect and do not necessarily sterilise the surface under treatment. An ideal antiseptic should destroy bacteria, spores, fungi, viruses and other infective agents without harming the tissues of the host.

Classification of Local Anti-Infective Agents

Class	Examples
I) Alcohols and related compounds	Alcohol, formaldehyde
II) Phenolic compounds	Phenol, chloroxylenol hexachlorophene, chlorocresol,
III) Halogen containing compounds	Iodophors, Povidone-iodine
IV) Cationic surfactants	Benzalkonium chloride
V) Dyes	Gentian violet
VI) Mercury compounds	Nitromersol
VII) Nitrofuran derivatives	Nitrofurantoin
VIII) Acridine derivatives	Proflavine

I] Alcohols and related compounds

1) Alcohol

CH_3CH_2OH (Ethanol)

Alcohol is a mixture of 95 per cent ethanol and 5 per cent water (by volume).

Properties : It is a clear, colourless, mobile, volatile liquid with a characteristic spirituous odour and a burning taste. It is readily inflammable. It burns with a blue smokeless flame. it is miscible with water, with ether and with chloroform. When mixed with water, contraction of volume and rise of temperature occur. Specific gravity is about 0.81 and boiling point is about 78°C. Dilute alcohols of various strengths can be prepared by diluting alcohol with water. Proof spirit has a specific gravity of 0.92 and contains about 57.1 per cent $^{v}/_{v}$ of C_2H_6O. The strength of an alcoholic preparation may be given as number of degrees, proof spirit being taken as 100°. Absolute alcohol contains 99.0 to 100 per cent $^{v}/_{v}$ of C_2H_6O.

Storage : It should be stored in airtight containers, in a cool place away from fire.

Labelling - The label on the container should state 'Flammable'.

Actions and Uses : Alcohol is a valuable solvent and preservative. It is used in the manufacture of tinctures, spirits and many other galenical preparations. For external use, industrial methylated spirit may be used. Alcohol has a bactericidal action against most vegetative organisms in concentrations from 60 to 95 per cent $^{v}/_{v}$ but it is not effective against bacterial spores.

A concentration of 70 per cent $^v/_v$ is optimum for bactericidal action.

2) Formaldehyde solution (Formalin)

It is an aqueous solution containing about 36 per cent $^w/_w$ of formaldehyde, HCHO. Methanol is added to prevent polymerisation of formaldehyde to solid paraformaldehyde $(CH_2O)_n$.

Properties : It is a colourless liquid with a characteristic irritating odour and a burning taste. It is miscible with water and with alcohol. On standing, for long especially in the cold, a white cloudy deposit is formed due to separation of paraformaldehyde. This deposit disappears when the solution is warmed.

Storage : It should be stored in airtight containers in a moderately warm place (at temperature above 15°C).

Incompatibility : It is incompatible with ammonia, with gelatin and with oxidising agents.

Actions and Uses : Formaldehyde is a powerful antiseptic. However, it irritates the mucous membrane. It reacts with and precipitates proteins and hardens the skin. It is used in antiseptic mouth washes and gargles. A 1:5,000 dilution effectively inhibits any microbial growth. In gaseous form, it has been used to disinfect rooms, instruments and clothing, but it is used little these days. A 1:10 dilution with saline solution is used as a preservative for pathological specimens.

Preparations : Formaldehyde lotion, gel and tooth paste.

II] Phenolic compounds

1) Phenol

(Carbolic acid) C_6H_5OH

Properties : Phenol occurs as colourless to light pink needle shaped deliquescent crystals or crystalline masses. It has a characteristic odour and in dilute solution, has a sweetish pungent taste. It has a melting point of 40°C and boiling point of 181°C. It is soluble in water (1:15) and very soluble in alcohol, glycerin, fixed and volatile oils. It is soluble in petrolatum and liquid petrolatums (1:70). Phenol is readily soluble in alkalis, forming solutions of alkali phenoxides. With sodium hydroxide, it forms sodium phenoxide which is soluble in water. Though phenol is more stable than the other phenols, it gets slightly oxidised on exposure to air.

Storage : It should be stored in airtight containers, protected from light, in a cool place.

Actions and uses : Phenol is one of the oldest antiseptics. It was introduced in surgery by Sir Joseph Lister in the year 1867. Phenol has moderate bactericidal activity. It destroys to tissues and has caustic action. It is corrosive to the skin. A concentration of 1 per cent of phenol in water kills most vegetative bacteria within a few minutes. Phenol is used commonly in 0.1 to 1 per cent concentrations as an antipruritic in phenolated calamine lotion or as ointment or as aqueous solution. Solutions containing greater than 2 per cent of phenol should not be applied to body surfaces.

Preparations : Included in B.P.C. are alkaline phenol mouth wash, liquefied phenol, oily phenol injection, phenol and glycerol injection, phenol ear-drops, phenol gargle and phenol glycerin.

Liquefied Phenol : It contains 80 per cent $^w/_w$ of phenol. Phenol - 800 gm, purified water - to make 1000 gm.

The phenol is melted by warming on a water bath. Sufficient water is added to produce the required weight and it is mixed thoroughly.

Properties : It is a colourless liquid which may become pinkish blue on storage. It has a characteristic odour and is caustic.

Storage : It should be stored in a well closed container, protected from light. It may congeal or deposit crystals, if stored below 4°C. In such cases, it should be completely melted before use.

Incompatibility : Liquefied phenol should not be mixed with collodion, fixed oils or paraffins. In such cases, melted phenol should be used.

Actions and uses : Its applications are similar to those for phenol.

2) Hexachlorophene

2,2' Methylene bis (3,4,6 trichlorophenol)

Properties : It is a white or pale buff crystalline powder. It is odourless or has a slight phenolic odour. but It is practically insoluble in water, soluble in alcohol, acetone and lipid solvents. It is stable in air.

Storage : It should be stored in airtight containers, protected from light.

Actions and uses : Hexachlorophene is a useful antiseptic. It is effective against Gram-positive bacteria but is less effective against Gram-negative bacteria. It is used in soaps, creams, oils and other vehicles for topical application in a concentration of 0.25 to 3 per cent. On repeated use, it accumulates on the skin and gives a prolonged effect. Skin sensitisation may occur: being used repeatedly. It may get absorbed into the blood stream and damage the central nervous system. Hence, it should not be applied on broken skin and to infants.

Preparations : Concentrated hexachlorophene solution B.P.C.

Hexachlorophene dusting powder B.P.C.

Hexachlorophene mixture B.P.C.

3) Chlorocresol

Tineafax

4-Chloro-3-methyl phenol

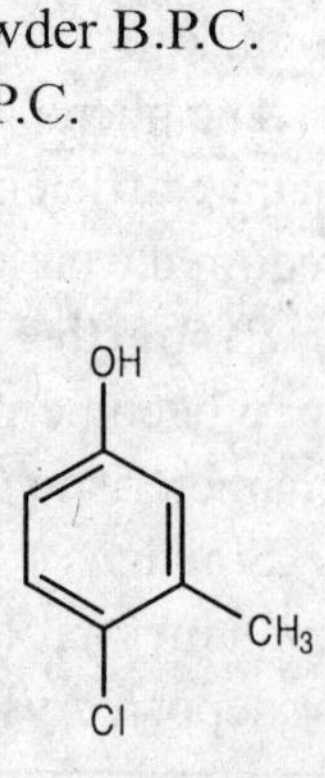

Properties : Chlorocresol occurs as colourless or faintly coloured crystals with a characteristic phenolic odour. It is volatile in steam. It is slightly soluble in water, soluble in hot water and readily soluble in alcohol. It is soluble in ether, in terpenes, in fixed oils, and in solutions of alkali hydroxides. It has a pKa of 9.2 and melting range of 64 to 66°C.

Storage : It should be stored in tightly closed containers.

Actions and uses : Chlorocresol is a powerful bactericide and fungicide of low toxicity. It is more active in acidic solution than in alkaline solutions. It is used in concentration of 0.2 per cent in the process of sterilising aqueous solutions and suspensions by heating with a bactericide. It is used in a concentration of 0.1 per cent as a bacteriostat. It can be used as a preservative in eye-drops at a concentration of 0.05 per cent. Concentrations greater than this should not be used in ophthalmic preparations. Chlorocresol is used as a preservative in creams and other externally used preparations. Its effectiveness is reduced if oils, fats or non-ionic surfactants are present.

Preparations : Solution containing 10 per cent of chlorocresol.

4) Chloroxylenol (Parachlorometaxylenol)

4-Chloro-3, 5-xylenol.

Properties : Chloroxylenol occurs as white or creamy white crystals or crystalline powder. It has a characteristic odour. It is volatile in steam. It is slightly soluble in water and is readily soluble in alcohol. It is soluble in ether, terpenes, fixed oils and in solutions of alkali hydroxides. It has a melting point of 115°C.

Actions and uses : Chloroxylenol is a relatively non-toxic and non-irritating antiseptic. It has useful antifungal properties. It is used topically in the treatment of tinea infections such as athlete's foot and jock itch. A 5 per cent solution is commonly used. Chloroxylenol solution is used as an antiseptic for the skin in surgical and obstetrical practise and also for cuts, wounds and abrasions.

Preparations : Included in the B.P.C. are chloroxylenol solution (Roxenol). This is an aqueous solution of chloroxylenol also containing soap (potassium oleate), terpinol and alcohol. It contains 5 per cent of chloroxylenol. Other preparations include cream, mouthwash and solution.

Chloroxylenol solution I.P.

Brand Names : Dettol®

III] Cationic surfactants

1) Benzalkonium chloride

Properties : It is a white, bitter tasting gel. It is freely soluble in benzene and very soluble in water and alcohol. Its aqueous solution is a clear, colourless or slightly yellow syrupy liquid. It has an aromatic odour and a very bitter taste. The solution is alkaline, turning litmus blue and foams strongly.

Benzalkonium chloride is a cationic surfactant belonging to the class of quaternary ammonium compounds. Its solution is official in I.P.

Storage : It should be stored in tightly closed, light resistant containers.

Incompatibility : It is incompatible with soaps and similar anionic compounds and alkali hydroxides. Incompatibilities have been reported with aluminium salts, fluorescein sodium, hydrogen peroxide, kaolin and some sulphonamides.

Actions and uses : Benzalkonium chloride possesses wetting, detergent and emulsifying actions. It is used as a surface antiseptic for intact skin and mucosa. For application to skin and to wounds and burns, dilutions of 1:500 to 1:2000 may be used. Dilutions of 1:20,000 are employed for irrigation of the bladder, urethra and vagina. It is used as a preservative for eye drops in a concentration of 0.01 per cent $^{w}/_{v}$. It is used in the form of lozenges to treat infections of the mouth and throat. Benzalkonium chloride solution, I.P. contains 50 per cent of benzalkonium chloride. Prolonged contact with skin leads to irritation.

Preparations : Benzalkonium lozenges B.P.C. Other preparations are cream, gel and solutions.

Brand Names : Ciplox® eye drops, Cifran® eye drops, Ciprobid® eye drops, Fairgenol-H®, Iteol-H®

IV] Nitrofuran derivatives

1) Nitrofurantoin

1-(5-Nitrofurfurylidene amino) imidazolidine 2-4, dione

Properties : Nitrofurantoin occurs as odourless lemon yellow crystals or fine powder. It has a bitter taste. It is very slightly soluble in water, alcohol and glycerol. It is soluble in dimethyl formamide. Melting point is 271°C.

Storage : It should be stored in tightly closed, light resistant containers in a cool place.

Actions and uses : Nitrofurantoin is a broad spectrum antibacterial agent. It is used in the treatment of urinary infections. It is well absorbed after oral administration.

Dose : 50 to 150 mg four times a day.

Preparations : Nitrofurantoin Tablets I.P., B.P.C.

Tablets containing 50 and 100 mg of nitrofurantoin.

Nitrofurantoin mixture B.P.C. This is a suspension of nitrofurantoin in a suitable flavoured vehicle. It is administered orally.

Other preparations include capsules and veterinary powder.

Brand Names : Furadantin®, Trifuran®

2) Cetrimide

It consists chiefly of tetradecyltrimethyl ammonium bromide along with small amounts of dodecyl and hexadecyl trimethylammonium bromide.

Properties : Cetrimide occurs as a white to creamy-white, voluminous, free-flowing powder. It has a faint characteristic odour and a bitter soapy taste. It is a quaternary ammonium compound freely soluble in water, soluble in alcohol and practically insoluble in ether. Melting range is 232°C to 247°C. At 20°C, at relative humidities of 40 to 50 per cent, it absorbs moisture causing caking of the powder. It is chemically stable in the dry state and in aqueous solution.

Storage : It should be stored in well-closed containers.

Incompatibility : It is incompatible with soaps and similar anionic compounds, with iodine, and with alkali hydroxides.

Actions and uses : Cetrimide is a relatively non-toxic antiseptic with detergent properties. Like other quaternary ammonium compounds, it is active against Gram-positive organisms but is less active against Gram-negative organisms. Aqueous solutions and creams containing 0.1 to 1 per cent may be used for treating wounds and burns, and cleaning skin. For cleansing and disinfection of vessels and apparatus, 0.5 to 1 per cent solutions may be used. Rubber articles are adversely affected by prolonged immersion. The presence of soaps, anionic compounds and organic matter greatly reduces the activity of quaternary compounds. Cetrimide is used in the preparation of cetrimide emulsifying wax, which is used as an emulsifying agent for preparing oil-in-water creams. Cetrimide is also used as a preservative in pharmaceutical and cosmetic preparations.

Preparations : Included in B.P.C. are

Cetrimide cream.

Cetrimide emulsifying ointment.

Cetrimide solution.

Strong cetrimide solution.

Brand Names : Aceptik®, Cetrim®, Iteol-3®, Scanbex® lotion, Ascabiol® emulsion, Scarab® cream

V] Acridine derivatives

1) Proflavine hemisulphate

Acridine - 3,6 - diamine sulphate dihydrate

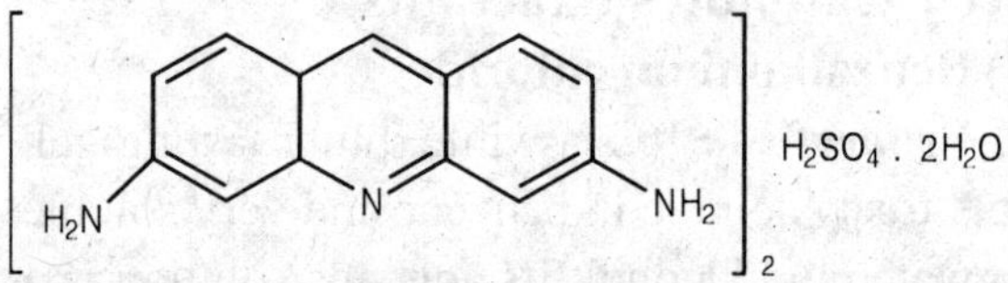

It is also called neutral proflavine sulphate.

Properties : It occurs as an orange to red crystalline powder. It is odourless and hygroscopic. It is slightly soluble in water at 20°C, but is freely soluble in boiling water. It is sparingly soluble in glycerol, very slightly soluble in alcohol and practically insoluble in ether and in chloroform.

Storage : It should be stored in airtight containers, protected from light.

Actions and uses : Proflavine is an acridine derivative. The acridine derivatives are slow-acting antiseptics which are effective against many Gram-positive and Gram-negative bacteria. They are used in the treatment of wounds and burns. For the dressing of wounds or burns, a 0.1 per cent solution of proflavine is used. Local infections of external ear, mouth, throat and skin may be treated using 0.1 to 1 per cent $^{w}/_{v}$ aqueous or alcoholic solutions. Acridine compounds stain the skin These stains are removed by washing with dilute hydrochloric acid.

Preparations : Proflavine cream B.P.C.

Drugs For Further Study

1) Povidone-Iodine - Betadine®, Povicidal®, Povid®, Wokadine®
2) Nitrofurazone - Emfurazone®, Furacin®
3) Sodium fusidate - Fucidin®, Fucinex®, Fusiwal®
4) Mupirocin - Bactroban®, Mupinova®, Mupirax®
5) Dichloroxylenol - Fairgenol® plain
6) Chlorhexidine - Microshield®, Newiteol-3®, Skeen® soap
7) Glutaraldehyde - Cadicide®, Cidex®
8) Triclosan - Gamophen®, Microshield-T®

Exercise

Q1. Write short note on - Antiseptics and disinfectants. (Kachchh Univ. 06)

Q2. Define antiseptics and disinfectants. Classify with examples. (Karnataka Univ.)

Q3. Write structures of - i) Proflavine and ii) Chlorocresol. (Winter 04)

Q4. Give uses of Cetrimide. (Winter 04)

Q5. Differentiate between "Disinfectants and Antiseptics" with suitable examples. Draw the structure of chloroxylenol. (Summer 03)

Q6. What are antiseptics and disinfectants? Give two examples from each. Discuss specific uses of ethanol and formaldehyde. (May-June 04)

Q7. Specify dosage forms (tablet, capsule etc..) for - Chloroxylenol. (May-June 04)

Q8. Write short note on - Antiseptics and disinfectant. (May 05)

■

3 Sulphonamides

Antimicrobial drugs have played a major role in reducing mortality rate due to communicable diseases. From the discovery of antimalarial properties of Peruvian bark in early seventeenth century to Ehrlich's magic antisyphilitic drug, Salvarsan, in 1909, little progress had been made in antimicrobial therapy. In 1933, Domagk introduced a bright red-coloured azo dye named Prontosil which showed good activity *in vivo* against staphylococcal and streptococcal infections. It was inactive *in vitro*. The activity *in vivo* was attributed to the metabolic conversion of prontosil to the active form, sulphanilamide. Observing the dramatic activity of prontosil, several sulphanilamide derivatives were synthesised. By the year 1948, more than 4500 sulphonamides were synthesised, of which, about 24 were introduced in medicine.

Sulphonamides are derivatives of sulphanilamide (p-aminobenzene sulphonamide).

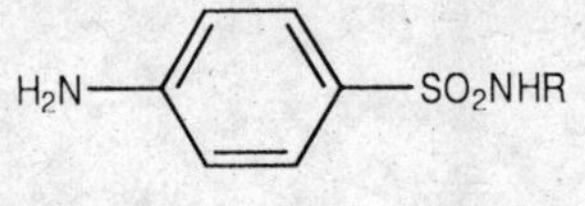

One of the hydrogen atoms of sulphonamido group is substituted by some other group.

After their invention, the sulphonamides were used indiscriminantly leading to the appearance of resistant strains. Also, sulphonamides caused toxic reactions in many patients. This led to the supercession of sulphonamides by modern antibiotics.

Mode of Action

Folic acid and its derivatives are essential for several biosynthetic pathways in the form of folate coenzymes. While human beings obtain folic acid from diet, bacteria must form it from p-aminobenzoic acid (PABA). The sulphonamide and sulphone antibacterials act as competitive inhibitors for the incorporation of PABA in folic acid biosynthesis. Blocking the biosynthesis of folate coenzymes in bacteria stops their growth and cell division. Sulphonamides and trimethoprim are bacteriostatic.

Stability

Sulphonamides darken in colour when exposed to light and heat, especially in the presence of traces of heavy metals. Oxygen and moisture accelerate the degradation. Aqueous solutions of salts eg. sulphacetamide sodium require stabilisation by the addition of a suitable antioxidant such as 0.1 per cent sodium metabisulphite. For parenteral products, the air in the container should be replaced by nitrogen or other suitable gas. A chelating agent such as disodium edetate may be added to inhibit the action of heavy metal ions. Aqueous solutions of sulphadimidine sodium are most stable in the pH range 10 to 11. A fall in pH below 10 leads to precipitation of sulphadimidine. Hydrolysis of water soluble sulphonamides may occur, especially when heated. The process of hydrolysis is accelerated by the presence of sodium metabisulphite. Sulphacetamide sodium is hydrolysed in aqueous solution to sulphanilamide. Hence, in aqueous solutions of sulphonamides, the degradative processes of oxidation and hydrolysis have to be controlled by a delicate balance.

Storage

Sulphonamides should be stored in airtight containers and should be protected from light.

Classification of Sulphonamides

I) Well absorbed, short and intermediate acting sulphonamides eg. Sulphadiazine, sulphamethoxazole, sulphacetamide.

These have plasma half-lives below 12 hours.

II) Well-absorbed, long-acting sulphonamides eg. sulphadimethoxine, sulphadoxine.

These have plasma half-lives from 17 to 200 hours.

III) Poorly absorbed sulphonamides for treating intestinal infections eg. Phthalylsulphathiazole, succinylsulphathiazole.

IV) Sulphonamides for ophthalmic infections eg. Sulphacetamide sodium, sulphisoxazole diolamine.

V) Sulphonamides for burn therapy eg. Mafenide acetate, silver sulphadiazine.

I] Well absorbed, short and intermediate acting

1) Sulphadiazine

N^1 - (2 - pyrimidinyl) sulphanilamide.

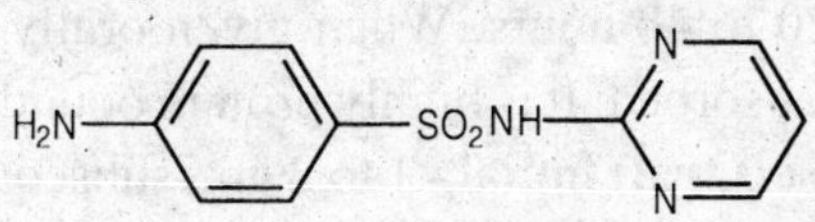

Properties : Sulphadiazine occurs as white or yellowish white or pinkish white crystals or crystalline powder. It is almost odourless and tasteless. It is practically insoluble in water and sparingly soluble in alcohol and in acetone. It is freely soluble in dilute mineral acids and in aqueous solutions of alkali hydroxides and carbonates. It melts at about 255°C, with decomposition.

Actions and uses : Sulphadiazine is effective in the treatment of infections due to haemolytic streptococci, pneumococci, meningococci, gonococci, Escherichia coli, and to a lesser extent, staphylococci. It is used for treating systemic infections as well as urinary tract infections. Sufficient fluid should be given to maintain a large urinary output. The urine should be kept alkaline to prevent crystallisation of the drug or its metabolite. Sodium bicarbonate may be given to increase urine pH. Sulphadiazine may be administered intravenously to patients for emergency treatment.

Dose : Initial dose - 3 gm.

Maintenance dose - 1 gm every 6 to 8 hours.

Preparations : Sulphadiazine tablets I.P. - usually of 0.5 gm strength.

Sulphadiazine Tablets B.P.C. - veterinary tablets containing 250 mg of drug.

Sulphadiazine and trimethoprim dispersible powder B.P.C.

Sulphadiazine and trimethoprim injection B.P.C.

Sulphadiazine and trimethoprim mixture B.P.C.

- an aqueous suspension of the drugs.

Sulphadiazine and trimethoprim tablets B.P.C.

Sulphadiazine injection B.P.C. - a sterile solution of sodium sulphadiazine.

Brand Names : Aubril®, Triglobe forte®, Silizine®

2) Sulphamethoxazole

N^1-(5- methyl isoxazol-3-yl) sulphanilamide.

Properties : Sulphamethoxazole occurs as a white or yellowish white, crystalline powder. It is almost odourless and has a slightly bitter taste. It is very slightly soluble in water and slightly soluble in alcohol. It is soluble in acetone and in solutions of alkali hydroxides. Melting point is about 170°C.

Storage : It should be stored in well-closed, light resistant containers.

Actions and uses : Sulphamethoxazole is well absorbed after oral administration and peak blood levels are reached within 4 hours of administration. It is commonly used in combination with trimethoprim under the name of cotrimoxazole.

Dose : Initial dose - 2 gm, followed by 1 gm every 12 hours.

Preparations : See under cotrimoxazole.

Brand Names : Antrima®, Bactrim®, Septran®

3) Cotrimoxazole

This is a synergistic combination of the drugs trimethoprim and sulphamethoxazole.

Actions and uses : Sulphonamides block the biosynthesis of folic acid from p-aminobenzoic acid. Trimethoprim inhibits the enzyme folate reductase and blocks the conversion of folic acid to tetrahydrofolic acid (THF). THF is the form required for coenzyme synthesis. The combination of sulphamethoxazole and trimethoprim, by synergism, produces a bactericidal effect.

Cotrimoxazole is used in the treatment of many infections, especially urinary tract infections due to Gram-negative rods and respiratory infections due to pneumococci or *Haemophilus influenzae.* Species of *Klebsiella, Proteus, Salmonella and Shigella* are usually sensitive.

Dose (Oral) : 160 mg of trimethoprim and 800 mg sulphamethoxazole, two or three times a day.

Preparations : Trimethoprim and sulphamethoxazole tablets I.P. -

Usually contain 80 mg trimethoprim + 400 mg sulphamethoxazole

or 160 mg trimethoprim + 800 mg sulphamethoxazole

Cotrimoxazole tablets B.P.C. - contain

20 mg trimethorpim + 100 mg sulphamethoxazole.

Cotrimoxazole injection B.P.C.

Cotrimoxazole mixture B.P.C.

Dispersible cotrimoxazole tablets B.P.C.

Paediatric cotrimoxazole mixture B.P.C.

Strong sterile cotrimoxazole solution B.P.C. - It is used for the preparation of cotrimoxazole injection.

Sulphamethoxazole and trimethoprim oral suspension I.P.

Brand Names : Ciplin®, Trisulfose®, Tprim forte®, Tabrol®, Bactrim®, Septran®, Sepmax®, Oripim®

II] Well absorbed, long acting

1) Sulphadimethoxine

N[1]-(2,6-Dimethoxypyrimidin 4-yl) sulphanilamide

Properties : Sulphadimethoxine occurs as a white or creamy white crystalline powder. It is odourless and tasteless. It is very slightly soluble in water and alcohol. It is soluble in dilute mineral acids and in solutions of alkali hydroxides and carbonates. pKa is 5.9. Melting point is about 201°C.

Storage : It should be stored in well closed, light resistant containers.

Actions and uses : Sulphadimethoxine is a long acting sulphonamide, having a serum half life of 20 to 40 hours. When given orally, it is rapidly absorbed. It is highly protein bound.

Dose : (Oral) Initial - 1 to 2 gm, subsequently 0.5 gm a day.

Preparations : Sulphadimethoxine tablets

B.P.C. - contain 500 mg of sulphadimethoxine.

2) Sulphamethoxypyridazine

N^1-(6-Methoxypyridazin-3-yl) sulphanilamide.

Properties : Sulphamethoxypyridazine occurs as a white or yellowish white crystalline powder. It is odourless and is tasteless at first, but has a bitter after taste. It is very slightly soluble in water and in alcohol. It is soluble in acetone, in dilute mineral acids and in solutions of alkali hydroxides. pKa is 7.2. Melting point is about 181°C.

Actions and uses : It is a long acting sulphonamide, with a serum half life of about 37 hours. Its action and uses are similar to those of sulphadimethoxine. It is given orally in the treatment of urinary tract infections.

Storage : It should be stored in airtight, light-resistant containers.

Dose (Oral) : Initial - 1 to 2 gm, subsequently 0.5 gm a day.

Preparations : Sulphamethoxypyridazine injection B.P.C. - a sterile solution of the sodium salt of the drug.

Sulphamethoxypridazine tablets B.P.C. - contain 500 mg of the drug.

III] Poorly absorbed

1) Sulphaguanidine

2-(4-Aminobenzene sulphonyl) guanidine monohydrate

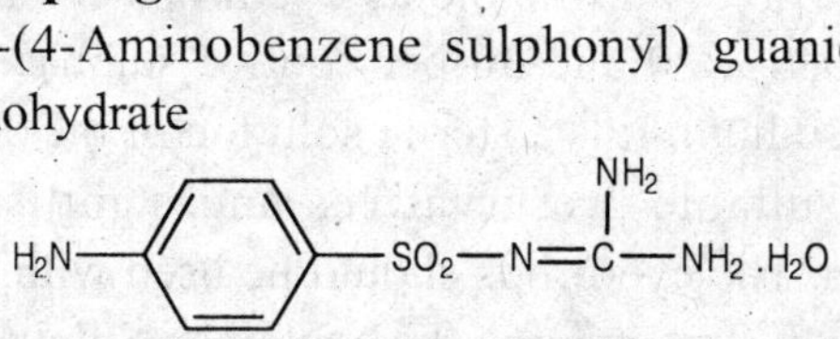

Properties : Sulphaguanidine occurs as odourless white crystals or powder. It darkens slowly on exposure to light. It is slightly soluble in water and alcohol. It is soluble in boiling water and in dilute mineral acids. It is very slightly soluble in acetone and practically insoluble in solutions of alkali hydroxides. Melting point is about 191°C.

Storage : It should be stored in airtight and light resistant containers.

Actions and uses : Sulphaguanidine is not readily absorbed from the gastrointestinal tract. It is therefore used in the treatment of local intestinal infections such as bacillary dysentery. It may also prove useful in refractory cases of amoebic dysentery by controlling secondary bacterial infections. Succinylsulphathiazole and phthalylsulphathiazole are preferred to this drug as their absorption into blood stream is much less.

Dose (Oral) : 3 gm, three to four times a day, for 3 days.

Preparations : Sulphaguanidine tablets B.P.C. - contain 500 mg of sulphaguanidine.

2) Phthalylsulphathiazole

Thalazole

4'[N-(Thiazol-2-yl) sulphamoyl] phthalanilic acid.

Phthalylsulphathiazole and succinylsulphathiazole may be considered to be prodrugs which are designed to be poorly absorbable. In the large intestine, the N^4-protecting group is cleaved and the free sulphonamide antibacterial is released.

Properties : Phthalylsulphathiazole occurs as white or yellow-white crystals or powder. It is odourless and has a slightly bitter taste. It is very slightly soluble in water and chloroform. It is slightly soluble in alcohol, soluble in aqueous solutions of alkali hydroxides and carbonates and in hydrochloric acid. Melting point is about 275°C, with decomposition.

Storage : It should be stored in airtight containers, protected from light.

Actions and uses : Phthalylsulphathiazole is a relatively insoluble compound. When given orally, it is slowly broken down in the gastrointestinal (GI) tract and most of the dose reaches the large intestine. A proportion of the dose gets absorbed as sulphathiazole. Phthalylsulphathiazole is used to treat bacterial dysentery and to reduce the bacterial flora of the large intenstine before surgery. Vitamins of the B-complex group should be administered to replace those normally synthesised by sensitive intenstinal microbes. Its prolonged use may lead to overgrowth of *Candida* species.

Dose : 5 to 10 gm a day, in divided doses.

Preparations : Phthalylsulphathiazole tablets I.P., B.P.C. - contain 500 mg of the drug.

3) Succinyl Sulphathiazole

4`[N-(Thiazol-2-yl) sulphamoyl] succinanilic acid monohydrate.

Properties : It occurs as white or yellowish-white crystals or powder. It is odourless and has a slightly bitter taste. It is very slightly soluble in water, sparingly soluble in alcohol and practically insoluble in chloroform. It is soluble in solutions of alkali hydroxides. It dissolves in sodium bicarbonate solution with the evolution of carbon dioxide. Melting point is about 190°C, with decomposition.

Storage : It should be stored in airtight and light resistant containers.

Actions and uses : Succinylsulphathiazole has actions and uses similar to those of phthalyl sulphathiazole. It is used in the treatment of bacillary dysentery.

Dose : 10 to 20 gm a day, in divided doses.

Preparations : Succinylsulphathiazole tablets I.P., B.P.C. - contain 500 mg of the drug.

Paediatric Succinylsulphathiazole mixture B.P.C. - This is a flavoured and coloured suspension of the drug.

IV] Sulphonamides for ophthalmic infections

1) Sulphacetamide sodium

N[1] - Acetylsulphanilamide sodium salt.

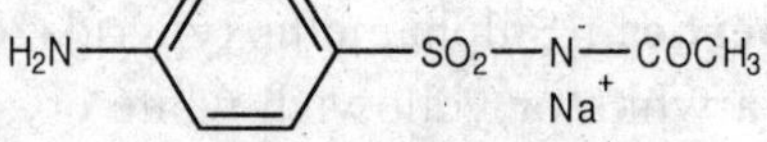

Properties : Sulphacetamide sodium is obtained as the monohydrate. It occurs as white or yellowish-white crystals or microcrystalline powder. It is odourless and has a slightly bitter taste. It is freely soluble in water and sparingly soluble in alcohol. It is practically insoluble in benzene, in chloroform and in ether. pKa is 5.4

Storage : It should be stored in tightly closed, light resistant containers.

Actions and uses : Sulphacetamide sodium is highly soluble in water at the physiological pH of 7.4. It is used mainly for local application in ophthalmic infections and injuries of the conjunctiva. In the treatment of acute conjunctivitis and other ocular infections, a 10 per cent solution is applied every 2 hours, or a 30 per cent solution twice a day.

Preparations : Sulphacetamide eye ointment, I.P. usually contains 5 per cent or 10 per cent of the drug. Sulphacetamide eye ointment B.P.C. - available as ointment containing 2.5 and 6 per cent of the drug. Sulphacetamide eye drops B.P.C. - available as eye drops containing 10, 15, 20 and 30 per cent of sulphacetamide sodium. It is a sterile solution of the drug with suitable preservatives and stabilising agents. The eye-drops should be used within 4 weeks of first opening the container, Sulphacetamide eye drops I.P.

Brand Names : Albucid® eye drops, Andremide®, Nebasulf® skin oint., Setride® eye drops, Locula®, Phenosulf®

Drugs For Further Study

1) Sulphamoxole (+ Trimethoprim) - Supristol®
2) Silver sulphadiazine - Argisept®, Silverex®, Silvindon®, Siofin®, Slozin®
3) Sulphacytine
4) Sulphisoxazole
5) Sulphamethizole
6) Sulphadoxine

Exercise

Q1. Write a note on Cotrimoxazole. (Karnataka Univ.)

Q2. Write the name, draw structure, chemical name and properties of sulphonamide used for the treatment of eye infections. (Winter 04).

Q2. Draw the structure from given chemical name - 4-Chloro-N-furfuryl-5-Sulphonamide Anthranilic acid. (Winter 04)

Q3. Describe the uses, official preparations and popular brand names of 'Cotrimoxazole'. (Summer 03)

Q4. Name the Sulphonamides used in - i) Urinary tract infection, ii) Eye infection Give the structure of - i) Sulphadiazine, ii) Sulphaguanidine. (Summer 03)

Q5. Write notes on antibacterial sulphonamides.(May-June 04)

Q6. Specify dosage forms (tablet, capsule etc..) for - Sulphaguanidine.(May-June 04)

Q7. Discuss with structure use of various sulphonamides.(May 07)

Q8. Write a note on sulphonamides used in the treatment of eye infections.(Nov 06)

4 Antitubercular Drugs

Tuberculosis is acute or chronic communicable disease caused by the Gram-positive, acid fast organism *Mycobacterium tuberculosis*. It usually affects the respiratory tract. The disease may spread to the lymphatic, urogenital and nervous systems and the gastrointestinal tract. It is a destructive process which replaces normal tissues with tubercles. It is characterised by inflammatory infiltrations, tubercle formation, caseation (formation of soft masses) fibrosis and calcification.

The tubercle bacillus usually enters the body by inhalation or ingestion. It commonly affects the lungs leading to pulmonary tuberculosis. The infection by tubercle bacillus is insidious and there are no symptoms in the first few weeks. The disease can be detected only by X ray examination. The tuberculin test is also a useful diagnostic aid. In the advanced stages of tuberculosis, the most common symptom is cough. Progressive pulmonary tuberculosis is characterised by fatigue, weight loss, anorexia, fever, weakness and malaise. other symptoms are cough, sputum formation, dyspnoea and chest pain, which is increases on respiratory effort. When tuberculosis occurs in the gastrointestinal tract, it may cause ulceration, perforation or obstruction. Tuberculosis in other organs leads to their destruction and loss of function. Tuberculous lesions which have been inactivated by drugs, may later spread due to reinfection or reactivation.

Chemotherapy of Tuberculosis

Until about 1945, no really effective antitubercular drug was available and patients were treated by prolonged isolation in a sanatorium and physical and mental rest. Surgery was performed if required. Major advances in the chemotherapy of tuberculosis were, first, the discovery of the antitubercular activity of streptomycin by Waksman in 1944, next, of the usefulness of p-aminosalicylic acid, followed by the discovery of the activity of isoniazid in 1952. The introduction of rifampicin in 1971 is a major milestone in the treatment of tuberculosis. Several chemotherapeutic agents have been developed over the recent years and now, patients need not be hospitalised. The previously dreaded disease can now be cured with a judicious choice of drugs.

Resistance frequently develops during the treatment of tuberculosis. To prevent the emergence of resistant strains, combination therapy is used. The treatment must include at least two drugs (usually 2 to 4 drugs) to which the bacteria are sensitive. Rifampicin and isoniazid are the most effective drugs presently available.

A commonly prescribed regimen is as follows: For the first two months the combination used is

Rifampicin - 450 to 600 mg daily, single dose.
\+ Isoniazid - 300 mg daily, single dose.
\+ Pyrazinamide - 1500 mg daily, single dose
\+ Ethambutol - 1.5 gm daily, in two doses.

Streptomycin may be used in place of rifampicin. Pyridoxine 15 to 50 mg daily should be administered.

For the next 7 months or more, the combination used is Rifampicin - 450 to 600 mg a day. + Isoniazid - 300 mg a day.

Therapy should be continued for nine months or more. The duration of treatment is decided by roentgenographic examination after every two months.

a) First line Drugs

These drugs combine the greatest efficacy with an acceptable level of toxicity and are the drugs of choice. These include isoniazid, rifampicin, ethambutol, pyrazinamide and streptomycin.

b) Second line Drugs

These are used in cases of microbial resistance or patient related factors.

These include ethionamide, cycloserine, p-amino salicylic acid etc. Thiacetazone is used in poor countries as it is cheap.

Classification of Antitubercular Drugs

I) Synthetic agents

p-Aminosalicylic acid, ethambutol, ethionamide, isoniazid, pyrazinamide, thiacetazone

II) Antibiotics

Streptomycin, cycloserine, rifampicin

I] Synthetic agents

1) p-Aminosalicylic acid (PAS)

4-Aminosalicylic acid

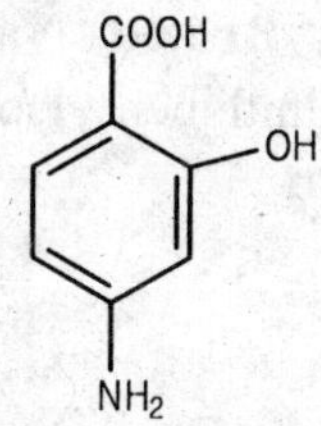

Previously, p-aminosalicylic acid was considered a first line antitubercular drug and was included in combination therapy along with streptomycin and isoniazid. However, with the introduction of more effective agents like ethambutol and rifampicin, it is now used only as a second line drug.

Properties : p-Aminosalicylic acid occurs as odourless, white or yellowish white crystals. It darkens on exposure to light and air. It is slightly soluble in water but is more soluble in alcohol, methanol and isopropyl alcohol. Solubility is increased with alkaline salts of alkali metals, eg. sodium bicarbonate, and in weak nitric acid. The amine salts of hydrochloric and sulphuric acids are insoluble. When aqueous solutions of the drug are heated, it decomposes.

The drug is also available as its sodium, potassium and calcium salt. The salts occur as white to slightly yellow crystalline powders with a saline and unpleasant taste. The salts are freely soluble in water. Their aqueous solutions are unstable and darken on standing. Hence, such solutions should be used within 24 hours after their preparation. They are incompatible with acids, ferric salts and oxidising agents.

Storage : It should be stored in tightly closed, light resistant containers.

Mechanism of Action : The tuberculostatic activity of p-aminosalicylic acid can be reversed by the administration of p-aminobenzoic acid. Hence, it has a mechanism of action similar to that of sulphonamides. It blocks the biosynthesis of folic acid in the tubercle bacillus by competitive antagonism with p-aminobenzoic acid.

Actions and uses : p-Aminosalicylic acid is rapidly and almost completely absorbed after oral administration. High concentrations of the drug are found in the lungs, liver and kidneys. Often, the use of p-aminosalicylic acid or its sodium salt, leads to severe gastrointestinal irritation. This problem may be overcome by using coated tablets, capsules and granules. An antacid such as aluminium hydroxide may be prescribed concurrently. The use of calcium salt also reduces gastrointestinal irritation.

Dose (Oral) : 10 to 20 gm a day, in divided doses.

Preparations :

Sodium aminosalicylate granules I.P.

Sodium aminosalicylate tablets I.P.

Sodium aminosalicylate powder B.P.C.

Sodium aminosalicylate and isoniazid granules B.P.C.

Sodium aminosalicylate and isoniazid powder B.P.C.

Brand Names : Inapas®, Monopas®, Q-Pas®

2) Isoniazid (INH)

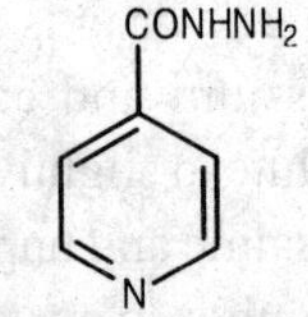

Isonicotinic acid hydrazide

Isoniazid was first prepared as an intermediate in the synthesis of a thiosemicarbazone derivative. On subjecting it to a routine study for antitubercular activity, it's excellent activity was discovered in 1952. Isoniazid has a bacteriostatic action against *Mycobacterium tuberculosis*. It is a first line drug in the treatment of tuberculosis.

Properties : Isoniazid occurs as colourless crystals or white crystalline powder. It is odourless and has a taste which is sweet at first and then bitter. It is freely soluble in water, sparingly soluble in alcohol, slightly soluble in chloroform and very slightly soluble in ether. Melting point is about 172°C.

Storage : It should be stored in airtight containers, protected from light.

Mechanism of Action : Isoniazid is a bacteriostatic which acts only on the growing bacilli and not on the resting forms. Its mechanism of action is not yet clear. Isoniazid may be interfering with enzymes requiring pyridoxal phosphate and nicotinamide as coenzymes. Inactive drug enzyme complexes may be formed resulting in changes in metabolism. Mycolic acid synthesis is inhibited thus disrupting normal cell wall synthesis.

Actions and uses : Isoniazid is a highly effective drug and is indispensable in chemotherapy of tuberculosis. It is readily and completely absorbed after oral administration. One of the major metabolic reactions is acetylation of the primary hydrazine nitrogen. On the basis of the capacity to acetylate isoniazid, humans are divided into fast acetylators (plasma half-life is about 1.2 hours) and slow acetylators (plasma half-life is about 3.5 hours). Isoniazid is used mainly in the treatment of pulmonary tuberculosis. It also appears to be effective in the treatment of extrapulmonary lesions, including meningitis and genitourinary infection.

If isoniazid is used alone, then within a few weeks, resistant strains of tubercle bacillus appear. To prevent this, isoniazid is commonly given in combination with rifampicin and ethambutol. The major side effects of isoniazid are peripheral neuritis and gastrointestinal disturbances. The peripheral neutritis appears to be caused by pyridoxine deficiency. Hence, fairly large doses of pyridoxine are administered to tuberculosis patients.

Dose : 300 mg a day.

Preparations : Isoniazid tablets I.P. - contain 50, 100 and 300 mg of isoniazid.

Isoniazid elixir B.P.C.

Isoniazid injection B.P.C.

Isoniazid tablets B.P.C. - contains 50 and 100 mg of isoniazid

Sodium aminosalicylate and isoniazid granules B.P.C.

Sodium aminosalicylate and isoniazid powder B.P.C.

Brand Names : Ipcazide®, Isonex®, Unithiben®, Isokin-300®, Siozide®

3) Ethambutol

(+)-N, N`-Bis(1-hydroxy methyl propyl) ethylene diamine

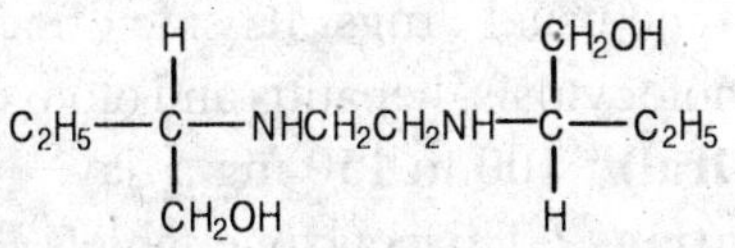

Properties : Ethambutol hydrochloride occurs as a white crystalline powder. It is odourless. It is freely soluble in water and in methanol. It is sparingly soluble in alcohol, slightly soluble in chloroform and very slightly soluble in ether. The molecule contains two asymmetric centres. The dextro isomer is much more active than the meso and laevo isomers. Its 10 per cent solution has a specific rotation of +5.8° to +6.6° at 25°C. Melting point is about 201°C.

Storage : It should be stored in airtight containers.

Mechanism of Action : Ethambutol prevents the synthesis of protein and DNA and reduces RNA synthesis. It complexes with divalent cations and inhibits the function of amines eg. spermidine, which maintain the integrity of nucleic acids.

Actions and uses : Ethambutol has good anti-mycobacterial activity. Combination therapy is recommended, as resistance may develop slowly. Ethambutol is also active against leprosy. It is rapidly absorbed after oral administration, and peak blood levels occur in about 2 hours. It has a plasma half-life of about 8 hours. It is almost free of side effects. A serious toxic effect which is sometimes observed is a decrease in visual acuity with inability to distinguish between colours.

Dose : 0.5 to 1.5 gm a day.

Preparations : Ethambutol tablets I.P. - contain 200 and 400 mg of ethambutol hydrochloride.

Ethambutol tablets B.P.C. - contain 100 and 400 mg of the drug.

Brand Names : Albutol®, Combutol®, Ebutol®, Emtb®, Etibi®, Themibutol®

4) Pyrazinamide

Pyrazine-2-carboxamide

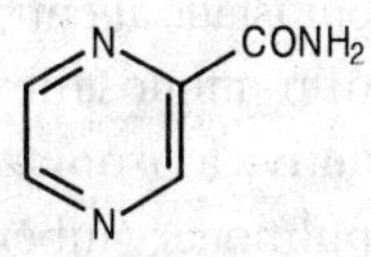

It is the pyrazine analogue of nicotinamide.

Properties : Pyrazinamide occurs as a white, crystalline powder. It is odourless and has a slightly bitter taste. It is sparingly soluble in water and slightly soluble in alcohol. It is soluble in ether and in chloroform. Melting point is about 189°C.

Storage : It should be stored in airtight containers.

Actions and uses : Pyrazinamide is a fairly active tuberculostatic drug. It is used in combination with the other drugs in treating tuberculosis. It causes a rather high incidence of liver damage. Hence, it is used only in infections which are resistant to other tuberculostatic drugs.

Dose : 1 to 3 gm a day, in divided doses.

Preparations : Pyrazinamide tablets I.P. - contain 250, 500 and 750 mg of pyrazinamide.

Pyrazinamide tablets B.P.C. - contain 500 mg of pyrazinamide.

Brand Names : Actizid®, Cavizide®, Mzide®, P-zide®, Pyzina®, Pza-Ciba®

5) Ethionamide

2-Ethylpyridine-4-carbothioamide

Properties : Ethionamide occurs as a bright yellow crystalline powder. It has a slight odour and an unpleasant sulphurous taste. It is practically insoluble in water. It is soluble in alcohol and slightly soluble in ether and in chloroform. It is soluble in hot acetone and in dichloroethane. Melting point is about 163°C.

Storage : It should be stored in light resistant containers.

Mechanism of Action : Ethionamide

inhibits protein biosynthesis in Mycobacteria. It blocks the incorporation of amino acids containing sulphur such as cysteine and methionine.

Actions and uses : Ethionamide is a tuberculostatic agent with applications similar to those of p-aminosalicylic acid. It is only one tenth as active as isoniazid. It is used in the treatment of pulmonary tuberculosis resistant to isoniazid or when the patient is intolerant to other drugs. Ethionamide is readily absorbed after oral administration. It has a half life to 2 to 4 hours. It is not well tolerated when given orally. It commonly causes severe gastrointestinal reactions.

Dose (Oral) : 0.5 to 1 gm a day.

Preparations : Ethionamide tablets I.P., B.P.C. - these usually contain 125 mg of ethionamide.

Brand Names : Myobid-250®, Ethide®, Mycotuf®, Ethiocid®

6) Thiacetazone

(Amithiozone, Thioacetazone)

4-Acetamidobenzaldehyde thiosemicarbazone.

It is a thiosemicarbazone which is chemically related to sulphathiazole.

Properties : Thiacetazone occurs as odourless pale yellow crystals or crystalline powder. It is very slightly soluble in water, slightly soluble in alcohol and sparingly soluble in propylene glycol. Melting point is about 227°C, with decomposition.

Storage : It should be stored in airtight containers, protected from light.

Actions and uses : Thiacetazone inhibits the growth of *M.tuberculosis* and *M.leprae*. It is used in the treatment of tuberculosis and leprosy. Its antitubercular activity was discovered in 1947. It was introduced into clinical practice and then abandoned, because of its toxic effects. It has now been reintroduced in Africa and India. It is less effective and as safe as p-aminosalicylic acid. It is cheap drug and therefore, widely used in poor countries. In the developed nations, it is used only in those cases which are resistant to the usual drugs. Its side effects include agranulocytosis, hepatitis and ototoxicity.

Dose (Oral) : 100 to 150 mg a day.

Preparations : Thiacetazone tablets B.P.C. - contain 75 mg of thiacetazone.

Thiacetazone and isoniazid tablets I.P.

- these are available in three strengths.

Thiacetazone 37.5 mg + Isoniazid 75 mg

Thiacetazone 75 mg + Isoniazid 150 mg

Thiacetazone 150 mg + Isoniazid 300 mg

Brand Names : Isokin-T Forte®, Unithiben®

II] Antibiotics

1) Streptomycin

Streptomycin is an aminoglycoside antibiotic. It was first isolated from *Streptomyces griseus* by Waksman and his associates in 1944. It became the first drug used clinically in the treatment of tuberculosis. On acid hydrolysis, streptomycin gives streptidine and streptobiosamine. Streptobiosamine is a combination of L-streptose and N-methyl-L-glucosamine.

Properties : Streptomycin sulphate occurs as a white or almost white hygroscopic powder. It is odourless or with a slight odour, and with a slightly bitter taste. It is very soluble in water and slightly soluble in alcohol. It is practically insoluble in chloroform and in solvent ether.

Storage : It should be stored in well closed containers, protected from moisture and at a temperature not exceeding 30°C. If it is intended for parenteral administration, the container should be sterile and sealed so as to exclude microorganisms.

Incompatibility : Streptomycin is incompatible with acids and alkalis. It is also inactivated by oxidising and reducing agents and urea. Precipitation is seen with amaranth, sodium alginate and sodium lauryl sulphate.

Stability : Streptomycin salts are stable when dry for at least 2 years at room temperature. Deterioration occurs due to moisture and high temperatures. Aqueous solutions may be stored at room temperature for one week without loss of potency. They are more stable if the pH is adjusted between 4.5 and 7.0. When sterlised by heating, the solutions decompose. Hence, sterile solutions are prepared by adding sterile distilled water to the sterile powder.

Mechanism of Action : The aminoglycoside antibiotics are bactericidal in action. The antibacterial activity of the aminoglycoside antibiotics is due to direct action on ribosomes through interaction with 30S ribosomal subunit. Protein biosynthesis is inhibited and abnormal protein may be formed. Inhibition of enzymatic polymerisation of amino acids leads to bactericidal activity.

Actions and uses : The aminoglycosides are generally classified as broad spectrum antibiotics, but they are more effective against Gram negative bacteria. Streptomycin is active against *Mycobacterium tuberculosis* and Gram negative bacteria including *Escherichia coli, Klebsiella pneumoniae*, Enterobacter species and some species of *Proteus, Salmonella and Shigella.* Streptomycin is used in the treatment of tuberculosis, bacterial endocarditis, tularemia and plague.

Streptomycin is used mainly in the treatment of tuberculosis, in combination with isoniazid, ethambutol and rifampicin. It is a first line or primary antitubercular agent. Streptomycin is not appreciably absorbed or inactivated in the gastrointestinal tract. Most of the dose administered orally is excreted unchanged in the faeces. Streptomycin is administered parenterally for treating systemic infections while it is given orally in the treatment of intestinal infections. The most serious toxic effects of the antibiotic arise from its toxic action on the eighth cranial nerve, especially the vestibular branch. This leads to vertigo and tinnitus, and sometimes, deafness, which may be permanent.

Dose : Streptomycin sulphate equivalent to 1 gm of the base is dissolved in water for injection and injected intramuscularly. The intramuscular dose is 1 gm a day or at longer intervals. The oral dose is 0.5 gm of streptomycin, every 8 hours.

Preparations : Streptomycin Injection I.P.,B.P. It is a sterile solution of streptomycin sulphate in water for injection. It is prepared by dissolving the contents of a sealed container in water for injection. The usual strength is the equivalent of 0.75 gm and 1 gm of streptomycin base.

Streptomycin Tablets I.P. - contain streptomycin sulphate equivalent to 0.5 gm of streptomycin base.

Paediatric streptomycin Elixir B.P.C.

Streptomycin sulphate Injection B.P.C. - a sterile solution, with suitable stabilising agents, in water for injection. It is prepared by an aseptic technique and may contain a buffering agent.

Brand Names : Ambistryn-S®, Merstrep®, Isos®

2) Rifampicin (Rifampin)

The rifamycins are a group of chemically related antibiotics obtained from *Streptomyces mediterrani.* They belong to the class of antibiotics called ansamycins. The rifamycins have a broad spectrum of antimicrobial activity. Rifampicin, a semisynthetic derivative of rifamycin B, is highly effective against *Mycobacterium tuberculosis*.

Properties : Rifampicin occurs as an odourless, brick-red to reddish-brown crystalline powder. It is very slightly soluble in water and slightly soluble in alcohol and in ether. It is soluble in chloroform and in methanol.

Storage : It should be stored in tightly closed,

light resistant containers in an atmosphere of nitrogen. It should be stored at a temperature not exceeding 15°C.

Stability : Rifampicin is unstable to moisture and a desiccant like silica gel should be included in containers of rifampicin capsules. Rifampicin is stable in the solid state but undergoes many reactions in solution, which are pH and temperature dependent. In alkaline pH, and in the presence of oxygen, it oxidises to the quinone. In acidic solutions, it hydrolyses to 3-formylrifamycin -SV. Even at neutral pH, a slow hydrolysis of the ester functions occurs.

Mechanism of action : Rifampicin is bactericidal in nature. It is a potent inhibitor of DNA-directed RNA polymerase in bacteria. Thus, it interferes with RNA synthesis in bacteria but it does not affect the mammalian enzyme. Its antiviral activity is because of inhibition of formation of virus particle by preventing a specific polypetide conversion.

Actions and uses : Rifampicin is effective against *Mycobacterium tuberculosis*. Though it is active against many Gram-positive and Gram-negative organisms including staphylocci and bacteroides, it is generally reserved for use in tuberculosis. Resistance to rifampicin develops rapidly in many bacteria. Hence, it is used in combination with other antitubercular drugs. Rifampicin is readily absorbed after oral administration. Food reduces its absorption and the drug should be administered on an empty stomach. It is excreted mainly through bile and faeces.

Rifampicin is also used in the prophylaxis of meningitis. It has low toxicity and may interfere with liver function in some patients.

Dose : 450 to 600 mg once a day.

Preparation : Rifampicin capsules I.P., B.P.C. these contain 150 and 300 mg of rifampicin.

Brand Names : Coxid-450®, Macox®, R-cin®, Rimpacin®, Ramactane®

3) Cycloserine

(R)-4-Aminoisoxazolidin-3-one

Cycloserine is an antimicrobial substance produced by the growth of *Streptomyces orchidaceous* or *Streptomyces garyphalus* or obtained by synthesis.

Properties : It occurs as a white or pale yellow crystalline powder. It is odourless and has a slightly bitter taste. It is hygroscopic. It is soluble in water and sparingly soluble in alcohol. It is slightly soluble in water and in chloroform. The compound shows keto-enol isomerism. It is quite stable in alkali but is unstable in acid. In aqueous solutions, it may form a dimer on standing. Melting point is about 154°C.

Storage : It should be stored in airtight containers at a temperature not exceeding 25°C.

Mechanism of action : The antibacterial activity of cycloserine results from its interference with bacterial cell wall synthesis. Cycloserine acts as an antimetabolite for D-alanine and inactivates the enzyme alanine racemase. This inhibits the incorporation of D-alanine in bacterial cell wall.

Actions and uses : Cycloserine shows antibiotic activity against many Gram-positive and Gram-negative bacteria including *Mycobacterium tuberculosis, streptococci, staphylococci, Klebsiella* species and *Escherichia coli*. However, its relatively weak potency and frequent toxic reactions limit its use to the treatment of tuberculosis. It is used as a second line drug in case of resistance. It is administered in combination with isoniazid and other drugs. It is well absorbed after oral administration and is excreted mainly in the urine.

Dose : 250 - 500 mg a day.

Preparations : Cycloserine capsules I.P., B.P.C. - contain 125 and 250 mg of cycloserine.

Cycloserine tablets I.P., B.P.C. - contain 250 mg of cycloserine.

Brand Names : Coxerin®, Cyclorin®, Myser®

Brand Names (with drug combinations):

1) Rifampicin + INH + Pyrazinamide - 3 FD®, Gocox-3®, RHZ®, Rifacept-3®, Tricox®
2) Rifampicin + INH + Ethambutol - AKT-3®, Akurit-3®, Auticox-3®, Coxina-3®, Rcinex-E®, RHE®
3) Rifampicin + INH + Pyrazinamide + Ethambutol - 4D®, AFB-4®, AKT-4®, Akurit-4®, Anticox-4®, RIPE®

Drugs For Further Study

1) Prothionamide - Pethide®, Prothicid®, Protomid®
2) Capreomycin - Kapocin®
3) Rifabutin

Exercise

Q1. Classify antitubercular drugs and write the structure of ethambutol. (Karnataka Univ., Winter 04)

Q2. Give uses of rifampicin. (Winter 04)

Q3. What are anti-mycobacterial agents? Classify them and draw the structure of Pyrazinamide. (Winter 04)

Q4. Give the uses of - i) PAS & ii) Isoniazid. (Summer 03)

Q5. What are mycobacterial infections? Discuss specific problems of the infections. Enlist currently used drugs for the infections. (May-June 04)

Q6. Write a note on Antitubercular agents. (May 07)

■

5 Antileprotic Drugs

Leprosy

Leprosy (Hansen's disease) has been known from time immemorial. It is a chronic disease caused due to infection with the acid fast bacterium, *Mycobacterium leprae*. Leprosy is characterised by lesions of the skin, mucous membranes and peripheral nerves. The lesions show hypesthesia and many are anaesthetic. The disease is only moderately communicable and the afflicted patients should not be made social outcasts.

Five clinical types of leprosy are recognised. At the two extreme ends are tuberculoid leprosy and lepromatous leprosy, there are three intermediate types.

Tuberculoid leprosy

It develops in patients with pronounced tissue reaction to the infection. The skin lesions are clearly demarcated and the peripheral nerves are involved early resulting in motor and sensory changes in the affected areas.

Lepromatous leprosy

It develops in those patients with little resistance to the organisms. They are able to multiply and disseminate freely in the tissues resulting in a generalised disease. The skin lesions may become extensive and indefinitely demarcated. The shiny skin later becomes thickened and oedematous and painless nodular lesions occur. The lesions may become necrotic and ulcerate, releasing large numbers of mycobacteria. There is little neurological damage until late in the disease.

Leprosy may also affect the eyes, testes, lymph nodes, bones and other structures.

Chemotherapy of leprosy

Leprosy is treated with suitable antibacterials. The disease is slow to respond. Treatment has to be given for many years and sometimes for life. A rapid destruction of *Mycobacterium leprae* is unadvisable as the breakdown products are toxic and may cause extensive tissue reaction. WHO recommends multi-drug therapy for all leprosy patients. The reasons for using combinations of drugs are reduction in development of resistance, need for adequate therapy when primary resistance exists and reduction in duration of therapy. The following regimen is suggested.

Dapsone - 50 to 100 mg a day

+ Clofazimine - 50 mg a day + 300 mg once monthly.

+ Rifampicin - 600 mg once monthly

or 450 to 600 mg a day.

The minimum duration of therapy is of two years. Treatment should be continued until acid fast bacilli are not detected in lesions.

1) Dapsone
(DDS, 4,4` Diaminodiphenylsulphone)

Dapsone belongs to the class of sulphones. The sulphones are chemically related to the sulphonamides.

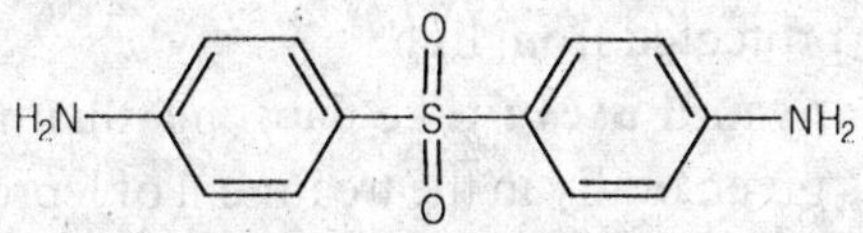

Bis (4-aminophenyl) sulphone.

Properties : Dapsone occurs as white or creamy white, crystalline powder. It is odourless and has a slightly bitter taste. It is very slightly soluble in water, sparingly soluble in alcohol, soluble in acetone and in dilute mineral acids. Melting point is about 175°C-181°C.

Stability : The pure compound is light stable. However, traces of impurities, including water, make it photosensitive. It gets discoloured on exposure to light.

Storage : It should be stored in airtight and light resistant containers.

Mechanism of action : Dapsone is an antibacterial with mode of action similar to the sulphonamides. It prevents the use of essential metabolites by certain bacteria. Its action is antagonised by p-aminobenzoic acid.

Actions and uses : Dapsone is mainly used in the treatment of leprosy. It is also used in treating dermatitis and malaria. It is usually given orally, twice a week. A suspension of dapsone in a sterile vehicle such as arachis oil or chaulmoogra oil may be administered intramuscularly for prolonged effect but the injections may cause pain and abscess formation.

In tuberculoid leprosy, skin lesions usually disappear in 3 to 9 months and in lepromatous leprosy in 1 to 5 years. Viable bacilli may persist in the peripheral nervous system for a longer time. Therefore, it is advisable to continue giving maintenance doses of dapsone for at least 18 months after disappearance of skin lesions or of granular bacilli from the skin.

Dose : 25 mg twice weekly, gradually increased to 200 mg twice weekly.

Preparations : Dapsone tablets I.P. - contain 25, 50 and 100 mg of dapsone.

Dapsone tablets B.P.C. - usual strength is 100 mg of dapsone.

Brand Names : Dapsone® (GSK)

2) Solapsone (Solasulphone)

Tetrasodium salt of bis [4-(3-phenyl- 1,3- disulphopropylamino) phenyl] sulphone.

Properties : Solapsone occurs as a white, amorphous powder. It is almost odourless and has an alkaline taste. It is very soluble in water and practically insoluble in most organic solvents. It is stable in neutral or alkaline solution but decomposes in acid solution.

Storage : It should be stored in airtight containers.

Actions and uses : Solapsone is partially metabolised to dapsone and has, therefore, a similar pharmacological profile. It can be given orally but is more commonly given by subcutaneous or intramuscular injection.

Dose : Injection 1.25 to 2.5 gm twice weekly.

Oral - 1.5 gm a day, gradually increased to 3 gm a day.

Preparations : Solapsone tablets (B.P. 1968)
Strong solapsone injection (B.P.C. 1968).

3) Clofazimine

3-(4 Chloro anilino)-10-(4-chlorophenyl)-2, 10 -dihydro-2-phenazin-2-ylidene isopropylamine.

Clofazimine is a phenazine dye. It is now considered as a secondary drug for the treatment of leprosy.

Properties : It occurs as dark red crystals or an orange red microcrystalline powder. It is practically insoluble in water, very slightly soluble in alcohol and in glycols and soluble in dimethylfomamide. Melting point is about 215°C.

Actions and uses : Clofazimine has antibacterial actions against species of *Mycobacterium* and certain other species such as *Actinomyces, Streptomyces* and *Nocardia*. It is used in the treatment of leprosy, especially when resistance to dapsone has been encountered. The dose is adjusted for each patient according to body weight and severity of the disease. The side effects include gastrointestinal disturbances and discolouration of skin and urine.

Dose : 100 mg weekly, gradually increased to 600 mg weekly

Maximum daily dose = 1.2 gm

Preparations : Clofazimine capsules, I.P., B.P.C. - contain 100 mg of clofazimine.

Brand Names : Clofaz® (soft gel capsule), Nansepran®, Clofozine®, Fazim®, Hansepran®

4) Thiambutosine

1-(4- Butoxyphenyl) 3(4-dimethylaminophenyl) thiourea.

Properties : Thiambutosine occurs as a white or creamy white crystalline powder. It is odourless and has a bitter taste. It is very slightly soluble in water, slightly soluble in ether, soluble in acetone and freely soluble in chloroform. Melting point is about 125°C.

Storage : It should be stored in airtight containers, protected from light.

Actions and uses : Like dapsone, thiambutosine is given orally in the treatment of leprosy. It is particularly useful in dimorphous cases with considerable tissue damage and in tuberculoid cases. It has been used in combination with sulphones or with isoniazid. It is more valuable when used alone in patients who react strongly to dapsone. It is useful in patients showing intolerance to sulphones.

Dose : 500 mg a day; dose may be increased, if necessary to 2 gm a day.

Preparations : Thiambutosine tablets, B.P.C. - contain 500 mg of thiambutosine.

Exercise

Q1. Name the two important drugs used in the treatment of leprosy. Draw structure and give chemical name of any one. (Winter 04)

Q2. Enumerate 'Leprostatic agents' from different classes and draw the structure, chemical name of a drug from 'Sulphone group'. (Summer 03)

Q3. Write note on Analeptics. (May 07)

Q4. Write category and use of Dapsone. (May 07)

6 Antiamoebics and Anthelmintics

Antiamoebics

Amoebiasis is caused by infection due to protozoan parasite *Entamoeba histolytica*. It is a disease primarily of the tropics but it has a worldwide occurrence. It also occurs in villages in temperate areas where sanitation is poor. Infection is transmitted by the faecal oral route.

Amoebae present in the lumen or wall of the gut may give rise to dysentery (intestinal amoebiasis) while those present in the liver give rise to liver abscesses (hepatic amoebiasis). The most common clinical symptom of amoebiasis is dysentery. An infection of the intestine or liver may lead to a chronic debilitating condition. Intestinal amoebiasis is characterised by a bloody diarrhoea along with mucus. The diarrhoea may occur intermittently separated by periods of constipation. In severe amoebic dysentery, intestinal ulceration may even cause perforation, haemorrhage and death. A majority of the carriers are symptom free with only cysts appearing in their stools. Amoebic liver abscess is caused by death and liquefaction of liver cells surrounding the amoebae. The amoebae are taken up via the hepatic portal system from the gut to the liver. Rarely, amoebic abscesses may develop in the lungs and brain.

Many drugs are available for the treatment of amoebiasis, and most of them are suitable for use in both intestinal and hepatic forms. They include acetarsol, chloroquine, clioquinol, diiodohydroxyquinoline, diloxanide furoate, emetine, haloquinol, metronidazole and tetracyclines.

Life Cycle of *Entamoeba Histolytica*

Infection is caused by the ingestion of viable cysts through food or drink contaminated with infected faeces. Motile amoebae are destroyed in the stomach and are not infective. The infective cyst contains four nuclei which divide once to form eight nuclei. In the intestine, the parasite develops into a metacyst. The cyst hatches in the small intestine and liberates eight trophozoites which grow into mature amoebae in the large intestine. The amoebae multiply by fission. These colonies cause the diarrhoea associated

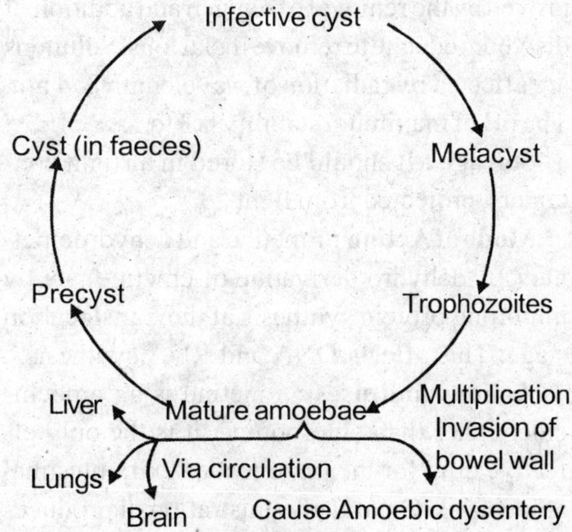

with the infection. They live on bacteria but may invade the intestinal wall causing ulcers. Some organisms enter the portal circulation and reach the liver causing liver abscesses while some may reach the brain or lungs.

The parasites form precysts in the dehydrated environment of the large intestine. Cyst formation enables the amoebae to survive the hardships during transfer from one host to another. The cysts are egested along with the excreta and are now capable of infecting a new host.

Chemotherapeutic Agents

1) Emetine hydrochloride

It is an alkaloid obtained from ipecacuanha and may be prepared by methylating cephaeline.

Properties : It occurs as a white, crystalline powder. It is odourless and has a bitter taste. It becomes faintly yellow on exposure to light. It is soluble in water, alcohol and chloroform. It is practically insoluble in ether. A solution in water is dextrorotatory.

Stability : Solutions of emetine hydrochloride buffered in the pH range 2 to 3.5 are sufficiently stable to be heat sterilised. Stability to heat is improved by the removal of oxygen and addition of disodium edetate to remove metal ions. Solutions are affected by radiation of wavelength 254 nm. The pH of maximum stability is 3 to 7.

Storage : It should be stored in airtight containers, protected from light.

Mode of Action : Emetine and dehydroemetine (2,3-dehydro derivative of emetine) act by inhibiting protein synthesis at the translocation stage. This affects DNA and RNA synthesis.

Actions and uses : Emetine is an amoebicide. Other than chloroquine, it is the only effective drug for the treatment of extraintestinal amoebiasis. On oral administration, it produces an emetic effect. Hence, it is used only as subcutaneous or intramuscular injections. It rapidly relieves the symptoms of amoebic dysentery but it does not eliminate cysts and does not effect a cure. For eradicating intestinal infection, emetine is recommended in combination with another amoebicide such as bismuth iodide, diloxanide furoate or metronidazole. Dehydroemetine is equally effective as emetine but is less toxic.

Emetine produces gastrointestinal, neuromuscular and cardiovascular side effects. Hypotension, tachycardia and arrhythmia may be observed.

Dose : 60 mg a day for 4 to 10 days by intramuscular (IM) or subcutaneous (SC) injection.

Preparations : Emetine injection I.P. It contains 60 mg of emetine hydrochloride in 1 ml.

Emetine injection, B.P., B.P.C.

Emetine hydrochloride injection, U.S.P.

All these indicate a sterile solution of emetine hydrochloride in water for injection, pH adjusted to 3. The usual strength is 60 mg per ml.

2) Metronidazole

2-(2-Methyl-5-nitroimidazol-1-yl) ethanol.

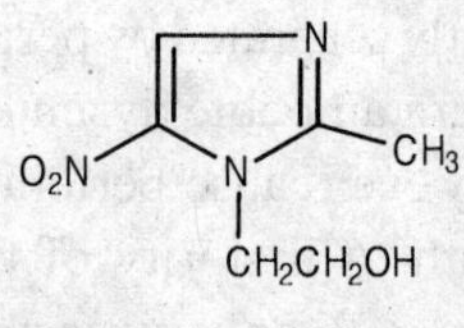

Metronidazole is a nitroimidazole derivative. Another drug belonging to this class and having similar activity is tinidazole.

Properties : Metronidazole occurs as a white or creamy white crystalline powder. It has a slight odour and a bitter, saline taste. It is sparingly soluble in water and slightly soluble in alcohol and chloroform. It is very slightly soluble in ether. Melting point is about 160°C. It darkens on exposure to light.

Storage : Store in airtight containers, protected from light.

Mode of action : The mechanism of action is not established. Activity may be due to 1-acetic acid metabolite.

Actions and uses : Metronidazole has antiprotozoal and antibacterial actions. It is effective against *Trichomonas vaginalis, Entamoeba histolytica, Giardia lamblia* and against anaerobic bacteria. It is a drug of choice for severe intestinal amoebiasis and is the primary drug in hepatic abscess. It is effective at all sites of infection in amoebiasis and also for eradication of *E. histolytica* from patients passing cysts. It is also used in the treatment of trichomoniasis of the genito-urinary tract and of giardiasis and Vincent's angina. It is a bactericidal drug used to treat infections by anaerobic bacteria such as Bacteroides and Fusobacterium species. The drug is well absorbed when given orally.

Dose : In amoebiasis 500 mg three times a day for 5 to 10 days.

Preparations : Metronidazole tablets, I.P., B.P., B.P.C., U.S.P. usual strength is 200 and 400 mg of metronidazole.

Metronidazole injection, I.P.

Metronidazole benzoate oral suspension, I.P.

Brand Names : Aldezol®, Aristogyl®, Flagyl®, Metrogyl®, Unimezol®

3) Iodochlorhydroxyquin

(Clioquinol, Chinoform, Quiniodochlor)

5 - Chloro - 8 - hydroxy-7 - iodoquinoline.

8-Hydroxyquinoline (oxine) has antibacterial and antifungal properties due to its ability to chelate metal ions. The substitution of halogen atoms on the quinoline nucleus produces compounds with a broad spectrum of antimicrobial properties.

Diiodohydroxyquin and iodochlorhydroxyquin are such halogenated hydroxyquinolines.

Properties : Iodochlorhydroxquin occurs as a yellowish-white to brownish-yellow, voluminous powder. It has a faint characteristic odour and is tasteless. It is very slightly soluble in water and alcohol. It is soluble in dimethylformamide and in pyridine. Melting point is about 180°C, with decomposition.

Storage : It should be protected from light.

Actions and uses : Iodochlorhydroxyquin is an antiseptic and amoebicide. It is poorly absorbed from the gastrointestinal tract and is therefore ineffective in extraintestinal amoebiasis. It is used in the treatment of intestinal amoebiasis and bacillary dysentery. It is also used as a suppository or cream for the treatment of intestinal trichomoniasis. For the treatment of skin infections, it is available in lotions, creams and ointments, usually in a concentration of 3 per cent. Toxic effects of the drug include optic and peripheral neuropathy. It stains the skin & clothes.

Dose : In intestinal amoebiasis 250 mg, 3 to 6 times a day for 10 days, course repeated after a gap of 10 days.

Preparations : Quiniodochlor tablets, I.P. - contain 250 mg of iodochlorhdroxyquin.

Iodochlorhydroxyquin tablets, U.S.P.

Clioquinol cream, B.P., B.P.C.

Hydrocortisone acetate and clioquinol cream, B.P.

Iodochlorhydroxyquin cream, U.S.P.

Hydrocortisone and clioquinol ointment, B.P., B.P.C.

Compound Iodochlorhydroxyquin powder, U.S.P.

Brand Names : Enteroquinol®, Quinoform®

4) Diiodohydroxyquinoline

(Diiodohydroxyquin, iodoquinol).

5, 7 - Diiodo - 8 - hydroxyquinoline.

Properties : It occurs as a pale yellowish to yellowish-brown, microcrystalline powder. It is practically insoluble in water and very slightly soluble in alcohol and in ether. Melting point is about 200° to 215°C, with decomposition.

Storage : It should be protected from light.

Actions and uses : Di-iodohydroxyquinoline is an amoebicide. It is poorly absorbed when given orally; and hence a large proportion of the dose reaches the large intestine and acts on the amoebae there. It is used chiefly to treat chronic infections. It is frequently used to supplement emetine therapy in amoebic dysentery. It has been used for the treatment of infections by *Giardia lamblia* and *Balantidium coli*. Pessaries of the drug are used to treat trichomonal and candidal vaginitis. The side effects include abdominal pain and optical neuritis.

Dose : In amoebiasis 300 to 600 mg, 3 to 4 times a day for 21 days.

Preparations : Diiodohydroxyquinoline tablets I.P., B.P. - contain 300 mg and 650 mg of diiodohydroxyquinoline.

Iodoquinol tablets, U.S.P.

Diiodohydroxyquinoline pessaries, B.P.C.

Brand Names : Diodoquin®

5) Diloxanide furoate

2,2-Dichloro-4-hydroxy-N-methylacetanilide -2-furoate.

Properties : It occurs as a white, crystalline powder. It is odourless and tasteless. It is slightly soluble in water and ether, sparingly soluble in alcohol and freely soluble in chloroform. Melting point is about 115°C.

Storage : It should be protected from light.

Mode of action : The mechanism is not yet clear. It probably interferes with the biosynthesis of protein, like chloramphenicol. Drug metabolism studies indicate that hydrolysis of the ester is required for amoebicidal effect.

Actions and uses : On oral administration, diloxanide furoate is hydrolysed and the free base is absorbed. It is used in the treatment of amoebiasis. It has a direct effect upon the amoebae in the gut and has no antibacterial action. It is used in the treatment of acute and chronic intestinal amoebiasis and of asymptomatic carriers. It is also used together with chloroquine in the treatment of amoebic hepatitis.

Dose : 500 mg three times a day for 10 days.

Preparations : Diloxanide furoate tablets I.P., B.P. contain 500 mg of diloxanide furoate.

Brand Names : Amicline®, Entamizole®, Dyrade-M®, Furamide®

6) Paromomycin sulphate

Aminosidin sulphate (crestomycin sulphate), an antibiotic obtained from *Streptomyces chrestomyceticus* and Monomycin, an antibiotic isolated from *Streptomyces circulatus* var. *monomycini*, are considered to be identical with paromomycin. Paromomycin sulphate is a mixture of the sulphates of the antimicrobial substances produced by the growth of certain strains of *Streptomyces rimosus* forma *paromomycinus*. It is an aminoglycoside antibiotic.

Properties : It occurs as a creamy-white to light yellow, hygroscopic and amorphous powder. It is odourless and has a saline taste. It is very soluble in water, soluble in dilute acids and solutions of alkali hydroxides. It is practically insoluble in alcohol, chloroform and ether. Its solution in water is dextrorotatory. The drug contains 750 units per mg.

Actions and uses : Paromomycin sulphate is directly amoebicidal against *Entamoeba histolytica*. It acts by interfering in DNA replication, leading to errors in transcription. It is poorly absorbed from the gastrointestinal tract. It is used orally in the treatment of intestinal amoebiasis. Its antimicrobial spectrum is similar to that of neomycin sulphate and it is also used to treat enteritis and to suppress intestinal flora preoperatively. It is also effective in tapeworm infestation.

Dose : The equivalent of 25 mg of paromomycin per kg body weight daily in 3 doses for 5 to 10 days.

Preparations : Paromomycin sulphate capsules U.S.P. - contain drug equivalent to 250 mg of paromomycin.

Anthelmintics

Anthelmintics are drugs used to rid the body of worms known as helminths. An anthelmintic may act either locally to expel worms from the gastrointestinal tract or systemically to eradicate different forms of helminths that invade organs and tissues.

Helminthiasis or worm infestation afflicts billions of people every year and its prevalence is increasing. A human patient may carry an infestation throughout his life. The most serious infestation is that due to *Schistosoma* or blood fluke. Effective drugs are now available that can cure infections caused by intestinal helminths. However, improved drugs are still needed to control systemic infections such as filariasis, trichinosis and schistosomiasis which are caused by tissue dwelling helminths.

Helminths parasitic to man and other animals are derived from two families Platyhelminthes - eg. cestodes (tapeworms) and trematodes (flukes).

Nemathelminthes - eg. nematodes (round worms).

Ascariasis is one of the most common helminth infections of the intestine. It is caused by Ascaris lumbricoides, commonly called roundworm, which is 15-25 cm long. It is transmitted by the faecal-oral route. Swallowed ova, hatch in the intestine. The larvae pass into the bloodstream and travel to the lungs from where they migrate via trachea and oesophagus to mature in the small intestine. Larvae which die on the way lead to foreign tissue reaction, giving rise to fever, cough, expectoration and dyspnoea. Though intestinal infection is usually symptomless, heavy infection may cause intestinal obstruction. Drugs used in the treatment of ascariasis include mebendazole, pyrantel pamoate, ivermectin, bephenium and piperazine.

1) Piperazine citrate

The adipate, citrate and phosphate salts of piperazine besides the hydrate, are official in I.P.

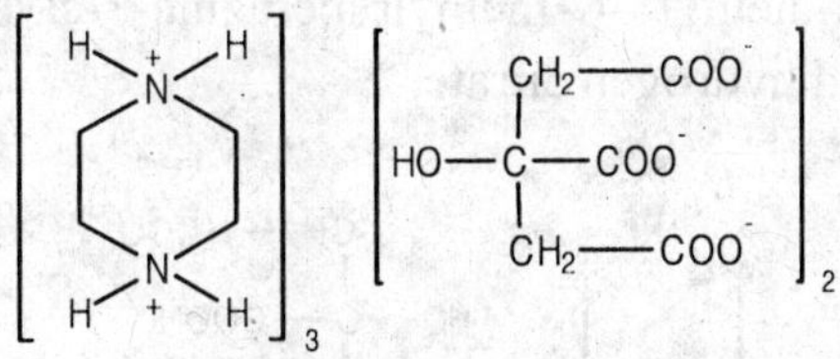

Properties : Piperazine citrate occurs as a white, crystalline powder. It is odourless. It is freely soluble in water, very slightly soluble in alcohol and ether. Melting point is about 190°C.

Storage : It should be protected from light.

Mode of action : Piperazine acts by selective neuromuscular blocking action on the parasites. It blocks the action of acetylcholine. The worms are paralysed and narcotised and thus expelled with the stools.

Actions and uses : Piperazine is effective against roundworms and threadworms. Narcosis of roundworms in the gut, at all stages of maturity occurs, but the larva forms in the tissues are not affected. Piperazine and its salts are readily absorbed after oral administration. If the patient has normal bowel movement, a purgative is not necessary. For who get constipated patients who get, a purgative should be given along with anthelmintic so that the worms are expelled before the effect of the drug wears off.

Dose : Against ascaris : 3.5 gm once a day for 2 days. Against enterobius (pinworms) : 2 gm once a day for 7 days.

Preparations : Piperazine adipate tablets I.P. - contain 300 mg of the drug.

Piperazine citrate elixir I.P., B.P.C.

Piperazine citrate syrup I.P.

Piperazine citrate oral suspension I.P.

Piperazine phosphate tablets I.P., B.P. - contain 260mg, 520mg of the drug.

Brand Names : Piperazine citrate 500®, Piperazine citrate® syp.

2) Diethylcarbamazine citrate (D.E.C.)

N,N-diethyl - 4 - methylpiperazine-1-carboxamide dihydrogen citrate.

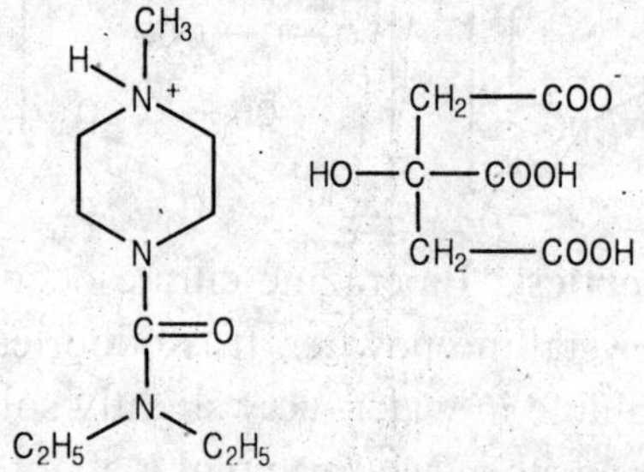

Properties : It occurs as a white, crystalline powder. It is odourless and has a bitter, acidic taste. It is soluble in water, sparingly soluble in alcohol and practically insoluble in ether, chloroform and acetone. Melting point is about 137°C.

Storage : It should be stored in airtight containers.

Actions and uses : Diethylcarbamazine is used in the treatment and prophylaxis of filariasis and tropical eosinophilia. It is lethal to the microfilaria of *Wuchereria bancrofti, Loa loa* (infection-loaiasis) and *Onchocerca volvulus* (infection-onchocerciasis).

In the treatment of *W. bancrofti* infections the microfilariae are rapidly eliminated from the blood stream. The drug modifies the larvae in such a way that they are trapped by reticuloendothelial cells in the liver sinusoids. This action on larvae limits the spread of the disease through the insect vector. The action of the drug on adult worms is much slower and several months may be required for eliminating them. In loaiasis, both microfilaria and adult worms are killed. In onchocerciasis, the microfilariae may be killed but the adult parasites are less affected by the drug.

Diethylcarbamazine is readily absorbed after oral administration. It has mild toxicity. The side effects include anorexia, drowsiness, headache, nausea, vomiting and allergic reactions.

Dose : 6 mg per kg body weight a day for 3 or 4 weeks.

Preparations : Diethylcarbamazine citrate tablets, I.P. - contain 50 mg and 100 mg of the drug.

Diethylcarbamazine citrate tablets, B.P. - contain 50, 100 & 200 mg of the drug.

Brand Names : Banocide®, Carbamyl®, Dicarb®, Hetrazan®

3) Mebendazole

Methyl-5-benzoylbenzimidazole-2-carbamate.

Mebendazole is a broad spectrum anthelmintic.

Properties : It occurs as a white to slightly yellow, odourless, amorphous powder. It is practically insoluble in water, alcohol, chloroform, ether and dilute mineral acids. It is freely soluble in formic acid. Melting point is about 290°C.

Storage : It should be stored in well-closed containers.

Mode of action : Mebendazole acts by inhibiting the uptake of glucose in the helminths. This leads to a lethal decrease in their energy reserves.

Actions and uses : Mebendazole is an anthelmintic effective against threadworms (*En-*

terobius), roundworms (*Ascaris*), whipworms (*Trichuris*) and hookworms (*Ancylostoma* and *Necator*). It is also used in the treatment of capillariasis and is possibly effective against tapeworms. There is evidence that mebendazole may be used as an alternative to diethylcarbamazine in the treatment of onchocerciasis. Mebendazole is poorly absorbed from the gastrointestinal tract. Adverse effects such as nausea, vomiting, abdominal pain and diarrhoea may occur occasionally.

Dose : For hookworm, roundworm and whipworm infections - 100 mg twice a day for 3 days.

Preparations : Mebendazole tablets I.P. - contain 100 mg of mebendazole.

Mebendazole tablets U.S.P.

Brand Names : Eben®, Mendazole®, Mebazole®, Mebex®, Wormin®

Drugs For Further Study

Antiamoebics

1) Dehydrometine
2) Satranidazole - Satrogyl®
3) Tinidazole - Cozit®, Fasigyn®, Tiniba®, Tinibid®
4) Secnidazole - Entosec®, Flagentyl®, Secnil®, Seczol®
5) Ornidazole - Dazolic®, Giro®, Oniz®, Orni®
6) Enteroquinol - Entrozyme®

Anthelmintics

1) Levamisole - Dewormis®, Dicaris®, Vermisol®
2) Pyrantel pamoate - Expent®, Nemocid®, Pymolar®
3) Ivermectin - Ivermectol®
4) Niclosamide - Niclosan®
5) Praziquantel - Prazine®
6) Albendazole - Alzad®, Combantrin-A®, Sioban®
7) Nitazoxanide - Nitarid®, Nizonide®, Zimdax®

Exercise

Q1. What are Anti-amoebic agents? Classify them with suitable examples. (Winter 04, Summer 03, May-June 04)

Q2. Draw structure and give chemical name, uses and official preparations of Metronidazole. (Winter 04)

Q3. Define Anthelmintics and name the drugs used for its treatment and is the properties of D.E.C. (Winter 04)

Q4. In what dosage form the the following drug is given - Metronidazole. (Summer 03)

Q5. Give dose, official preparation, uses and one brand name of - i) Mebendazole, ii) Metronidazole. (Summer 06)

Q6. Specify dosage forms (tablet, capsule etc..) for the following - i) Emetine HCl, ii) Mebendazole. (May-June 04)

Q7. Write category and use of - Diloxanide. (May 07)

Q8. Write the brand names of the following drugs - i) Diloxamide furoate, ii) Metronidazole. (Nov 06)

Q9. What do you understand by ameobiasis? Classify antiameobic drugs. Write a note on emetine hydrochloride. (Nov 06)

Q10. Write the structure and use of Metronidazole. (Nov 06)

Q11. What is DEC? Give it's structure, chemical name and uses. (Summer 06)

■

7 Antibiotics

Antibiotics are substances produced by microorganisms during growth, which in high dilution can destroy or inhibit the growth of other species of microorganisms. Antibiotics are a category of antimicrobials, the other category being chemotherapeutic substances. The term 'antibiotic' was introduced by Waksman in 1942. Though the term technically includes only microbial metabolites, it has been now extended to include chemically related and derived substances which are produced entirely or partly by chemical synthesis. There are some antibiotics which have little or no antimicrobial activity but show a cytotoxic effect on mammalian tumour cells and are used as antineoplastic drugs.

Antimicrobial Action

Based on their *in vitro* effects on certain strains of microorganisms, antibiotics are divided into two types - bacteriostatic and bactericidal. The results should be obtained using antibiotic concentrations which are attained in human body by the administration of therapeutic doses. Bacteriostatic antibiotics reversibly inhibit the growth of susceptible microorganisms while bactericidal antibiotics kill the organisms. Given in high therapeutic doses, penicillins, cephalosporins, aminoglycosides and polymyxins are bactericidal, whereas tetracyclines, chloramphenicol and erythromycin are usually bacteriostatic. An antibiotic which is bactericidal in higher concentration may become bacteriostatic at lower concentrations. The maintenance of a bactericidal effect depends upon adequate dosage and tissue penetration.

The sensitivity of a specific microorganism to an antibiotic is shown by the parameter, minimum inhibitory concentration (MIC). This is the lowest concentration of antibiotic which will inhibit the growth of a given strain of microorganism under controlled conditions. It is expressed as mcg of antibiotic per ml of medium. Similarly, the minimum bactericidal concentration (MBC) may also be used.

The mechanisms of action of different antibiotics are discussed for the separate classes.

Antimicrobial Spectrum of Antibiotics

Bacteria may be divided into Gram-positive and Gram-negative types and may be coccal or rod-shaped. Gram-positive genera include *Bacillus, Clostridium, Corynebacterium, Micrococcus and Streptococcus, Gram-negative genera include Brucella, Escherichia, Haemophilus, Klebsiella, Pseudomonas, Salmonella, Shigella* and *Neisseria.*

Classification According to Antimicrobial Spectrum

A) Those active against Gram-positive Bacteria and Gram-negative Cocci

Standard penicillins (penicillin G and penicillin V), antistaphylococcal penicillins (cloxacillin), erythromycin, rifampicin and spectinomycin.

B) Those active against Gram-negative Bacilli

For systemic use-aminoglycosides, penicillins (ampicillin, amoxycillin), polypeptides (bacitracin).

For topical use - neomycin.

C) Broad spectrum antibiotics

Cephalosporins (cephalexin, cephaloridine), chloramphenicol, tetracyclines.

D) Antibiotics used for specific infections

a) Anaerobic organisms - lincomycin.

b) Tuberculosis - rifampicin, streptomycin, cycloserine.

c) Antifungals - amphotericin, griseofulvin, nystatin.

d) Antivirals - cytarabine (synthetic drug).

Classification According to Chemical Structures

I) Penicillins

eg. penicillin G , penicillin V, ampicillin, amoxycillin, cloxacillin, dicloxacillin.

II) Cephalosporins

eg. cephalexin, cephaloridine, cephalothin.

III) Aminoglycosides

eg. streptomycin, gentamycin, amikacin.

IV) Tetracyclines

eg. tetracycline, chlortetracycline, oxytetracycline, doxycycline.

V) Polypeptides

eg. bacitracin, capreomycin, colistin, polymyxin B, dactinomycin, viomycin.

VI) Macrolides

eg. erythromycin, leucomycin, oleandomycin, spiramycin.

VII) Lincosamides

eg. clindamycin, lincomycin.

VIII) Rifamycins (ansamycins)

eg. rifampicin, rifamycin SV.

IX) Steroids

eg. fusidic acid.

X) Polyenes

eg. nystatin, amphotericin B, candidicin.

XI) Miscellaneous

eg. chloramphenicol.

I] Penicillins

Penicillin was discovered by Sir Alexander Fleming in 1928. It was first used clinically in 1941. In the earlier years, penicillin G (benzylpenicillin) was obtained from strains of *Penicillium notatum*. It is now obtained from strains of *Penicillium chrysogenum* which are more productive.

Only two clinically useful penicillins are produced naturally by fermentation which are penicillin G and penicillin V (phenoxymethylpenicillin). These two penicillins on enzymatic or chemical hydrolysis, give the microbial metabolite, 6-aminopenicillanic acid (6 APA). From this intermediate, a series of semisynthetic penicillins has been prepared by acylation eg. ampicillin, amoxycillin, cloxacillin.

Mode of action of penicillins and cephalosporins

Penicillins and cephalosporins are β-lactam antibiotics and have a similar mode of action. They produce a bactericidal effect by interfering with cell wall synthesis. The cell wall of bacteria is essential for their normal growth and development. It is composed of peptidoglycan. The biosynthesis of peptidoglycan involves about 30 bacterial enzymes of which transpeptidase enzyme is inhibited competitively by penicillins and cephalosporins. The enzyme is acylated by penicillin resulting in formation of penicilloyl enzyme.

Besides inhibiting transpeptidase, the β-lactam antibiotics also act at penicillin binding proteins (PBP) and on autolytic enzymes, i.e., autolysins. These antibiotics increase the activity of the autolysins leading to lysis of bacteria.

Classification of Penicillins

Penicillins may be classified according to their spectrum of antimicrobial activity as -

a) Penicllin G and its close congeners penicillin V and phenethicillin : These are highly active against Gram-positive cocci but are readily hydrolysed by penicillinase produced by *Staphylococcus aureaus* and other organisms.

b) Penicillinase resistant penicillins : methicillin, nafcillin, oxacillin, cloxacillin and dicloxacillin. These are effective against penicillinase producing *Staphylococcus aureaus*.

c) Broad spectrum penicillins : ampicillin, amoxycillin and hetacillin. These are active against Gram-positive bacteria and also Gram-negative bacteria such as *Haemophilus influenzae*, *Escherichia coli* and *Proteus mirabilis*.

d) Extended spectrum antibiotics : carbenicillin, ticarcillin. These are active against Gram-positive bacteria and some Gram-negative bacteria such as *Pseudomonas, Enterobacter* and *Proteus* species.

e) Other extended spectrum penicillins : mezlocillin and piperacillin. These have an extended spectrum against Gram-negative bacteria such as *Pseudomonas* and *Klebsiella.*

Stability of penicillins

Penicillins are degraded by strong acids and alkalis and by bacterial enzymes called penicillinases. Bacterial resistance to penicillins is commonly due to the production of β-lactamases (penicillinases and amidases). Strong mineral acids or mercuric chloride cause breakdown of penicillin to penicillamine and penaldic acid. Penaldic acid loses carbon dioxide on heating to produce penilloaldehyde. In dilute acid solutions (pH 5), at room temperature, penicillin undergoes molecular rearrangement to give penillic acid.

Alkalis and the enzyme penicillinase attack the β-lactam ring to yield penicilloic acid. On heating, penicilloic acid loses carbon-dioxide to give penilloic acid. On treatment with mercuric chloride, this acid gives penicillamine and penilloaldehyde. The role of amidases in causing bacterial resistance is less important because of their less frequent occurrence. Amidases or acylases hydrolyse penicillin to produce 6-aminopenicillanic acid (6 APA).

General pharmacological properties of penicillins

The penicillins which are stable to gastric acid are well absorbed after oral administration. Following absorption, the penicillins are widely distributed throughout the body. Therapeutic concentrations are readily achieved in tissues and in secretions such as joint fluid and bile. Concentration in cerebrospinal fluid, pleural fluid, are low and are between 1 to 5 per cent of the plasma concentration in the normal patient. When there is inflammation of the meninges and a proteinaceous exudate, the levels are the same as in blood. Penicillins are rapidly eliminated by the kidneys and have short half-lives of 30 to 60 minutes.

Untoward reactions

All penicillins carry a risk of causing hypersensitivity which develops most readily as a result of topical application. Penicillins should be avoided being administered to patients with a history of allergy to any form of penicillin. Allergic reactions observed include skin rashes, dermatitis, fever, serum sickness and angioedema. Anaphylactic shock may develop rapidly and is characterised by cardiovascular collapse, bronchospasm and angioedema. It may lead to severe hypotension and rapid death.

Products

1) Benzylpenicillin (Penicillin G, Penicillin)

Potassium or sodium salt of (6R)-6-phenylacetamido-penicillanic acid.

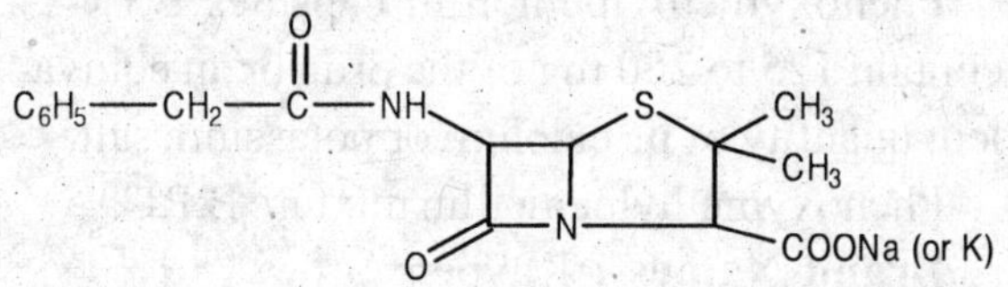

Benzylpenicillin is an antibiotic produced by growing certain strains of *Penicillium notatum* or related organisms under appropriate conditions in a suitable culture medium. The international unit (I.U.) of penicillin is the specific activity contained in 0.6 mcg of the crystalline sodium salt of benzylpenicillin. 1 mg of the pure drug equals 1667 units, 600 mg equals 1 mega unit (10 lakh units).

Properties : Benzylpenicillin sodium (or potassium) occurs as a white, finely crystalline, hygroscopic powder. It has a faint characteristic odour. It is very soluble in water, practically insoluble in fixed oils and liquid paraffin. Its solution is dextrorotatory.

Stability : The stability of benzylpenicillin depends mainly on its moisture content. When moisture is less than 0.5 per cent, it can be stored at room temperature for 2 to 3 years without significant loss of potency. For maximum stability, aqueous solutions of benzylpenicillin should be buffered at pH 6 to 7 and kept at a low temperature.

Incompatibility : Acids, alkalis, penicillinase and many other substances inactivate benzylpenicillin at varying rates. Traces of heavy metals, high concentrations of glycerol and propylene glycol have a deleterious action on penicillin solutions. Benzylpenicillin salts are incompatible with sympathomimetic amines and hydrochlorides of tetracyclines. Other incompatible substances are oxidising agents, organic peroxides, wool alcohols, paraffins, macrogols, cocoa butter and many surfactants. Benzylpenicillin should not be given as intravenous infusion in dextrose injection, because the acidity of the dextrose solution will bring about its rapid decomposition.

Storage : It should be stored in airtight containers at a temperature not exceeding 30°C.

Actions and uses : Benzylpenicillin is a highly potent antibiotic and is widely used even today. It is the antibiotic of choice for several infections. It is useful in infections caused by *Streptococcus pneumoniae (pneumococcal pneumonia), Streptococcus pyogenes*, species of *Neisseria, Actinomyces, Clostridium, Corynebacterium and Erysipelothrix, Bacillus anthracis* and the spirochaetes. It is also used to treat infections caused by anaerobes, in meningococcal infections, in gonococcal infections and in syphilis. It is used prophylactically to prevent infections caused by *Streptococcus pyogenes*, recurrences of rheumatic fever, gonorrhoea, syphilis and infections during certain surgical procedures. Many Gram-negative bacteria and resistant strains of *staphylococci* produce enzymes called penicillinases which destroy penicillin by opening the β - lactam ring.

On oral administration, gastric acid rapidly destroys benzylpenicillin. About 30 per cent of the oral dose is absorbed from the intenstine. Its potassium and sodium salts are administered by oral and parenteral routes. Since excretion is rapid, injection of salt solution has to be given frequently. Its excretion by renal tubular secretion can be blocked by administering probenecid. This prolongs its action. More commonly, repository preparations such as procaine penicillin and benzathine penicillin are used to get a prolonged effect.

Dose : 2.5 to 10 lakh units (150 to 600 mg),

2 to 4 times a day by IM injection or orally.

Preparations : Benzylpenicillin injection, I.P. - usual strengths are 2.5 lakh, 5 lakh and 10 lakh units. It is prepared immediately before use by dissolving the contents of a sealed container in water for injection.

Benzylpenicillin injection, B.P.C. - Powder in vials containing 0.2 lakh, 5 lakh and 10 lakh units, in bottles containing 5 and 10 megaunits. Bottles contain sodium citrate as buffering agent.

Brand Names : Pentids®, Benzyl PEN®, Bistrepen® inj., Sodicillin®

2) Phenoxymethylpenicillin (Penicillin V)

(6R) -6-(2-Phenoxyacetamido) penicillanic acid

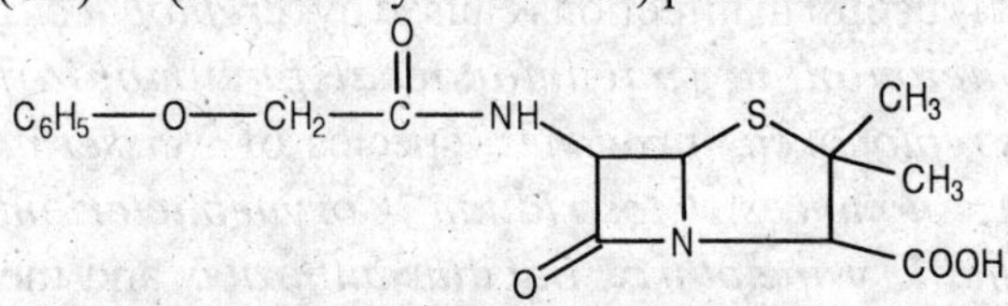

Properties : Phenoxymethylpenicillin occurs as a white, finely crystalline powder. It is freely soluble in alcohol, very slightly soluble in water, practically insoluble in fixed oils and liquid paraffin. It is dextrorotatory.

Storage : It should be stored in airtight containers.

Actions and uses : It resists hydrolysis by the acidic gastric juice and therefore, is well absorbed after oral administration. Its spectrum of activity and uses are similar to those of benzylpenicillin. The free acid is relatively insoluble in water. For preparing parenteral solutions, its potassium salt is usually employed. Solutions are made from the dry salt at the time of administration. The salt of phenoxymethylpenicillin with hydrabamine, Compocillin V, provides a very long-acting form of this compound. Aqueous suspensions of this drug are used as liquid oral dosage forms.

Dose : 125 to 500 mg (2 lakh to 8 lakh units) every 6 to 8 hours.

Preparations : Phenoxymethylpenicillin potassium tablets I.P. - contain the equivalent of 62.5 mg, 125 mg, 250 mg and 500 mg of phenoxymethylpenicillin.

Phenoxymethylpenicillin tablets, B.P.C. - contain 125, 250 and 300 mg of phenoxymethylpenicillin or an equivalent amount of its calcium or potassium salt.

Phenoxymethylpenicillin capsules B.P.C. - contain 125 to 250 mg of the drug or an equivalent quantity of its calcium or potassium salt.

Phenoxymethylpenicillin mixture B.P.C.

Brand Names : Kaypen®

3) Benzathine penicillin

(Benzathine Penicillin G)

It is the N,N`-dibenzylethylenediamine salt of benzylpenicillin. 1.2 mega units of penicillin is contained in approximately 900 mg of benzathine penicillin.

Properties : It occurs as a white, crystalline powder. It is hygroscopic and odourless. It is very slightly soluble in water, alcohol, ether and in chloroform. It is freely soluble in formamide and dimethylformamide. Melting point is about 131°C with decomposition.

Stability : When stored protected from moisture at room temperature, the dry material retains its potency for upto 5 years. Aqueous suspensions buffered to pH 6 to 7 and stored at a low temperature (below 25°C), retains potency up to 2 years.

Storage : It should be stored in airtight containers at a temperature not exceeding 25°C, protected from light, in a dry place.

Actions and uses : Benzathine penicillin is a derivative of benzylpenicillin having low solubility. Its action is due to release of benzylpenicillin. When given by mouth, it is hydrolysed in the gut with the formation of benzylpenicillin which is absorbed. Therapeutic doses give an effective concentration for 6 hours or more. Intramuscular injections of benzathine penicillin are used to provide a prolonged effect and avoid the need for repeated injections. A dose of 900 mg provides therapeutic blood levels for 2 weeks.

Dose : Oral - 450 mg (6 lakh units) every 6 hours.

Intramuscular injection - 225 mg (3 lakh units) to 750 mg (1 mega unit)

Preparations : Benzathine Penicillin injection, I.P. - usual strength is 6 lakh units. It is prepared by dissolving the contents of a sealed container in water for injection. The constituted suspension should be stored in a cool place and used within 7 days. When a buffering agent is present and the suspension is stored in a cold place, it should be used within 14 days.

Fortified benzathine penicillin injection, I.P., B.P.C. - it is a sterile suspension of benzathine penicillin (6 lakh units) and procaine penicillin (3 lakh units), with appropriate adjuvants, in a solution of benzylpenicillin potassium or sodium (3 lakh units) in water for injection. It is prepared by adding water for injection to the contents of a sealed container. The injection should be used immediately after preparation or within 7 days, if stored at 2°C to 4°C.

Benzathine penicillin tablets, I.P. - usually contain 2 lakh units of penicillin.

Brand Names : Pencom® inj., Penidux® inj., Longacillin®

4) Ampicillin

(6R)-6-(α-D-Phenylglycylamino) penicillanic acid.

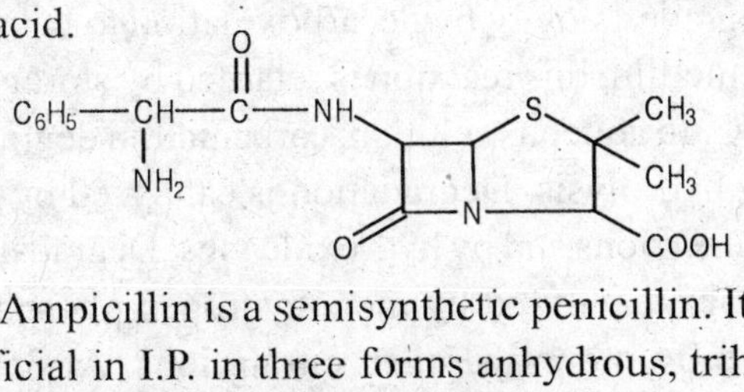

Ampicillin is a semisynthetic penicillin. It is official in I.P. in three forms anhydrous, trihydrate, and sodium salt.

Properties : Ampicillin occurs as a white, microcrystalline powder. It is odourless and has a bitter taste. It is sparingly soluble in water, slightly soluble in alcohol and practically insoluble ether, in chloroform, acetone and fixed oils. It is dextrorotatory. Melting point is about 200°C.

Storage : It should be stored in tightly closed containers in a cool place.

Actions and uses : Ampicillin belongs to the category of broad spectrum penicillins. These are active against both Gram-positive and Gram-negative bacteria. Sensitive organisms include meningococcus, *pneumococcus, gonococcus, enterococcus* and *Haemophilus influenzae*. The therapeutic applications include gonococcal infections; upper respiratory tract infections caused by *H. influenzae* and *Streptococci*, urinary tract infections caused by *Enterobacter* and *Escherichia coli*, meningitis and *Salmonella* infections.

Ampicillin is stable to acid and 30 to 60 per cent of an oral dose is absorbed. It is destroyed by penicillinase produced by resistant strains of microorganisms.

Dose : 2 to 6 gm a day, in divided doses.

Preparations: Ampicillin trihydrate dispersible tablets, I.P.

Ampicillin capsules, I.P. - contain 250 and 500 mg of ampicillin or equivalent quantity of ampicillin trihydrate.

Ampicillin capsules, B.P. - contain 50, 250 and 500 mg of the drug.

Ampicillin for oral suspension, I.P., Ampicillin mixture, B.P.C. - A mixture which, when reconstituted, contains 125 and 250 mg to ampicillin, or the equivalent amount of ampicillin trihydrate, in 5 ml.

Paediatric ampicillin tablets, B.P.C

Ampicillin injection, I.P. - it is a sterile solution of ampicillin sodium equivalent to 100, 250, 500 and 1000 mg of ampicillin. It is prepared by dissolving the contents of a sealed container in water for injection immediately before use.

Brand Names : Ampilin®, Aristocillin®, Campicilin®, Ampidil®

5) Ampicillin sodium

It is freely soluble in water and practically insoluble in ether and fixed oils.

Stability : In aqueous solution, ampicillin sodium degrades by hydrolysis. Degradation is catalysed by hydrogen ions and by hydroxyl ions. Maximum stability at 35°C is at about pH 5.9. Citrate ions and phosphate ions also catalyse degradation. When stored at 5°C, 90 per cent of the potency is retained for 7 days for 1 per cent aqueous solution and for 24 hours for 5 per cent solution.

Incompatibility : In aqueous solution, ampicillin sodium is compatible with streptomycin sulphate but not with its stabilised injection. Ampicillin is incompatible with adrenaline, atropine sulphate, calcium salts, chloramphenicol, heparin, tetracyclines, thiopentone sodium, sodium, solutions of vitamins B and C and many other drugs.

Brand Names : Propen® inj., Unicilin® inj.

6) Cloxacillin sodium

Sodium (6R)-6-[3-(2-chlorophenyl)-5-methylisoxazole-4-carboxamido] penicillanate monohydrate.

Properties : Cloxacillin sodium occurs as a white, crystalline, hygroscopic powder. It is odourless and has an intensely bitter taste. It is freely soluble in water, soluble in alcohol and slightly soluble in chloroform. It is dextrorotatory.

Stability : In aqueous solution, cloxacillin sodium degrades by hydrolysis. Degradation is catalysed by hydrogen ions and by hydroxide ions. Degradation is considerably accelerated by lactate ions. At 25°C, solutions are most stable at pH 6.3, such solutions may lose 10 per cent of their potency after 12 days.

Storage : It should be stored in airtight containers in a cool, dry place.

Actions and uses : Cloxacillin is a semisynthetic penicillin which is not decomposed by staphylococcal penicillinase. It is destroyed by other penicillinases produced by Gram-negative bacteria. It is mainly used in the treatment of penicillinase producing staphylococcal infections. It is acid stable and is used by both oral and parenteral routes.

Dose : Equivalent to 500 mg of cloxacillin, 4 times daily.

Preparations : Cloxacillin capsules I.P., B.P. - contain the sodium salt equivalent to 250 and 500 mg of cloxacillin.

Cloxacillin injection, I.P., B.P., prepared shortly before use, sodium salt equivalent to 250 and 500 mg of cloxacillin.

Cloxacillin elixir, B.P.C.

Brand Names : Bioclox®, Clopen®, Klox®, Neoclox®

7) Carbenicillin disodium

Disodium salt of (6R)-6-(2-carboxy-2-phenylacetamido) penicillanic acid.

It is an extended spectrum penicillin.

Properties : Carbenicillin disodium occurs as a white hygroscopic powder. It is odourless and has a bitter taste. It is freely soluble in water, soluble in alcohol, practically insoluble in chloroform and in ether. It is dextrorotatory.

Stability : In a moist atmosphere, the drug degrades slowly by decarboxylation to benzylpenicillin, this reaction is retarded by storage at 5°C. In aqueous solution, carbenicillin degrades by hydrolysis. Degradation is catalysed by hydrogen ions and by hydroxide ions. Degradation is also catalysed by monohydrogen phosphate and by monohydrogen citrate ions. At 35°C, solutions are most stable at pH 6.5.

Storage : It should be stored in sterile containers, at a temperature not exceeding 5°C, protected from light.

Actions and uses : Carbenicillin is a semisynthetic penicillin which resembles ampicillin. It is not absorbed orally and is given parenterally. It has an extended spectrum of activity against *Pseudomonas aeruginosa, Enterobacter* and *Proteus* species. It is used primarily for the treatment of infections caused by these organisms. It is sometimes given in conjunction with aminoglycosides for synergistic antibacterial activity and to retard the development of resistance during treatment. It is useful in urinary tract infections. The 5-indanyl ester of the drug, carbenicillin indanyl, is orally effective.

Dose : 1 to 2 gm 4 times a day, by IM injection.

Preparations : Carbenicillin injection, I.P., B.P. - available as powder in vials containing sodium salt equivalent to 1 and 5 gm of carbenicillin. The contents are dissolved in water for injection, immediately before use.

Brand Names : Carbelin® inj.

II] Cephalosporins

Cephalosporins have a ring structure closely related to that of the penicillins. In penicillins a thiazolidine ring is fused with the β-lactam ring. In cephalosporins, the thiazolidine ring of penicillins is expanded to a six-membered ring and this is fused with a β-lactam ring. Their mode of action on the bacterial cell wall is similar to that of penicillin and they are bactericidal in nature. They tend to promote allergy in patients allergic to penicillin. They have a broader spectrum of activity than benzylpenicillin. They are relatively resistant to penicillinases. Some of the cephalosporins can be given orally while others have to be given parenterally. The important drugs are cephalexin, cephaloridine and cephalothin.

1) Cephalexin

(7R)-3-Methyl -7- (α-D-phenylglycylamino) ceph-3-em-4, carboxylic acid monohydrate.

Properties : Cephalexin occurs as a white to cream coloured crystalline powder. It has a characteristic odour. It is soluble in dilute acid; sparingly soluble water; very slightly soluble in alcohol, ether, chloroform and acetone.

Stability : Aqueous solutions and suspensions degrade rapidly in neutral or alkaline systems. In acid conditions, the solutions are stable for several days, if refrigerated. Stability is optimum at pH 4.5.

Storage : It should be stored in airtight containers, at a temperature not exceeding 30°C; protected from light.

Actions and uses : Cephalexin is a cephalosporin antibiotic. Cephalexin is not affected by penicillinases produced by Gram-negative organisms. Blood levels of the drug may be increased by blocking tubular excretion with probenecid. Cephalexin is well absorbed after oral administration. It is used to treat infections of respiratory tract, urinary tract, skin and soft tissues, and also in bone and joint infections.

Dose : 500 mg, 4 times a day.

Preparations : Cephalexin capsules, I.P., B.P. - contain 250 and 500 mg of cephalexin.

Cephalexin tablet, I.P. - contain 250 mg of the drug.

Cephalexin tablets, B.P. - contain 250 and 500 mg of the drug.

Cephalexin mixture, B.P.C.

Brand Names : Alcephin®, Cefalex®, Oriphex®, Phexin®, Rofex®, Sporidex®, Sepexin®

2) Cephaloridine

(7R)-3-(1-Pyridiniomethyl)-7-[(thien-2-yl)acetamido-]-ceph-3-em-4-carboxylate

Properties : Cephaloridine occurs as a white, crystalline powder. It is odourless and has a bitter taste. It is freely soluble in water; slightly soluble in alcohol; slightly soluble in ether and in chloroform. It is dextrorotatory.

Stability : Cephaloridine discolours on exposure to light. It is unstable in acidic solutions and in solutions which contain both dextrose and sodium bicarbonate.

Storage : It should be stored in sterile, airtight containers, in a cool place, protected from light.

Actions and uses : It is a cephalosporin antibiotic having some resistance to staphylococcal penicillinase. It is used in the treatment of infections of respiratory tract, urinary tract, soft tissue, bone, joint and other infections. It is used as prophylactic in surgery, dialysis and dental procedures. It is not absorbed when given orally due to its acid labile nature. It is administered by intramuscular injection.

Dose : 0.5 to 1 gm, 2 to 3 times a day by IM injection.

Preparations : Cephaloridine injection, I.P. - available as powder in vial containing 0.5 and 1 gm of cephaloridine.

Cephaloridine injection, E.P.

Brand Names : Ceproan® inj

3) Cephalothin Sodium

Sodium (7R)-7-(thien-2-ylacetamido) cephalosporanate.

Properties : It occurs as a white, crystalline powder. It is almost odourless. It is freely soluble in water; slightly soluble in alcohol; practically insoluble in ether and chloroform.

Stability : Aqueous solutions may retain their potency for 2 days when stored at 2-10°C. It is unstable towards acid.

Storage : It should be stored in sterile, airtight containers, in a cool place, protected from light.

Actions and uses : Cephalothin is a cephalosporin antibiotic with a pharmacological spectrum similar to that of cephaloridine. It is mainly used to treat infections due to organisms which have become resistant to benzylpenicillin and ampicillin. It is the most active of the cephalosporins against staphylococci. It is acid labile and is poorly absorbed when given orally. It is given parenterally.

Dose : Equivalent to 2 to 6 gm of cephalothin daily, in divided doses, by IM or IV injections.

Preparations : Cephalothin injection, B.P. - available as powder in ampoules containing sodium salt equivalent to 1 and 4 gm of cephalothin.

III] Aminoglycosides

These are antibiotics which contain glycosides and aminosugars in their structure. Streptomycin, the first aminoglycoside antibiotic to be used clinically, was discovered by Waksman in 1944. Since then, several antibiotics have been isolated from *Actinomycetes,* particularly from the genus *Streptomyces*. Only the gentamycins are derived from Micromonospora species. Gentamycin, neomycin, kanamycin and paromomycin are closely related in structure to streptomycin.

These antibiotics are poorly absorbed from the alimentary tract. Some of them eg. paromomycin, are used to treat local infections in the intestines. For treating systemic infections, they must be given parenterally. Though they have a broad antimicrobial activity, their use has been limited by serious side effects to the treatment of infections caused by Gram-negative bacteria.

Mechanism of action

The aminoglycoside antibiotics are rapidly bactericidal. They act on the 30S ribosomal subunit in bacteria and inhibit protein synthesis. They also induce misreading of the m-RNA code and incorporation of incorrect amino acids in the polypeptide chains.

Untoward effects

All aminoglycosides can produce ototoxicity and renal toxicity. Ototoxicity occurs due to damage to the eighth cranial nerve. Tinnitus followed by deafness may occur.

(For details of streptomycin, refer unit on antitubercular drugs. For details of paromomycin, refer unit on antiamoebic drugs).

1) Gentamycin Sulphate

Gentamycin sulphate is a complex mixture of the sulphates of gentamycin C_1, gentamycin C_{1A} and gentamycin C_2, antimicrobial substances produced by *Micromonospora purpurea*.

Properties : It occurs as a white to cream-coloured powder. It is soluble in water; practically insoluble in alcohol, ether and chloroform. It is dextrorotatory.

Storage : It should be stored in airtight containers.

Actions and uses : Gentamycin sulphate is a broad spectrum antibiotic which is effective against Gram-positive and Gram-negative bacteria, including *Staphylococcus aureus*, *Pseudomonas* and *Proteus* species and many coliform bacilli. It is bactericidal. It is mainly used to treat severe infections caused by *Pseudomonas aeruginosa* and other bacteria. It is indicated in septicaemia, infections of central nervous system, genitourinary tract, gastrointestinal tract, respiratory system, skin and soft tissue infections, including burns. It is also used in the form of eye drops and ear drops to treat local infections. To delay development of resistance, gentamycin may be given in conjunction with carbenicillin for synergistic action.

Dose : IM or IV - 3 to 5 mg of gentamycin (3000 to 5000 units, as sulphate) per kg body weight daily, in divided doses.

Preparations : Gentamycin injection I.P. - a sterile solution of gentamycin sulphate in water for injection, 80 mg in 2 ml.

Gentamycin eye drops, B.P.C

Gentamycin injection, B.P.C

Gentamycin ointment, B.P.C.

Brand Names : Bactigen® eye drops, Drep® ear drops, Garamycin®, Genka®, Genticyn® E/E drops, Mycin®, Tamiacin®

2) Neomycin Sulphate

Neomycin sulphate is a mixture of the sulphates of the antimicrobial substances produced by the growth of *Streptomyces fradiae*, 500 mg of neomycin sulphate is equivalent to 3.5 lakh units of neomycin.

Properties : It occurs as a hygroscopic, white or yellowish-white powder. It is almost odourless. It is freely soluble in water; very slightly soluble in alcohol and practically insoluble in ether, chloroform and in acetone.

Storage : It should be stored in airtight containers, protected from light, at a temperature not exceeding 30°C.

Actions and uses : Neomycin is an aminoglycoside antibiotic having a wide antibacterial spectrum similar to gentamycin. It is absorbed poorly when given by mouth. It is used typically for the control of staphylococcal infections. It may be used orally as an intestinal antiseptic in gastrointestinal infections. It is used as 0.25 per cent to 0.5 per cent creams and ointments to treat local infections.

Dose : In intestinal infections - 1 to 3 gm a day, in divided doses .

Preparations : Chlorhexidine and neomycin cream, B.P.C

Hydrocortisone and neomycin cream, B.P.C.

Hydrocotisone and neomycin ear-drops, B.P.C.

Hydrocortisone and neomycin eye-drops, B.P.C.

Neomycin elixir, B.P.C.

Neomycin tablets, B.P.

Brand Names : Neosporin® antibiotic powder, Nebasulf®, Betnovate-N® oint., Eldrem® cream

IV] Tetracyclines

The tetracyclines are a group of antibiotics obtained by fermentation procedures from Strep*tomyces* species or by chemical transformations of the microbial metabolites. These antibiotics are derivatives of naphthacene, a hydrocarbon made of four fused rings.

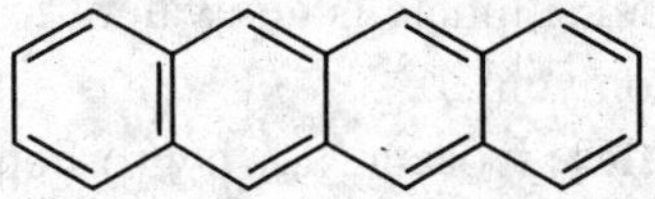

Important drugs from this class are tetracycline, oxytetracycline, chlortetracycline, doxycycline and minocycline. The tetracyclines have emerged as the most important broad spectrum antibiotics. They are active against many Gram-positive and Gram-negative bacteria and also against *rickettsiae, Mycoplasma, Chlamydiae, Plasmodium* and amoebae. Tetracyclines are useful for infections caused by *H.ducreyi* (chancroid), *Brucella* (brucellosis), *Vibrio cholerae,*(cholera) *Yersinia pestis* (plague) and *Francisella tularensis* (tularaemia). These drugs are widely used for the treatment of infections of the chest, soft tissues and for superficial infections. They also have application in treating malaria, typhus, pneumonia, Q fever and psittacosis. The tetracyclines and their hydrochlorides are quite stable as dry powders. Most of them lose activity rapidly in solution. The tetracyclines undergo epimerisation in solutions between pH 4 to 8 to give epitetracyclines which are inactive. The tetracyclines are also degraded by acids and bases. They form insoluble complexes with metals such as calcium, magnesium and aluminium, impairing absorption. Hence, tetracyclines should not be taken along with such antacids, iron salts and milk. They are adequately absorbed when taken orally.

Mechanism of action

Tetracyclines act by interfering with protein synthesis in bacteria, probably during formation of peptide linkages. They bind to the 30S subunits of bacterial ribosomes and inhibit protein synthesis. Their action is bacteriostatic and only multiplying organisms are affected.

Untoward effects

The tetracyclines may cause gastrointestinal disturbances with flatulence, nausea, vomiting and diarrhoea. Phototoxicity, hepatic toxicity (jaundice) and renal toxicity may occur. Deposition of these drugs on the surface of the teeth in children causes discolouration.

1) Tetracycline Hydrochloride

Tetracycline is official in I.P. as the free base and hydrochloride salt.

Properties : It occurs as an odourless yellow crystalline powder with a bitter taste. Tetracycline is very slightly soluble in water; sparingly soluble in alcohol, practically insoluble in ether and chloroform and soluble in dilute acids. Tetracycline hydrochloride is freely soluble in water; sparingly soluble in alcohol; very slightly soluble in ether and chloroform. It is laevorotatory.

Stability : Tetracycline, in powder form, darkens in strong sunlight in a moist atmosphere. In aqueous solutions, it degrades by epimerisation to 4-epitetracycline. It is rapidly inactivated below pH 2 and is slowly destroyed above pH 7. Citric acid increases the rate of degradation.

Storage : It should be stored in airtight containers, protected from light.

Actions and uses : The activities of tetracyclines are discussed earlier. Tetracycline is the drug of choice in infections of the central nervous system and urinary tract.

Dose : 250 to 400 mg, 4 times a day.

Preparations : All the following preparations contain tetracycline hydrochloride.

Tetracycline capsules, I.P., B.P. - contain 250 mg of the drug.

Tetracycline injection, I.P., B.P. - available as powder in vials, strength in I.P. are 100, 250 and 500 mg.

Tetracycline tablets, I.P., B.P. contain 250 mg of the drug.

Tetracycline eye ointment, I.P.

Brand Names : Achromycin®, Hostacycline®, Resteclin®, Subamycin®, Tetrastar®

2) Oxytetracycline Hydrochloride

Oxytetracycline is official in I.P. as the free base and the hydrochloride salt.

Properties : It occurs as an odourless, yellow crystalline powder with a bitter taste. Oxytetracycline is very slightly soluble in water; soluble in dilute acids and alkalis. The hydrochloride salt is freely soluble in water and sparingly soluble in alcohol. It is laevorotatory.

Storage : It should be stored in airtight containers, protected from light.

Actions and uses : These have been discussed earlier.

Dose : 1 to 2 gm a day, in divided doses.

Preparations : Contain the hydrochloride salt.

Oxytetracycline hydrochloride injection, I.P., B.P. available as powder in vials, equivalent to 250 and 500 mg of the base.

Oxytetracycline capsules, I.P. - contain 250 and 500 mg of the drug.

Oxytetracycline eye ointment, I.P.

Brand Names : Oxytetracyline® inj., Terramycin®, Betetra® inj., Oxyteracin®

VI] Macrolides

1) Erythromycin

Erythromycin is an antibiotic produced by certain strains of *Streptomyces erythreus*. It is a macrolide antibiotic having a large lactone ring. It is official in I.P. in three forms, as the free compound and as two esters which are estolate and stearate.

Properties : Erythromycin occurs as odourless, slightly hygroscopic, white or slightly yellow crystals or powder with a bitter taste. It is slightly soluble in water, freely soluble in alcohol and ether soluble in dilute acid. It is laevorotatory. Erythromycin estolate is a tasteless powder and is very slightly soluble in water. Erythromycin stearate has a slightly bitter taste and is very slightly soluble in water.

Storage : It should be stored in airtight containers, protected from light, at a temperature below 30°C.

Actions and uses : Erythromycin is a bacteriostatic at therapeutic concentrations. It acts by interfering with ribosomal protein synthesis within the bacterial cell. It is used mainly to treat infections in patients allergic to penicillin and infections caused by penicillinase producing *staphylococci.* It is also effective against leptospirae, entamoebae, *Diplococcus pneumoniae, Streptococcus pyogenes, Haemophilus influenzae* and *Bordetella pertussis*. It is also used for skin and eye infections.

Its major drawback is the ready development of resistance in bacteria.

Erythromycin is destroyed by gastric acid. Hence it should be given orally either as enteric coated tablets or in the form of a stable ester. The stearate ester is hydrolysed in the intestine and the free drug is absorbed, while, the estolate is absorbed as an ester and is then hydrolysed.

Dose : 1 to 2 gm a day, in divided doses.

Preparations : Erythromycin tablets, I.P., B.P. - 250 mg enteric coated tablets.

Erythromycin estolate tablets, I.P. - contain

the ester equivalent to 250 and 500 mg of erythromycin.

Erythromycin estolate capsules, B.P.

Erythromycin stearate tablets, I.P., B.P. - contain the ester equivalent to 100 and 250 mg of erythromycin (as per I.P.)

Erythromycin mixture, B.P.C. - a suspension of erythromycin stearate.

Brand Names : Althrocin®, Calthrox®, Eltocin®, Emthrocin®, Erythrocin®

XI] Miscellaneous antibiotics

1) Chloramphenicol

2,2-Dichloro-N-[(αR,βR)-β-hydroxy-α-hydroxy-methy-4-nitrophenethyl] acetamide.

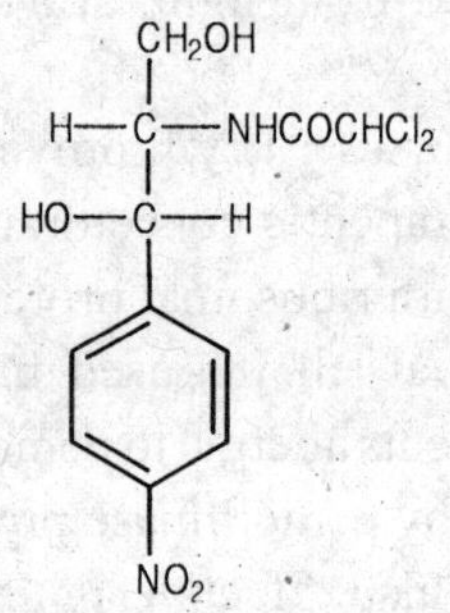

Chloramphenicol was first produced by the growth of *Streptomyces venezuelae*, but it is now produced synthetically. There are four possible stereoisomers of which only the (αR, βR) form or D - threo form is active. It is official in I.P. as the free alcohol and two esters prepared by esterification of terminal hydroxy group which are palmitate and sodium succinate.

Properties : Chloramphenicol occurs as a fine white to greyish-white or yellowish-white crystalline powder or crystals, needles or elongated plates, with a very bitter taste. It is slightly soluble in water; freely soluble in alcohol and in propylene glycol; soluble in acetone and very slightly soluble in ether. A solution in alcohol is dextrorotatory. Chloramphenicol palmitate exists in four polymorphic forms, of which, only polymorph B is active. It is practically insoluble in water and is, therefore, almost tasteless. It is preferred for preparing oral suspensions. Chloramphenicol sodium succinate is freely soluble in water and is used to prepare injectables.

Stability : In aqueous solution, chloramphenicol degrades by amide hydrolysis to give dichloroacetic acid which then releases chloride ions. Chloramphenicol also degrades by a photolytic reaction. Hydrolysis is catalysed by monohydrogen phosphate ions, mono and dihydrogen citrate ions.

Storage : It should be protected from light.

Mechanism of action : Chloramphenicol is a broad spectrum antibiotic with a bacteriostatic action. It inhibits the biosynthesis of proteins in bacteria by acting on 50S ribosomal subunit.

Actions and uses : Chloramphenicol has a wide range of antimicrobial activity similar to that given for tetracyclines. It is also effective against *Salmonella typhi* and *Salmonella paratyphi*. It is well-absorbed after oral administration. Chloramphenicol esters are hydrolysed in the gastrointestinal tract prior to absorption. Its most serious side effect is on the haemopoietic system, resulting in agranulocytosis, thrombocytopenic purpura or aplastic anaemia. Other side effects include renal toxicity, optic neuritis, jaundice and Stevens-Johnson syndrome. In infants, it causes Gray baby syndrome.

Due to the serious side effects, the use of chloramphenicol is restricted mainly to the treatment of typhoid and paratyphoid fevers. It is also used in the treatment of meningitis caused by *Hemophilus influenzae*. It is also used topically to treat infections of the skin, eyes and ears.

Dose : 500 mg, 4 times a day.

Preparations : Chloramphenicol capsules, I.P. - contain 250 and 500 mg of the drug.

Chloramphenicol capsules, B.P. - contain 250 mg of the drug.

Chloramphenicol eye ointment, I.P. - contains 1 per cent w/w of the drug.

Chloramphenicol eye-drops, B.P.C.

Chloramphenicol palmitate oral suspension, ,I.P., B.P.C.

Chloramphenicol sodium succinate injection, I.P., B.P. - available as powder in vial equivalent to 1 gm of chloramphenicol.

Brand Names : Chloromycetin® drops, Chlorocin®, Fencol®, Tycol®, Otocin® solution, Praxin® ear drops

Antibiotics used for specific infections :Griseofulvin

(2S, 6`R)-7-Chloro-2`,4,6-trimethoxy-6`-methyl-benzofuran-2-spiro-1'cyclohex-2`-ene-3,4`-dione.

It is produced by the growth of *Penicillium griseofulvum*.

Properties : Griseofulvin occurs as a white to pale cream powder. It is odourless and tasteless. The particles are generally upto 5 μm in maximum dimension. It is very slightly soluble in water; slightly soluble in alcohol; soluble in acetone and in chloroform. It is dextrorotatory. Melting point is about 221°C.

Storage : It should be stored in airtight containers.

Actions and uses : Griseofulvin is an antibiotic which has an antifungal action against a wide range of dermatophytoses. It is effective against infections caused by various species of *Trichophyton* (tinea, ringworm), *Epidermophyton* and *Microsporum*. It is ineffective against most systemic fungal infections. It is used orally to treat infections of the skin, nails and hair.

The absorption of griseofulvin depends upon particle size and dissolution rate. It is irregularly and incompletely absorbed after oral administration. Absorption is increased when given with fatty meals and milk.

Dose : 0.5 to 1 gm a day.

Preparations : Griseofulvin tablets, I.P. - contain 125 mg of the drug.

Griseofulvin tablets, B.P. - contain 125 and 500 mg of the drug.

Brand Names : Gris-OD-375®, Grisoral®, Grisovin-FP®

Drugs For Further Study

Pencillins

1) Bacampicillin - Penglobe®
2) Piperacillin - Pipracil®, Piprex®, Pracil®

Cephalosporins

3) Cefazolin - Azolin®, Cefadin®, Orizolin®, Reflin®
4) Cefadroxil - Acudrox®, Bludrox®, Cefadrox®
5) Cefuroxime - Bacticef®, Ceforim®, Furobid®
6) Cefaclor - Distaclor®, Eclor®, Vercef®
7) Cefotaxime - Bestax®, Blutax®, Haltax®, Taxim®
8) Ceftazidime - Cefazid®, Ceftidin®, Tazid®, Tizime®
9) Ceftriaxone - C-Tri®, Cefaxone®, Cefezone®, Xone®
10) Ceftizoxime - Cefizox®, Eldcef®, Epocelin®
11) Cefixime - C-Tax-O®, Cefi®, Cefic®, Ceftas®, Xim®
12) Cefoperazone - Cefomycin®, Cefpar®, Megacef®
13) Cefpirome - Bacirom®, Cefrom®, Forgen®, Tafrom®
14) Cefpodoxime - Cefective®, Cefoprox®, Doxcef®
15) Cefdinir - Adcef®, Cefdiel®, Sefdin®, Zinir®
16) Cefepime - Ceficad®, Cepime®, Forpar®, Novapime®

17) Cefetamet - Altamet®, Cepime-O®, Ultipime-O®

18) Aztreonam - Azenam®, Aztreo®

Aminoglycosides

19) Amikacin - Amcin®, Amikef®, Mikacin®, Nimicin®

20) Tobramycin - Tobacin®, Tobraneg®, Tobreb®

21) Kanamycin - Efficin®, Kancin®, Neokanyn®

22) Netilmicin - Neticin®, Netromycin®, Netspan®

Tetracyclines

23) Doxycycline - Avidox®, Doxina®, Doxt®

24) Minocycline - CNN®, Cynomycin®, Minolin®

25) Demeclocycline - Ledermycin®

Polymxyins

26) Polymyxin B - Aerosporin®, Poly®-B

27) Colistin (Polymyxin E) - Walamycin®

Macrolides

29) Roxithromycin - Ambroxit®, Arbid®, Ralrox®, Roxid®

30) Azithromycin - Azee®, Azithral®, Zathrin®, Zycin®

31) Spiramycin - Rovamycin®

32) Clarithromycin - Clamycin®, Clar®, Clarimac®

Miscellaneous

33) Clindamycin - Climycin®, Dalcinex®, Daltrex®

34) Lincomycin - Linkam®, Lynx®

35) Vancomycin - Cytovan®, Vancogen®, Vanlid®

36) Teicoplanin - Targocid®, Ticocin®

37) Spectinomycin - Myspec®, Spectin®, Trobicin®

38) Meropenem - Merocrit®, Meronem®, Merotrol®

Exercise

Q1. Write short note on β-lactam antibiotics (Kachchh Univ. 06)

Q2. Define and classify antibiotics. Write the structure and uses of ampicillin, benzyl penicillin & phenoxy methyl penicillin. (Karnataka Univ., Winter 04, Summer 06)

Q3. Give structure, properties and uses of benzyl penicillin. (Winter 04)

Q4. Give uses of griseofulvin & chloramphenicol. (Winter 04, Summer 03)

Q5. Draw the general structure of 6-amino penicillanic acid and name the antibiotics derived from amino acids. (Winter 04)

Q6. Classify the antibiotics with examples from each class. Write the structure of ampicillin. (Summer 03)

Q7. Write structures of - i) Penicillin-G & ii) Penicillin-V. (Summer 06)

Q8. Give uses of erythromycin. (Summer 06)

Q9. Define and classify antibiotics. Specify which antibiotic should - i) not be given with milk, ii) be parenterally used, iii) be used in enteric coated form, iv) be used in fungal infection. (May-June 04)

Q10. Write short note on β-Lactam antibiotics. (May 2005)

Q11. Define antibacterial and antibiotics. Write note on various types of antibiotics and draw the structure of atleast one drug from each class. (May 07)

Q12. What are β-Lactam antibiotics? Write an account of antibiotics derived from acetate or propionate units. (Nov 06)

■

8 Antifungal Drugs

Fungi are plant-like, nonphotosynthetic eukaryotes growing in colonies of single cells (yeasts) or in filamentous multicellular aggregates (moulds). Most fungi are saprophytes in soil or dead plants. Some species are parasites on plants and animals. The majority of fungal infections (mycoses) involve superficial infection of the skin or mucous membranes of body orifices. Fungal infections are of two types -

a) Contagious, nonsystemic infections

These are dermatophytoses (tinea infections) which are caused by *Epidermophyton, Microsporum* and *Trichophyton* species. These are epidermal infections affecting skin, hair and nails. The antifungal agents used to treat dermatophytoses are tolnaftate, griseofulvin, clotrimazole, miconazole and ketoconazole.

b) Noncontagious, systemic infections

These are caused by saprophytic yeasts such as *Aspergillus, Blastomyces, Candida, Coccidioides* and *Cryptococcus* species. These affect various organs and tissues such as lungs, eyes, testes, vagina, liver, skin and gastrointestinal tract. The drugs used in systemic fungal infections are amphotericin B, nystatin, 5- fluorocytosine, clotrimazole, miconazole and ketoconazole.

Treatment of fungal infections is determined by the nature of the infecting organisms. Tinea (ringworm) infections of the body, fingernails, groin, hands, head and soles of the feet can be treated with oral griseofulvin. Local treatments for tinea include fatty acids (eg. undecenoic acid) and their salts, econazole, miconazole, tolnaftate and other drugs. Superficial candidal infection may be treated with local applications of amphotericin or nystatin and systemic infections with amphotericin, flucytosine or miconazole.

Classification of Antifungal Drugs

I] Synthetic antifungal agents

a) Imidazoles

clotrimazole, miconazole, ketoconazole

b) Other compounds

tolnaftate, flucytosine.

II] Antifungal antibiotics

a) Polyenes

nystatin, amphotericin B, natamycin, hamycin.

b) Other antibiotics

griseofulvin.

I] Synthetic antifungal agents

1) Undecylenic acid (Undecenoic acid)

Undec-10-enoic acid

$CH_2=CH(CH_2)_8COOH$

Properties : Undecylenic acid occurs as a colourless or pale yellow liquid or a white or very pale yellow crystalline mass with a characteristic odour. It is practically insoluble in water; miscible with alcohol, ether and fixed and volatile oils. Zinc undecylenate occurs as a fine white powder which is practically insoluble in water and alcohol.

Storage : It should be stored in airtight containers, protected from light.

Actions and uses : Undecylenic acid and its zinc salt have similar fungicidal activities and similar applications. Undecylenic acid is used for the prophylaxis and treatment of superficial dermatophytoses of the head, ears, feet, axillae and groin and of candidiasis and mycotic infections of the vulva and vagina. For application to the skin ointments, emulsions and dusting powders containing 2 to 15 per cent of undecylenic acid, sometimes in conjunction with zinc undecylenate, are used. Drug concentration should not exceed 1 per cent for applications to mucous surfaces.

Preparations : Zinc undecenoate dusting powder, B.P.C

Zinc undecenoate ointment B.P.

2) Tolnaftate

O-2-Naphthylm,N-dimethylthiocarbanilate.

Tolnaftate is an ester of β-naphthol.

Properties : It occurs as an odourless white to creamy-white powder. It is very slightly soluble in water and alcohol, sparingly soluble in ether, freely soluble in chloroform and acetone.

Actions and uses : Tolnaftate is an antifungal agent used topically for the treatment of ringworm and other skin infections due to *Epidermophyton, Microsporum* and *Trichophyton* species. It is not active against species of *Candida* or bacteria. It is used topically as a 1 per cent solution, powder or cream to treat tinea infections and pityriasis versicolor. It is not suitable for the treatment of tinea of the nails and scalp, but it may be used as an adjunct with oral griseofulvin. Skin tolerance is good to the drug but irritation and allergic sensitisation may occur occasionally.

Preparations : Tolnaftate cream, U.S.P.

Tolnaftate gel, U.S.P.

Tolnaftate powder, U.S.P.

Tolnaftate topical aerosol powder, U.S.P.

Tolnaftate topical solution, U.S.P.

Brand Names : Quadriderm® cream, Tinaderm® solution, Tinasal® solution

II] Antifungal antibiotics

a) Polyenes

1) Nystatin

Nystatin is a polyene antibiotic. It is produced by the growth of *Streptomyces noursei*. 1 mg has a potency of 4400 units.

Properties : Nystatin occurs as a yellow to light brown, hygroscopic powder. It has a characteristic odour. It is very slightly soluble in water, alcohol and methyl alcohol. It is practically insoluble in ether and chloroform.

Storage : It should be stored in airtight containers, protected from light, at a temperature not exceeding 5°C.

Actions and uses : Nystatin is an antibiotic with a wide range of activity against fungi and yeasts. It is used mainly in the local treatment of candidal infections of the mucous membrane and of the skin and nails. It is poorly absorbed after oral administration and hence, it has no use in systemic infections. It is used orally in the treatment of gastrointestinal candidiasis. Skin infections are treated using ointments while pessaries are used in vaginal candidiasis.

Dose : 5 lakh to 10 lakh units, 3 times a day.

Preparations : Nystatin ointment, I.P., B.P.C

Nystatin tablets, I.P., B.P. - contain 5 lakh units of the drug.

Nystatin vaginal tablets, I

Nystatin pessaries, B.P.C.

Nystatin mixture, B.P.C.

Brand Names : Mycostatin®

2) Amphotericin B

Gold, et al isolated a polyene antibiotic from *Streptomyces nodosus* in 1956. The antibiotic material was found to contain two closely related substances which were named amphotericin A (a conjugated tetraene) and amphotericin B (a conjugated heptaene).

Properties : Amphotericin occurs as a yellow to orange powder. It is odourless and almost tasteless. It is practically insoluble in water, in alcohol and in ether. It is soluble in propylene glycol and in dimethyl sulphoxide.

Stability : It is inactivated at low pH values. Dilute solutions are light sensitive.

Incompatibility : It is precipitated from solution by sodium chloride. Its suspensions are sensitive to dissolved ions. It is incompatible with heparin.

Storage : It should be stored in airtight containers at a temperature of 2 to 10°C, protected from light.

Actions and uses : Amphotericin is a polyene antibiotic having a structure similar to that of nystatin. It has antifungal action against a wide range of yeasts and fungi. It is used in the treatment of candidiasis, crypttococcosis, blastomycosis, and histoplasmosis. For treating systemic infections, it is administered intravenously. It is poorly absorbed from the gastrointestinal tract. Local infections are treated using tablets, lozenges, creams, ointments, pessaries and other dosage forms. For systemic therapy, the dose should be gradually increased to avoid severe systemic reactions like renal dysfunction.

Dose : 60 mg on alternate days, IV infusion.

Preparations : Amphotericin cream B.P.C.
Amphotericin lozenges B.P.C.
Amphotericin ointment B.P.C.
Amphotericin injection B.P.C.

Brand Names : Amfocan®, Amphotin® inj. Fungizone® (IV) inj., Amfotex® inj.

3) Hamycin

Hamycin is a polyene antibiotic produced by the growth of *Streptomyces pimprina.*

Properties : It occurs as a yellow amorphous powder. It is practically insoluble in water.

Actions and uses : Hamycin has antifungal and antitrichomonal properties. It is administered topically and orally, in a variety of fungal infections including candidiasis, tinea, blastomycosis and madura foot. Hamycin is available as a suspension containing 2 lakh units per ml for topical application. Ovules containing 4 lakh units are used for local treatment of vaginal infections.

Brand Names : Hamycin® suspension

b) Other Antibiotics

1) Griseofulvin

Refer to chapter no.7 on antibiotics.

Drugs For Further Study

1) Clotrimazole - Canazole®, Candid®, Mycoderm-C®
2) Miconazole - Candistat®, Daktarin®, Micogel®, Zole®
3) Quiniodochlor - Cortoquinol®, Dermoquinol®, Millicorten-Vioform®
4) Ciclopiroxolamine - Batrafen®, Olamin®, Onylac®
5) Ketoconazole - Danclear®, Ketotar®, Ketorate®
6) Oxiconazole - Zoderm®
7) Bifonazole - Mycospor®
8) Terbinafine - Fungotek®, Hifen®, Terbofin®
9) Butenafine - Butop® Cream, Exebute®, Fintop® cream
10) Fluconazole - Flumed®, Flunova®, Fluzide®, Forcan®
11) Itraconazole - Candistat®, Cantitral®, Itaspor®
12) Griseofulvin - Fungal®, Grisomed®, Idifulvin®, Myconorm®

Exercise

Q1. Classify Antifungal agents with examples. Write the properties and uses of nystatin. (Winter 04, Summer 03, May 07)

Q2. In what dosage form the following drugs are given - i) Nystatin, ii) Zinc Undecylenate & iii) Tolnaftate. (Summer 03)

Q3. Give an account on antifungal agents. (Nov 06)

■

9 Antimalarial Drugs

Malaria

Malaria is mainly a disease of the tropics and sub-tropics. Its incidence is highest in warm, wet and marshy regions. Malaria is caused due to infection by protozoan parasites belonging to the genus Plasmodium. Four species infect man *Plasmodium vivax, P. falciparum, P. ovale* and *P. malariae*. They are transmitted by the bite of infected female Anopheles mosquito.

Malaria is characterised by paroxysms or periodic bouts of fever, chills and profuse sweating. These bouts of fever and chill occur when the erythrocytes of the patient rupture to release the merozoite forms of the parasite. The intervals between the malarial attacks are determined by the species of Plasmodium involved.

The terms tertian and quartan are used to indicate occurrence of malarial attacks after every 48 hours and 72 hours respectively. Benign tertian malaria (vivax malaria) is caused by *P. vivax*, Malignant tertian malaria (falciparum malaria) is the most severe form and is caused by *P. falciparum*. In this type, paroxysms occur at irregular intervals. Quartan malaria (malariae malaria) is caused by *P. malariae*. Mild tertian malaria, caused by *P. ovale*, is the least common form.

Life Cycle of Malaria Parasite

The life cycle of Plasmodium is composed of an asexual phase in humans and sexual phase in the vector, female Anopheles mosquito. The male Anopheles mosquito does not feed on vertebrate blood.

Life cycle in mosquito

When the female Anopheles mosquito bites an infected person, it ingests erythrocytes carrying plasmodia in various stages of development. The asexual forms are destroyed while the gametocytes develop into gametes. The male gamete (microgamete) and female gamete (macrogamete) undergo conjugation to produce a zygote. The zygote develops into the ookinete which forms a rounded cyst called oocyst. The oocyst undergoes nuclear division and then bursts releasing several motile sporozoites. The sporozoites migrate to the salivary glands and when the mosquito bites a healthy person, are transferred to him. This cycle in the mosquito, called sporogony, takes 7 to 11 days.

Life cycle in humans

In humans, the parasite first resides outside and then inside the red blood cells.

The exoerythrocytic phase : The sporozoites enter the hosts's liver cells and each sporozoite undergoes several nuclear divisions to form a schizont. The enlarged liver cells burst to release the parasites, now called merozoites, into the blood stream. They enter the erythrocytes. Some merozoites (except in *P. falciparum*) invade fresh liver cells and repeat the cycle.

The erythrocytic phase : Inside the erythrocytes, the merozoites grow into round vacuolated cells called trophozoites. Cell division occurs giving daughter cells called schizonts. Each schizont divides giving rise to upto 30 merozoites. These are liberated when the erythrocytes rupture (this corresponds to the malarial attack) and enter fresh erythrocytes. This cycle of asexual reproduction in the erythrocyte is called schizogony. It takes about 48 to 72 hours. Some of the erythrocytic merozoites develop into male and female gametocytes. These are ingested by the vector and undergo sexual phase there.

Chemotherapy of Malaria

The control and eradication of malaria is attempted in two ways which are eradication of the vector, mosquito, by maintaining sanitation and spraying insecticides regularly and carrying out effective prophylaxis and treating patients. Several drugs are now available for malaria chemotherapy and these act on various stages of the parasite.

Acute attacks of malaria occur when the schizonts are released in the body. Clinical cure in patients showing malarial attacks can be achieved by using erythrocytic schizonticides like 4-amino quinolines. Radical cure or complete cure can be achieved by eliminating both erythrocytic and exo-erythrocytic forms of the parasite. This requires a combination of 4-aminoquinolines and 8-aminoquinolines. Persons visiting areas where malaria is endemic, should take precautions against infection. They should take prophylactic treatment or suppressive treatment. Drugs which are not lethal to the parasite but suppress its growth are used for this purpose. Table 9.1 shows antimalarial drugs used for different purposes. Quinine, which had been largely replaced by synthetic antimalarials, has now staged a comeback, as many cases of parasites resistant to the synthetic compounds are occurring. In the past few years, many cases of chloroquine resistant *P. falciparum* have been observed.

Table 9.1 : Commonly used antimalarial drugs

Purpose	Drugs of First Choice	Reserve Drugs
Clinical Cure	4-Aminoquinolines (eg. chloroquine, amodiaquine) *Quinine, Pyrimethamine	Quinine, Mepacrine
Radical Cure	Combination Therapy- 4-aminoquinoline (eg. chloroquine) + 8-aminoquinoline (eg. primaquine)	
Prophylaxis	Pyrimethamine, Chloroquine *Pyrimethamine + sulphadoxine	Proquanil, Quinine

* For drug-resistant species

Classification of Antimalarials

According to their chemical structure, the antimalarial drugs may be classified as follows

I) Cinchona Alkaloids

quinine

II) 4-Aminoquinolines

chloroquine, amodiaquine, sontoquine

III) 8-Aminoquinolines

primaquine, pentaquine, isopentaquine

IV) 9-Aminoacridines

quinacrine

V) Pyrimidines

pyrimethamine, trimethoprim

VI) Biguanides

proguanil, cycloguanil

VII) Miscellaneous

mefloquine

I] Cinchona alkaloids

1) Quinine

Cinchona bark has been used medicine since ancient times. It contains several alkaloids, the important ones being quinine, quinidine, cinchonine and cinchonidine. The quinine structure consists of a quinoline ring attached through a hydroxymethylene bridge to a quinuclidine system. Quinine is official in I.P. as bisulphate, dihydrochloride and sulphate salts.

Properties : The quinine salts occur as odourless, white powders or crystals with a very bitter taste. The mono-acid salts of quinine are generally much less soluble in water than the di-acid salts. Quinine hydrochloride is soluble in water and is used as tablets while the dihydrochloride salt is very soluble in water and is also used in the form of injections. Quinine sulphate is only slightly soluble in water and is used as tablets. On exposure to light, the salts become yellowish in colour. The hydrate forms are efflorescent in dry air. The salts are laevorotatory.

Incompatibility : Quinine salts are incompatible with alkalis, alkali carbonates, iodides, tannic acid and mercuric chloride.

Storage : They should be stored in airtight containers, protected from light.

Actions and uses : The quinoline type antimalarials cause inhibition of protein synthesis, DNA replication and RNA transcription in the plasmodia. Quinine suppresses the erythrocytic asexual cycle of development of the malarial parasites. It has no action on the tissue forms of the parasite. Though quinine is a highly active blood its schizonticide, its applications have declined due to toxic effects like deafness, vertigo and visual disturbances. It is now mainly used in the treatment of falciparum malaria resistant to chloroquine and other antimalarial drugs. It is used in conjunction with primaquine in the radical cure of relapsing vivax malaria. Its use as prophylactic has been superseded by better drugs. Quinine is readily absorbed after oral administration.

Dose : 600 mg, 3 times a day, for 4 days or longer.

Preparations : Quinine bisulphate tablets I.P., B.P. - contain 300 mg of the drug.

Quinine dihydrochloride injection I.P., B.P.

Quinine dihydrochloride tablets B.P.C.

Quinine sulphate tablets I.P., B.P.

Brand Names : Cinkona® inj., Kwinil®, Qinarsol-300®, Quininga®, Rez-Q®

II] 4-Aminoquinolines

1) Chloroquine

7-chloro-4-4-(diethylamino)-1-methylbutyl amino quinoline

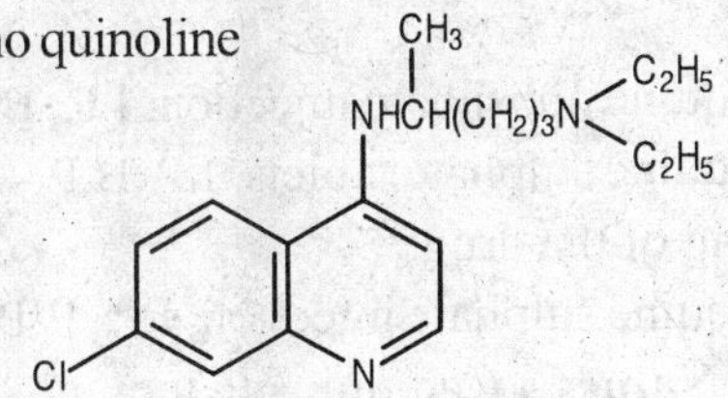

Chloroquine is official in I.P. as phosphate and sulphate salts.

Properties : Chloroquine phosphate and sulphate occur as odourless, white crystalline powders with a bitter taste. The salts are freely soluble in water, very slightly soluble in alcohol, ether and chloroform.

Stability : Solutions of chloroquine phosphate having pH 4 to 6 are stable when heated, but are sensitive to light.

Storage : It should be stored in well-closed containers, protected from light.

Actions and uses : Chloroquine has a rapid schizonticidal effect and it kills the erythrocytic forms of malarial parasites. It affects cell growth by interfering with DNA. Chloroquine is widely used to treat acute malarial attacks. However, it does not affect the sporozoites and tissue forms of the parasite. It may not eliminate the infection completely and overt malaria may develop after its withdrawal. To prevent such relapses and effect a radical cure, combination therapy of chloroquine and primaquine is given. Chloroquine is also used as a prophylactic.

Chloroquine is of value in the treatment of hepatic amoebiasis, liver abscess, giardiasis and rheumatoid arthritis.

Dose : Total dose equivalent to 1.5 gm of chloroquine base is used. Initial dose - 600 mg of base followed by 300 mg of base after 6 hours and further, 300 mg of base daily for two days. Salts equivalent to above amounts are used.

Preparations : Chloroquine phosphate tablets, I.P., B.P. - contain 100 and 250 mg of the drug.

Chloroquine phosphate injection, I.P., B.P.

Chloroquine sulphate tablets, I.P.,B.P. - contain 200 mg of the drug.

Chloroquine sulphate injection, I.P., B.P.

Brand Names : Cadiquin®, Cloquin®, Emquin®, Lariago®, Resochin®

2) Amodiaquine Hydrochloride

4-(7-Chloroquinol-4-ylamino)-2-(diethylaminomethyl) phenol dihydrochloride

Properties : It occurs as a yellow crystalline powder. It is odourless and has a bitter taste. It is soluble in water and sparingly soluble in alcohol.

Storage : It should be stored in airtight containers.

Actions and uses : Amodiaquine is an antimalarial with actions and uses similar to those of chloroquine. It is readily absorbed after oral administration.

Dose : Initial - Equivalent to 600 mg base; followed by equivalent of 400 to 600 mg of base daily for 3 days.

Preparations : Amodiaquine tablets I.P., B.P. - contain amodiaquine hydrochloride equivalent to 200 mg of base.

III] 8-Aminoquinolines

1) Primaquine Phosphate

8-[(4-Amino-1-methylbutyl)amino]-6-methoxyquinoline (dihydrogen phosphate)

Properties : It occurs as an orange-red crystalline powder. It is odourless and has a bitter taste. It is soluble in water and practically insoluble in organic solvents.

Stability : It is affected by light. Aqueous solutions are thermolabile.

Storage : It should be protected from light.

Actions and uses : Primaquine kills the exoerythrocytic stages of Plasmodium. It also kills the gametocytes but it has little action on other erythrocytic forms. Hence, it should not be used alone in the treatment of a malarial attack. It is rapidly absorbed and metabolised. It is mainly used for the radical cure of *P. vivax* infections in patients returning from areas where maleria is prevalent. First, a short course of chloroquine is given to kill the erythrocytic parasites. This is followed by primaquine for 14 days to kill the tissue forms. The major side effects are abdominal pain, methaemoglobinaemia and haemolytic anaemia.

Dose : 25 mg once a day, for 14 days.

Preparations : Primaquine tablets, I.P., B.P.

Brand Names : Malirid®, P-Quin®, Primalex®, PMQ-Inga®

IV] 9 - Aminoacridines

V] Pyrimidines

1) Pyrimethamine

5-(4-Chlorophenyl)-6-ethylpyrimidine-2,4-diamine.

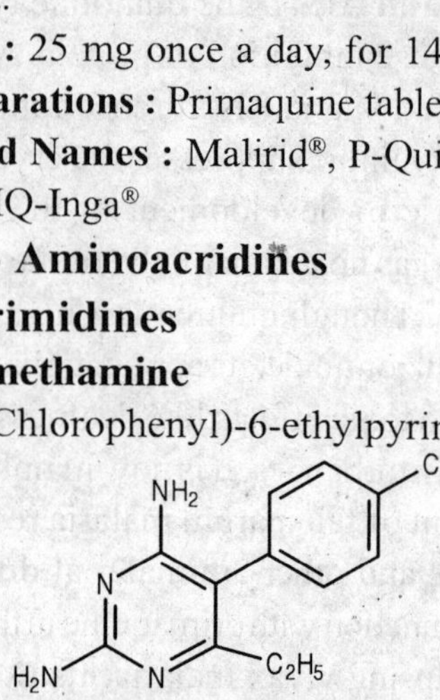

Properties : It occurs as a white, crystalline powder. It is odourless and tasteless. It is practically insoluble in water; slightly soluble in alcohol and soluble in warm, dilute mineral acids.

Mode of Action : Pyrimidine antimalarials affect the nucleoprotein metabolism of the parasite by interference in the folic-folinic acid system. This action is exerted mainly at the time when the nucleus divides. The last step in tetrahydrofolic acid (THF) biosynthesis is -

$$\text{Dihydrofolic acid} \xrightarrow{\text{Dihydrofolate reductase}} \text{Tetrahydrofolic acid}$$

THF cofactors are required as one-carbon donors in many biosynthetic pathways. The pyrimidines and biguanides are selective inhibitors of dihydrofolate reductase of malaria parasite.

Actions and uses : Pyrimethamine kills the primary exoerythrocytic forms of Plasmodium and affects the gametocytes rendering them incapable of complete development in the mosquito. It has less effect on the erythrocytic forms and is therefore slow in controlling a malarial attack. It acts as a suppressant. It is used to prevent relapses in benign tertian malaria. It is given in combination with chloroquine to patients during malaria eradication campaigns. Chloroquine rapidly kills the asexual parasites and pyrimethamine helps to prevent transmission by the mosquito. Sulphonamides (eg. sulphadiazine, sulphadoxine) and sulphones (eg. dapsone) enhance the action of pyrimethamine by blocking dihydrofolic acid synthesis. Combined courses of treatment may be used against chloroquine resistant strains of malarial parasite. The chief use of pyrimethamine presently is as a prophylactic.

Dose : Prophylactic 25 mg, once weekly.

Preparations : Pyrimethamine tablets, B.P. - contain 25 mg of the drug.

Brand Names (with a combination of Sulphadoxine) : Laridox®, Malcidal®, Malocide®, Pyralfin®

2) Trimethoprim

5-(3,4,5-Trimethoxybenzyl) pyrimidine-2,4-diamine.

Properties : Trimethoprim occurs as a white powder. It is odourless and has a very bitter taste. It is very slightly soluble in water; slightly soluble in alcohol and sparingly soluble in chloroform. Melting point is about 200°C.

Actions and uses : Trimethoprim is an antibacterial agent which acts by inhibiting dihydrofolate reductase in bacteria (for details, refer to the profile of pyrimethamine). Trimethoprim is used mainly in combination with sulphamethoxazole, under the name cotrimoxazole. It is also used in conjunction with a sulphonamide in the treatment of chloroquine resistant falciparum malaria.

Dose : 0.5 to 1.5 gm of trimethoprim + 0.75 to 1.5 gm of sulphametopyrazine.

Preparations : Cotrimoxazole tablets, I.P., B.P.

Cotrimoxazole injection, B.P.C.

Cotrimoxazole mixture, B.P.C.

Brand Names : Oriprim®, Tprim forte®, Trisulfose®

VI] Biguanides

1) Proguanil Hydrochloride

1-(4-Chlorophenyl)-5-isopropylbiguanide hydrochloride.

Properties : It occurs as a white, crystalline powder. It is odourless and has a bitter taste. It is slightly soluble in water and sparingly soluble in alcohol.

Actions and uses : Proguanil is used for the prevention and treatment of malaria. It acts through its active metabolite, cycloguanil. In falciparum malaria, proguanil kills the schizonts in erythrocytes and also in the tissues. It, thus, acts as a causal prophylactic and effects a radical cure. In vivax malaria, proguanil kills the erythrocytic parasites but may not always eradicate latent tissue infection. Acute attacks of malaria should be treated with more rapidly acting drugs. Proguanil is used mainly as prophylactic and suppressant. It is rapidly absorbed after oral administration.

Dose : Prophylactic - 100 mg a day.

Preparations : Proguanil tablets, I.P., B.P.

Brand Names : Laveran®, Progunal®

VII) Miscellaneous -

Drugs For Further Study

1) Mefloquine - Confal®, Falcital®, Mefax®, Mefloc®
2) Bulaquine - Aablaquin®
3) Mepacrine - Maladin®, Mepalex®
4) Arteether - Betamotil®, Cadither®, Falcy®
5) Artemether - Falcydol®, Larither®, Malither®
6) Artesunate - Dunate®, Falcigo®, Falcinil®, Ulteria®

Exercise

Q1. Write short note on antimalarial drugs. (Kachchh Univ. 06)

Q2. Classify antimalarials. (Karnataka Univ.)

Q3. Define and classify antimalarials giving examples from each class. (Winter 04)

Q4. Write the structure of : 7-Chloro, 4'-4 (diethylamino-1 methyl butylamino) - Quinoline. (Summer 03)

Q5. Explain life cycle of plasmodium. (Summer 06)

Q6. Give structure, properties, uses and dose of choloroquine. (Summer 06)

Q7. Give uses of quinine. (Summer 06)

Q8. Define and classify antimalarials. (Summer 06)

Q9. Draw structure of chloroquine.(Winter 06)

Q10. Write note on antimalarials. (May-June 04)

Q11. Write short note on antimalarial drugs.

Q12. What are antimalarials. Classify with examples. (May 07)

10 Tranquilisers

The term tranquilisers include anxiolytic sedatives and neuroleptics.

Anxiolytic sedatives

(Minor tranquilisers)

They are used to treat anxiety and include benzodiazepines, carbamates and other compounds. They are used in the symptomatic treatment of psychoneuroses to reduce anxiety, agitation and tension.

Neuroleptics

(Major tranquillisers, ataratics, antipsychotics)

They used in the treatment of psychoses and include phenothiazines, thioxanthenes, butyrophenones and oxypertine. They are used in the symptomatic treatment of psychoses such as schizophrenia, mania and senile dementia. Lithium salts are used in treating mania and are called antimanic agents.

The introduction of Rauwolfia alkaloid reserpine in 1953 and an antihistamine related compound, viz., chlorpromazine in 1954, revolutionised the treatment of certain mental disorders. First these agents were termed as ataraxic, neurosedative, etc. But then the term tranquilising agent was most suitable and was accepted.

They act differently than barbiturates and other sedatives, which act by producing general CNS depression. These agents act primarily in paleocortex and subcortical areas of the brain. They cause strong sedation and relieve the state of anxiety Sleep then comes naturally due to a state of indifference to the surroundings. They produce sleep, but the arousal response of the patient is still present. A person under sedation of barbiturates is difficult to awaken, but under tranquilisers, he still can be awakened from sleep, like a normal person. These drugs are useful in reducing excitement, agitation, aggressiveness and impulsiveness. These drugs however do not produce anesthesia even at a high dose, like some of the barbiturates do.

Some of the important agents of this class are as follows :

1) Chlorpromazine hydrochloride

2-Chloro-10[3-(dimethylamino) propyl] phenothiazine hydrochloride

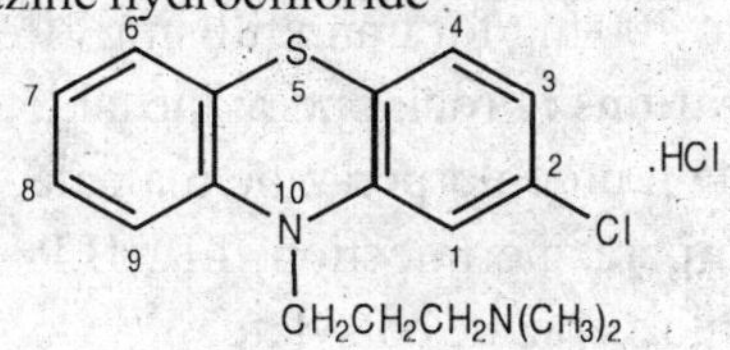

Properties : Chlorpromazine hydrochloride occurs as a white or cream-coloured powder with a slight odour. It is freely soluble in alcohol and very soluble in water.

Stability : Powder or aqueous solution of the drug decomposes by oxidation on exposure to light. Degradation is rapid in alkaline solution.

Incompatibility : In aqueous solution, it is incompatible with pentobarbitone sodium and phenobarbitone sodium.

Storage : It should be protected from light.

Actions and uses : This drug is used as its

hydrochloride, orally or parenterally in the treatment of nausea and vomiting. It is also used to potentiate effects of anesthetics, analgesics, hypnotics and sedatives, and in a variety of mental and emotional disturbances.

Dose : 75 to 800 mg a day, in divided doses.

Preparations : Chlorpromazine tablets, I.P., B.P.

Chlorpromazine injection, I.P., B.P.

Chlorpromazine elixir, B.P.C.

Brand Names : Cain®, Clozine®, Chlorpromazine®, Megatil®, Relitil®

2) Prochlorperazine maleate

2-Chloro-10-[3-(4-methyl, 1-piperazinyl) propyl] phenothiazine maleate.

Properties : It occurs as a white or pale yellow, crystalline powder. It is almost odourless and has a slightly bitter taste. It is very slightly soluble in water and in alcohol.

Actions and uses : Its action is similar to chlorpromazine, but in much smaller dose.

Dose : 5 mg to 40 mg for antiemetic effect.

10 mg to 200 mg for tranquillising effect.

Preparations : Prochloperazine tablets, I.P., B.P. - contain prochlorperazine maleate.

Prochlorperazine injection, I.P., B.P. - contains prochlorperazine edisylate.

Brand Names : Stemetil®, Emidoxyn®, Oset®

3) Trifluoperazine hydrochloride

10-[3-(4-Methyl-1-piperazinyl)propyl]-2-(trifluoromethyl) phenothiazine dihydrochloride.

There is a trifluoromethyl group (CF_3) instead of chloro. Other part of the structure is the same as in prochlorperazine.

Properties : It occurs as a white to pale yellow, crystalline powder. It is odourless, hygroscopic and has a bitter taste. It is freely soluble in water and very slightly soluble in alcohol.

Stability : In aqueous solution, it is readily oxidised by atmospheric oxygen.

Storage : It should be stored in airtight containers, protected from light.

Actions and uses : This a much more potent drug especially useful in chronic psychoses marked by hyperactivity. It controls, what is known in psychoses, as extrapyramidal symptoms. It is a useful antipsychotic drug.

Dose : Equivalent of 2 to 30 mg of trifluoperazine, daily in divided doses.

Preparations : Trifluoperzine tablets, B.P.

Brand Names : Neocalm®, Sycot®, Trazine®, Trinicalm plus®

4) Haloperidol

4-[4-(p-Chlorophenyl)-4-hydroxypiperidino] 4`-fluorobutyrophenone.

Properties : Haloperidol occurs as an odourless, tasteless, white to faintly yellowish powder. It is practically insoluble in water and sparingly soluble in alcohol.

Actions and uses : This is a very potent drug with similar actions as piperazine phenothiazine class of transquilisers, like prochlorperazine and trifluoperazine. It has less prominent sedative action. It has been claimed to be more effective in highly agitated and maniac patients. The incidences of extrapyramidal effects of this drug are high and it does not seem to be any superior to phenothiazines in the treatment of schizophrenia.

Dose : 1.5 to 7.5 mg three times a day.

Preparations : Haloperidol tablets, I.P.

Haloperidol injection, I.P.

Haloperidol oral solution, I.P.

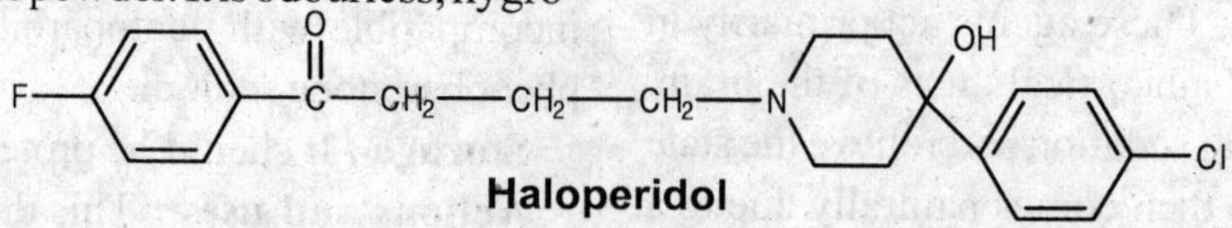

Haloperidol

Brand Names : Relinase®, Senorm®, Trancodol®

5) Trifluperidol

4`-Fluoro-4-[4-hydroxy-4-(m-trifluoromethyl phenyl) piperidino] butyrophenone.

Trifluperidol is like haloperidol, in its structure except that the chloro group is replaced by trifluoromethyl (CF_3).

Properties : Trifluperidol hydrochloride occurs as a white, amorphous or crystalline, flocculent powder. It is slightly soluble in water and soluble in alcohol. It is stable in air but darkens slowly on exposure to light.

Actions and uses : Its actions are just like haloperidol in the management of major psychoses, including schizophrenia and paranoia.

Dose : 1 to 2.5 mg a day.

Brand Names : Triperidol®

6) Chlordiazepoxide hydrochloride

7-Chloro-2-(methylamino)-5-phenyl-3H,1,4, benzodiazepine-4-oxide hydrochloride.

This drug was introduced in 1960 and was the first of the benzodiazepine series.

Properties : It occurs as a white crystalline powder with a slight odour and a very bitter taste. It is freely soluble in water and sparingly soluble in alcohol.

Stability : Chlordiazepoxide undergoes hydrolysis to demoxepam which further degrades into many compounds.

Storage : It should be stored in airtight containers, protected from light.

Actions and uses : It was shown to block the spinal reflexes at 1/10th of dose of meprobamate. The drug is rapidly absorbed from the GI tract and peak blood levels are reached in 2 to 4 hours. It has a long half life of 20 to 24 hours. The drug is classified as mild central depressant, with a centrally mediated skeletal-muscle-relaxant effect.

Dose : 15 to 60 mg a day, in divided doses.

Preparations : Chlordiazepoxide tablets, I.P.
Chlordiazepoxide capsules, B.P.

Brand Names : Librium®, Peace®, Smoothspas®

7) Diazepam

7-Chloro-1,3-dihydro-1-methyl-5 phenyl-2H-1,4- benzodiazepin-2 one

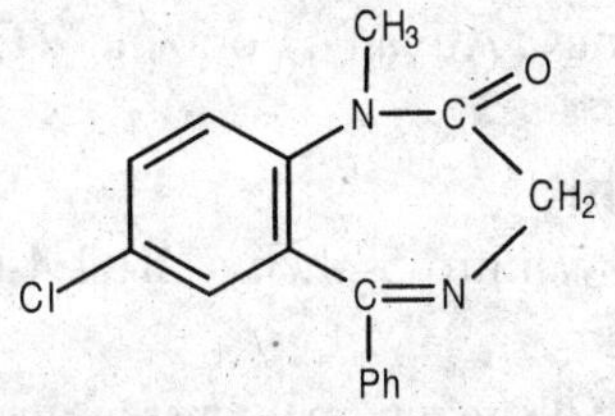

Properties : Diazepam occurs as a white, crystalline, odourless powder. It is very slightly soluble in water and soluble in alcohol.

Stability : Diazepam degrades by hydrolysis into several products.

Actions and uses : This drug was introduced in 1964 and is used for the control of anxiety and stress. It is also useful in the management of acute agitation during alcohol withdrawal. Diazepam also has significant anticovulsant properties. Diazepam is metabolised in liver and is converted to a 3-hydroxy derivative, oxazepam, which is also a sedative and muscle relaxant.

Dose : 2 to 15 mg orally. Not to exceed 30 mg in a day. 2 to 10 mg IM or IV repeated in 2-4 hours if needed.

Preparations : Diazepam capsules, I.P., B.P.
Diazepam tablets, I.P., B.P.
Diazepam injection, I.P., B.P.C.
Diazepam elixir, B.P.C.

Brand Names : Calmpose®, Valium®, Elcion-CR®

8) Lorazepam

7-Chloro-5-(2-chlorophenyl)-1,3-dihydro-3-hydroxy-2H-1,4-benzodiazepin-2-one.

Properties : Lorazepam occurs as an odourless, white powder. It is practically insoluble in water and soluble in alcohol.

Actions and uses : This drug is more potent than diazepam with a very low dose of 1-4 mg and effective half-life of 5-24 hours. All other actions are similar to diazepam. But the drug is used clinically only under special conditions.

Brand Names : Ativan®, Lorazine®, Trapex®

9) Nitrazepam

1,3-Dihydro-7-nitro-5-phenyl-2H-1,4-benzodiazepin-2-one

Properties : Nitrazepam occurs as an odourless, yellow crystalline powder. It is very slightly soluble in water and slightly soluble in alcohol.

Actions and uses : This drug is also more potent than diazepam, and is effective at a low dose of 5-10 mg. Its half life is 5 to 24 hours. It has more of hypnotic effect than sedative effect.

Preparations : Nitrazepam tablets, I.P., B.P.

Brand Names : Hypnoril®, Nitrosun®, Nitravet®

10) Meprobamate

2-Methyl-2-propyl-1,3-propanediol-dicarbamate

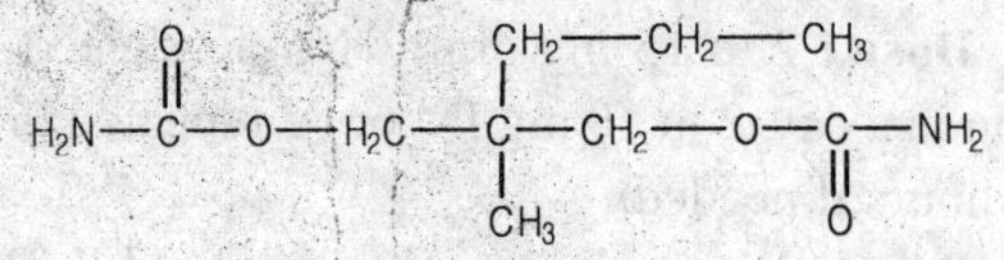

Properties : Meprobamate occurs as an odourless white, crystalline powder with a bitter taste. It is freely soluble in alcohol and slightly soluble in water.

Actions and uses : Meprobamate produces skeletal muscle relaxation by intraneural blockade at the spinal level. However, the popular use of this drug has been in the treatment of simple insomnia and to relieve anxiety and tension states. Meprobamate is also useful in the prevention of attacks of petitmal epilepsy. It is stable in dilute acid and alkali.

Dose : 400 mg, 3 times a day.

Preparations : Meprobamate tablets B.P.

11) Oxypertine

5,6-Dimethoxy-2-methyl-3[2-(4-phenylpiperazin-1-yl) ethyl]-indole

Properties : It occurs as a white crystalline powder. It is slightly soluble in water and in alcohol.

Actions and uses : Oxypertine has antipsychotic actions similar to those of chlorpromazine. The important side-effects are sedation and extrapyramidal symptoms. In lower doses (30 mg daily) it may be used for non-psychotic emotional disturbances such as anxiety and tension.

Dose : 80 to 120 mg a day, in divided doses.

12) Thiothixene hydrochloride

(Z)-N,N-dimethyl-9-[3-(4-methylpiperazin-1-yl) propylidene] thioxanthene-2-sulphonamide dihydrochloride

Properties : It occurs as a white crystalline powder with a slight odour. It is freely soluble in water; slightly soluble in alcohol.

Storage : It should be stored in airtight containers, protected from light.

Actions and uses : Thiothixene is a thioxanthene with general properties similar to those of the phenothiazine chlorpromazine. It is widely used as antipsychotic. Extrapyramidal symptoms, restlessness and insomnia are the important side effects.

Dose : 20 to 30 mg a day.

Preparations : Thiothixene capsules, U.S.P.

Thiothixene hydrochloride injection, U.S.P.

Thiothixene hydrochloride oral solution, U.S.P.

Drugs For Further Study

1) Thioridazine - Melozine®, Ridazin®, Sycoril®
2) Fluphenazine - Anatensol®, Prolinate®
3) Haloperidol - Combidol®, Halidol®, Hexidol®
4) Droperidol - Droperol®
5) Loxapine - Loxapac®
6) Clozapine - Lozapin®, Sizopin®, Skizoril®
7) Risperidone - Respidon®, Risnia®, Rispid®
8) Pimozide - Mozep®, Pimodac®
9) Quetiapine - Placidin®, Qutipin®, Socalm®
10) Penfluridol - Semap
11) Flupenthixol - Fluanxol®
12) Zuclopenthixol - Clopixol®
13) Olanzapine - Olan®, Olanzotic®, Oleanz®
14) Aripiprazole - Arilan®, Aripra®, Arip-MT®, Arzu®
15) Ziprasidone - Azona®

Exercise

Q1. Write structure and uses of diazepam. (Kachchh Univ. 06, Winter 06, May 05)

Q2. Write the structure and chemical name of chlorpromazine and diazepam. (Karnataka Univ.)

Q3. Define and explain the following term - Tranquilisers. (Winter 04, May-June 04, Summer 06)

Q4. Draw structure and describe skeletal structure, peripheral groups and linkage of diazepam. (Winter 04)

Q5. Give the structures and uses of haloperidol. (Summer 03, Nov 06)

Q6. Write structure, chemical name and uses of chlorpromazine or promethazine HCl. (Summer 03)

Q7. Classify 'Tranquilisers' with examples of each class. Write the structure of any one. (Summer 03)

Q8. What are tranquilising agents? Classify tranquilising agents with example. (May 07)

11 Hypnotics

Sedatives and hypnotics are general CNS depressants. A sedative produces mild depression and calms anxiety and excitation without causing drowsiness or impaired performance. A hypnotic induces sleep. The degree of depression depends on the potency of the drug and the dose used.

The indications for sedation are stressful conditions involving emotional strain and stress, control of convulsions and as adjuncts to anesthetics. Hypnotic doses are used in the treatment of insomnia. Prolonged administration of hypnotics is harmful as tolerance and drug dependance may occur, besides other side effects.

Classification of Hypnotics

I] Barbiturates

I] Barbiturates

Barbiturates are widely used hypnotic-sedative agents. Barbital, the first member of the class was introduced in 1903. Since then, reacting diethyl-malonate with various alkyl halides, produced several barbiturates with a range of degree of sedative action.

All barbiturates are colourless, crystalline solids, melting at 96 - 205°C. They are not soluble in water, but their sodium salts are quite soluble. The solutions are strongly alkaline and often hydrolyse to give precipitates of barbiturates.

Stability

The free barbituric acids are generally stable compounds. Stable aqueous solutions may be prepared by incorporating a solubilising agent such as alcohol or glycerol. The alkali and alkaline earth metal salts (soluble barbiturates) are hygroscopic. When exposed to air, they absorb carbon dioxide and free barbituric acid is liberated. Aqueous solutions of the soluble barbiturates decompose, decomposition increases with temperature. Propylene glycol and alcohol are used to stabilise such solutions.

Incompatibility

Solutions of sodium salts are incompatible with acidic substances owing to precipitation of the free barbituric acids. They are also incompatible with ammonium salts. When barbiturate solutions are mixed with solutions of weak bases (eg. calcium chloride, magnesium sulphate), complexes of low solubility may be formed.

Classification

Barbiturates are usually grouped as long acting (8 hrs or more), intermediate acting (3-6 hrs), short acting (less than 3 hrs) and ultra short acting (less than 30 minutes) Some of the important and frequently used barbiturates are as follows-

1) Phenobarbital

5-Ethyl-5-phenyl barbituric acid

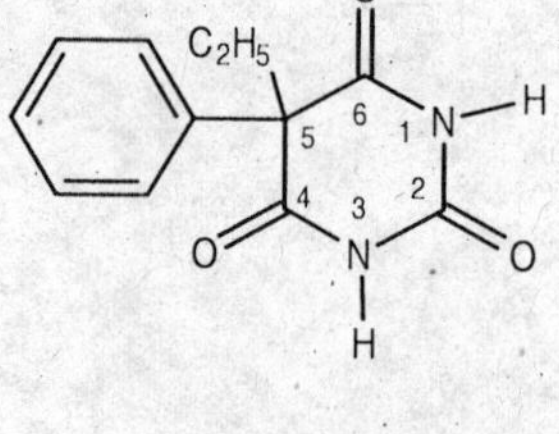

Properties : Phenobarbital occurs as an odourless white, crystalline powder or colourless crystals with a slightly bitter taste. It is very slightly soluble in water, freely soluble in alcohol, soluble in ether and in solutions of alkali hydroxides and carbonates. Phenobarbital sodium is freely soluble in water and soluble in alcohol.

Storage : It should be stored in airtight containers.

Actions and uses : Phenobarbital is a long acting barbiturate, more potent than its parent compound barbital. It has slow onset - about 1 hour - but long duration - about 10 to 16 hours. It is also effective for epilepsy, especially in grandmal and petitmal type. It is used as a sodium salt and is available either in oral or parenteral dosage forms.

Dose : 30 to 600 mg (oral), IM or IV 130 to 200 mg

As anti-convulsant : 200 - 320 mg IM/IV

Preparations : Phenobarbitone tablets, I.P., B.P.

Phenobarbitone elixir, B.P.C.

Phenobarbitone sodium tablets, I.P., B.P.

Phenobarbitone sodium injection, I.P., B.P.

Brand Names : Beetal®, Phenobarb®, Gardenal®, Luminal®

2) Butobarbital

5-Butyl-5-ethyl barbituric acid.

Properties : Butobarbital occurs as colourless crystals or white crystalline powder with a very slight odour and a slightly bitter taste. It is slightly soluble in water and freely soluble in alcohol, ether and chloroform. It is readily soluble in solutions of alkali hydroxides and carbonates.

Actions and uses : Butobarbital is an intermediate acting (3-6 hours) barbiturate. Sodium salt is usually used orally, in a dose of 8 to 60 mg as sedative and 100-200 mg as hypnotic. Sedative action lasts for about 5-6 hours.

Preparations : Butobarbitone tablets B.P.

3) Cyclobarbital

5-Ethyl-5-cyclohexenyl barbituric acid.

Both cyclobarbital and its calcium salt are official in I.P.

Properties : Cyclobarbital calcium occurs as white or slightly yellowish, odourless, crystalline powder with a bitter taste. It is sparingly soluble in water and very slightly soluble in alcohol.

Actions and uses : It is a short acting barbiturate of duration less than 3 hours. Onset of action is usually in 15-30 minutes.

Dose : Hypnotic dose is 100-300 mg.

Preparations : Cyclobarbitone tablets, I.P.

Cyclobarbitone calcium tablets, I.P., B.P.

II] Non-barbiturate hypnotics

II] Non-barbiturates

Benzodiazepines such as diazepam and nitrazepam are the hypnotics of first choice as they are safer than barbiturates.

1) Glutethimide

5-Ethyl-5-phenyl glutarimide

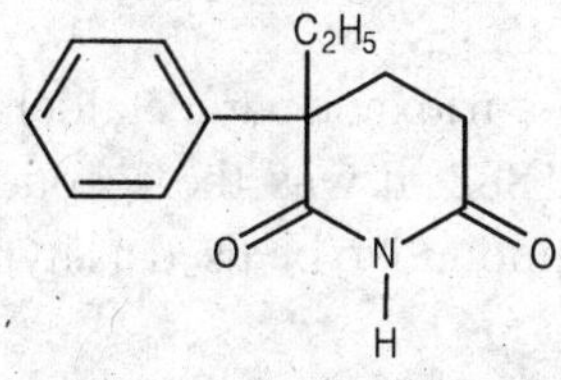

Properties : It occurs as odourless, colourless crystals or white powder, with a bitter taste. It is practically insoluble in water and freely soluble in alcohol.

Storage : It should be stored in airtight containers protected from light.

Actions and uses : It was first introduced in 1954 and is closely related in action to barbiturates. Its hypnotic effects begin in about 30 minutes after administration, and last for about 4 to 8 hours. The drug is useful for induction of sleep in simple insomnia and is also useful to relieve anxiety-tension states.

Dose : Sedative : 125 to 250 mg, 1-3 times a day.

Hypnotic : 500 mg to 1 gm

Preparations : Glutethimide tablets, B.P.

2) Methyprylon

3,3-Diethyl-5-methyl-2,4-piperidinedione

Properties : Methyprylon occurs as a white crystalline powder. It has a slight characteristic odour and a burning taste with bitter after taste. It is soluble in water and very soluble in alcohol.

Storage : It should be stored in airtight containers protected from light.

Actions and uses : Methyprylon is a hypnotic-sedative, structurally related to barbiturates and has similar actions. It induces sleep within 15-30 minutes, useful in simple insomnia.

Dose : Hypnotic dose is 50 to 400 mg at bedtime.

Preparations : Methyprylon tablets, B.P.

3) Paraldehyde

2,4,6-trimethyl-s-trioxane paracetaldehyde

Introduced in 1882, it was the second synthetic organic compound to be used as hypnotic sedative.

Properties : Paraldehyde occurs as a clear colourless liquid with a strong characteristic odour and an unpleasant taste. It is soluble in 9 parts of water and is miscible with alcohol.

Stability : Paraldehyde decomposes on storage by oxidation to acetic acid. Stored samples have been found to contain upto 98 per cent of acetic acid. It must not be used if it has a brownish colour or if an odour of acetic acid has developed.

Storage : It should be stored in small, well-filled, airtight bottles, in complete darkness, in a cool place. Its contact with cork and plastics should be avoided.

Actions and uses : The drug is more potent and toxic than alcohol, but less than chloral hydrate. With an oral dose of 10 ml, sleep is induced within 10-15 minutes. Because of its unpleasant taste, it is often given by rectal route. It is also used as anticonvulsant.

The main objection to paraldehyde is its disagreeable and potent odour which is exhaled with the breath of the patients. Although an excellent and safe drug, its unpleasant odour prevents its use as daytime sedative.

Dose : 5 to 10 ml

Preparations : Paraldehyde injection B.P.C.

4) Triclofos sodium

Sodium hydrogen 2,2,2-trichloroethyl phosphate

Properties : It occurs as an odourless, white, hygroscopic powder, with a saline taste. It is freely soluble in water and slightly soluble in alcohol.

Storage : It should be stored in airtight containers.

Actions and uses : Triclofos sodium has sedative and hypnotic actions similar to those of other chloral derivatives. It should be given along with fluid since chloral is a gastric irritant.

Dose : Sedative dose : 500 mg, once or twice a day.

Hypnotic dose : 1 to 2 gm

Preparations : Triclofos elixir, B.P.C.

Triclofos tablets, B.P.

Brand Names : Foskid® syp., Pediclory® solution, Silence®, Slep®, Tricloryl®.

Drugs for further study

1) Nitrazepam - Dormin®, Nigap®, Nitrosun®
2) Flurazepam - Fluracap®, Fluraz®
3) Zopiclone - Zolinox®, Zonap®, Zopicon®
4) Melatonin - Eternex®, Meloset®, Zytonin®

Exercise

Q1. What are barbiturates? Write an account of barbiturates used as hypnotics and sedatives. (Kachchh Univ. 06, May 05)

Q2. Write structures and uses of the following - 1) Phenobarbitone, 2) Paraldehyde and 3) Triclofos sodium (Kachchh Univ. 06, May 05)

Q3. Define and classify hypnotics and sedatives with suitable examples. (Winter 04, Summer 03, Summer 06, May-June 04)

Q4. Give structure, properties, uses and dose of phenobarbitone. (Summer 06)

Q5. What are barbiturates? Give name, structure and use of various barbiturate. (May 07)

Q6. Name hypnotic having a cyclic ureide structure. (Nov 06)

Q7. Define and classify anti-epileptic drugs. Write a note on non-barbiturates as hypnotics and sedatives. (Nov 06)

■

12 General Anesthetic Agents

General anesthetic agents belong to the class of drugs named Central Nervous System Depressants (CNS Depressants). In this class general anesthetics produce the highest order of CNS depression. The word 'anesthesia', meaning insensibility to the surroundings, was first used by Olive Holmes, after the first successful use of ether as a general anesthetic agent.

General anesthesia is the controlled, reversible depression of the functional activity of the CNS, producing loss of sensation and consciousness. The relief of pain through general anesthesia during surgery was first carried out in 1841 by using ether, nitrous oxide was used in 1844 and chloroform was used in 1847 as anesthetic agent. Later many more new and better agents were invented and used.

Classification of General Anesthetics

I] **Hydrocarbons**

II] **Halogenated hydrocarbons**

III] **Ethers**

IV] **Other Agents**

I] Hydrocarbons

1) Cyclopropane

It was first introduced in 1934 as a general anesthetic agent.

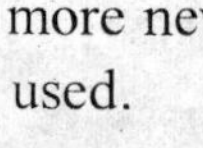

Properties : Cyclopropane is a colourless gas. Boiling point is about 33°C and is highly inflammable and explosive.

Incompatibility : Cyclopropane is liable to leach out some material from the walls of rubber or plastic tubing leading to leakage or bursting the tube.

Storage : It should be stored in metal cylinders in a cool place. The cylinders should be painted orange.

Actions and uses : It is the most potent gaseous agent currently in use. With the use of the premedications and depressant drugs, such as morphine or barbiturates, surgical anesthesia can be produced using cyclopropane within 2-3 minutes. A mixture of cyclopropane and oxygen (15:85) is used for anesthesia.

2) Ethylene

Ethene $H_2C{=}CH_2$

This is an unsaturated hydrocarbon, occurring as a colourless gas. It produces rapid anesthesia, but requires high concentration (90:10 mixture with oxygen). It is highly explosive and is not used any more.

II] Halogenated hydrocarbons

1) Trichloroethylene

1,1,2-Trichloroethene

Properties : It is a volatile liquid. Boiling point is about 88°C. Practically insoluble in water and miscible with ether, alcohol and chloroform.

Stability : It is stable in the presence of

moisture but undergoes decomposition on exposure to light in presence of air.

Storage : It should be stored in airtight containers, in a cool place, protected from light.

Actions and uses : It is an effective agent, but due to its serious side effects, especially cardiac irregularities and hepatic damage, it is not recommended as anesthetic.

2) Chloroform

$CHCl_3$

Chloroform was discovered in 1847.

Properties : It occurs as a colourless, heavy, volatile liquid. It has a characteristic odour and a sweet burning taste. It is slightly soluble in water and miscible with alcohol.

Stability : On exposure to air and light, chloroform decomposes by oxidation to chlorine and highly poisonous phosgene (carbonyl chloride). This decomposition can be retarded by adding a small quantity of alcohol.

Storage : It should be stored in airtight containers protected from light.

Actions and uses : It was used as general anesthetic agent for minor surgeries and ailments like bone-setting. Due to its serious side effect of liver damage, it could not make the rank of general anesthesia for surgical purposes. It may be used as an emergency anesthetic for major first-aid field surgery. It is used as a carminative and flavouring agent in pharmaceutical mixtures.

Preparations : Chloroform spirit, I.P., B.P. - a pharmaceutical aid.

3) Halothane

Fluothane Introduced in 1956.

2-bromo-2-chloro-1,1,1-trifluoroethane

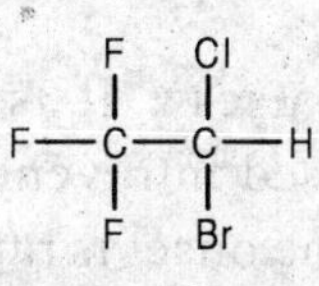

Properties : Halothane occurs as a colourless, mobile, heavy liquid. It has a characteristic odour. Boiling point is about 50°C. It is slightly soluble in water and miscible with alcohol.

Stability : When exposed to ultraviolet radiation for a long period, it decomposes with the formation of halogen acids and free halogens. 0.01 % $^{w}/_{w}$ of thymol is added as a preservative.

Storage : It should be stored in airtight containers at a temperature not exceeding 25°C, protected from light.

Actions and uses : Anesthesia is produced by 2-2.5 per cent of the liquid in vapourised form, given by inhalation.

Halothane is a good general anesthetic, four times more potent than ether. Due to its chemical inertness and low toxicity it was quickly developed into general anesthetic agent. Its solubility and vapour pressure were in the desirable range and its induction period was rapid for general anesthesia (2-10 minutes). Recovery of the patient was also good. Only side effect was hypotension and bradycardia.

Brand Names : Fluothane®

III] Ethers

1) Ether

Diethylether $CH_3.CH_2.O.CH_2.CH_3$

Properties : Ether occurs as a clear, colourless, very mobile liquid. Boiling point is about 35°C. It has a characteristic odour and a sweet burning taste. It is very volatile and highly inflammable. It is soluble in water, miscible with alcohol and chloroform.

Stability : Atmospheric oxidation leads to formation of explosive peroxides. 0.002 % $^{w}/_{v}$ of propyl gallate or hydroquinone is added to retard this degradation.

Storage : It should be stored in dry, airtight containers in a cool place, protected from light.

Actions and uses : It is a potent general anesthetic. With increase in knowledge regarding its handling, ether became quite safe to use. Along with other agents like nitrous oxide, ether can be used effectively, with its prolonged induction time shortened. Concentration used is usually 6 to 7 per cent by volume. Since better drugs are available now, it is no longer used.

2) Vinylether

Divinylether, Vinethene. $CH_2=CH-O-CH=CH_2$

Properties : It occurs as a clear, colourless liquid. Boiling point is about 28°C. It has a characteristic odour. It is slightly soluble in water, miscible with alcohol and ether. It is inflammable.

Stability : On exposure to air and light, it decomposes into formaldehyde and formic acid, finally polymerising into a jelly. Decomposition is retarded by adding 0.01 % $^{w}/_{v}$ of phenyl-α-naphthylamine as a stabiliser.

Storage : It should be stored in airtight containers of not more than 200 ml capacity, in a cool place, protected from light.

Actions and uses : It is a volatile anesthetic four times more potent than ether. It causes extensive liver damage on longer use. It is used only for induction of anesthesia to cut short prolonged induction time of ether. It is also used in minor operations of short duration.

IV] Other Agents

1) Ultrashort acting barbiturates

a) Methohexital Sodium

Sodium 5-allyl-1-methyl-5-(1-methyl-2-pentynyl) barbiturate.

Properties : It occurs as an odourless, hygroscopic white powder. It is soluble in water.

Stability : Aqueous solutions decompose on keeping. Solutions which have become discoloured or cloudy should not be used.

Storage : It should be stored in airtight containers.

Actions and uses : It was introduced in 1960 as intravenously administered anesthetic. It is a rapidly acting agent and recovery is also fast. It has no muscular relaxation properties. Therefore, it is used along with gaseous anesthetic agents like ether and other muscular relaxants like succinyl choline.

b) Thiopental Sodium

(Thiopentone Sodium)

Sodium 5-ethyl-5-(1-methylbutyl)-2-thiobarbiturate

Properties : It occurs as a hygroscopic, yellowish-white powder. It has a characteristic alliaceous odour and a bitter taste. It is freely soluble in water, partly soluble in alcohol.

Stability : Aqueous solutions decompose on keeping. Solutions should not be used if they have become cloudy or a precipitate has formed. Sodium carbonate is added to the powder to prevent conversion of salt to free acid by atmospheric carbon dioxide.

Incompatibility : Same as for barbiturates (See page 82)

Barbiturates are widely used hypnotic-sedative agents. Barbital, the first member of the class was introduced in 1903. Since then, reacting diethyl-malonate with various alkyl halides, produced several barbiturates with a range of degree of sedative action.

All barbiturates are colourless, crystalline solids, melting at 96 - 205°C. They are not soluble in water, but their sodium salts are quite soluble. The solutions are strongly alkaline and often hydrolyse to give precipitates of barbiturates.

Storage : It should be stored in airtight containers.

Actions and uses : It is available as a powder and is used intravenously (45mg/kg body weight). The onset is rapid (30 sec) and ing general anesthesia and as anesthetic for short durations.

Dose : 100 to 150 mg IV.

Preparations : Thiopentone injection I.P., B.P.

Brand Names : Pentothal®, Thiojex®, Thiosol®

2) Nitrous oxide

Nitrogen monoxide : N_2O

Properties : It occurs as an odourless, tasteless, colourless gas, which is heavier than air. It is freely soluble in water.

Storage : It should be stored in metal cylinders in a cool place. The cylinders should be painted blue.

Actions and uses : It is useful for rapid induction of anesthesia. It is a gas and its application is by inhalation (60-80 : 20-40 oxygen). It produces surgical anesthesia, but is not recommended for prolonged use. It is used as induction anesthetic. It is used in dental and obstetric procedures for producing analgesia and light anesthesia.

Balanced Anesthesia

Any of the single anesthetic agents, is rarely used alone. It is always used in combination with others or is followed after the use of other agents. Usually a patient is first given an ultrashort acting barbiturate (to induce unconsciousness) followed by muscular relaxing agent. Then he is a general anesthetic like halothane administered. In between, drugs like atropine are given to reduce internal secretions, followed by potent analgetics like morphine or pethidine.

Compounds such as thiopental sodium and ketamine hydrochloride are called basal anesthetics. These are used initially to induce anesthesia as they are quick and short acting. Anesthesia is then maintained by using an inhalation anesthetic.

Drugs For Further Study

1) Ketamine - Aneket®, Ketajex®, Ketalar®
2) Propofol - Cleofol®, Profol® 1%, Propovan®

Exercise

Q1. Classify the general anaesthetics by different methods and give their examples of each class. (Summer 03)

■

(13) Antidepressant Drugs

After the discovery of the therapeutic value of phenothiazines like chlorpromazine (major tranquilisers) many modifications were made in their structure, which resulted in dibenzazepine derivatives like imipramine, amitriptyline, nortriptyline which are now known as antidepressant drugs. Since they have three rings in their structure, they are known as 'Tricyclic antidepressants'.

Their major therapeutic actions are -

1. Effective in the treatment of emotional and psychiatric disorders in which major symptom is depression.

2. Removal of endogenous depression, thus resulting in elevation of mood of the patient.

3. Increase physical activity and mental alertness.

4. Increase appetite.

5. Useful in the treatment of enuresis in children, especially imipramine.

Some of the major side effects of these drugs are -

1. Dryness of mouth

2. Tachycardia.

3. Constipation and sweating.

4. Dangerous synergistic effect (additive effect) with monoamine oxidase inhibitors like isoniazid, phenelzine, etc.

Tricyclic Antidepressants

1) Imipramine hydrochloride

5-[3-(Dimethylamino)propyl]-10, 11-dihydro-5-H-dibenz[b,f]-azepine hydrochloride

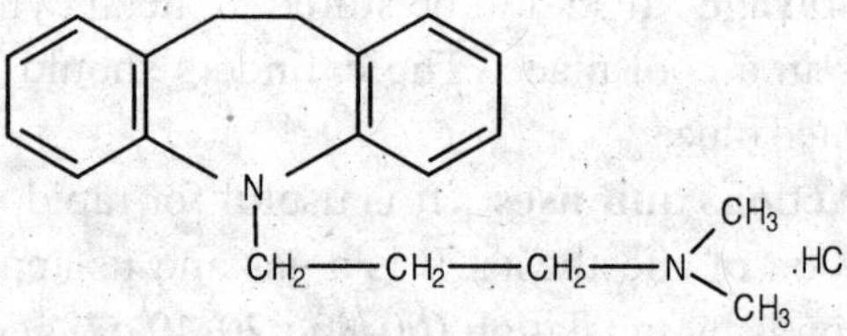

Properties : Imipramine hydrochloride occurs as a white or slightly yellow, crystalline powder. It is almost odourless with a bitter taste. It is freely soluble in water and alcohol.

Stability : In the presence of water and oxygen, degradation occurs. This is accelerated by light and increase in temperature.

Storage : It should be stored in airtight containers, protected from light.

Actions and uses : Imipramine was introduced in 1959. The drug is potent parasympatholytic and displays prominent atropine like side effects. It is most useful in the treatment of anxiety, the drug is often given along with phenothiazine tranquilising agent. Severe toxic reactions have occurred when imipramine is taken along with monoamine oxidase inhibitors like isoniazid or phenelzine.

Imipramine is available as 10, 25 and 50 mg tablets for oral use and in ampules of 25 mg for IM administration. Sometimes small crystals may form in the ampules, but these readily dissolve on shaking or holding the ampules in warm water. On N-demethylation, it gives desipramine.

Doses : 25 to 75 mg, 3 times a day.

Preparations : Imipramine tablets I.P., B.P.

Brand Names : Antidep®, Depsonil®, Diamin®, Depsol®, Microdep®

2) Amitriptyline hydrochloride

5-(3-Dimethyl aminopropylidene)-10,11-dihydro-5H-dibenzo(a,d) cycloheptene, hydrochloride

Properties : It occurs as odourless, colourless, crystals or white powder. It has a bitter and burning taste. It is freely soluble in water, alcohol and chloroform.

Stability : Oxidation of the drug in aqueous solutions is catalysed by metal ions. Disodium edetate is a suitable stabiliser.

Storage : It should be stored in airtight containers, protected from light.

Actions and uses : This drug is indicated for depression. It also has a tranquilising effect and is useful where anxiety accompanies depression. It also has sedative effect which manifests quickly. However, the antidepressant effect may onset in about 4 days. Improvement in mood and behaviour is seen in 2-3 weeks of treatment.

Some minor side effects like dry mouth, blurred vision are common. Amitriptyline is not to be used in conditions of glaucoma or cardiovascular complications. Like other tricyclic antidepressant drugs, it has serious potentiation effect with monoamine oxidase inhibitors.

Dose : 75 to 150 mg a day.

Preparations : Amitriptyline injection, B.P., Amitriptyline tablets, I.P., B.P.

Brand Names : Amitone®, Amline®, Amixide®, Eliwel®, Tryptomer®

3) Nortriptyline hydrochloride

5-(3-Methyl amino propylidene)-10,11-dihydro-5H-dibenzo(a,d) cycloheptene hydrochloride

Chemically, nortriptyline is closely related to amitriptyline. It is the N-demethylated derivative of amitriptyline, where one of the methyl groups on the dimethylamino propyl side chain is replaced by hydrogen.

Properties : It occurs as a white powder. It has a slight characteristic odour and a burning bitter taste. It is sparingly soluble in water and freely soluble in alcohol.

Storage : It should be protected from light.

Actions and uses : The drug has the same effects as its parent compound, amitriptyline, i.e., antidepressant and tranquillising effects. It also has the same side effects like dry mouth and other anticholinergic effects. However, these effects are little less for nortriptyline as compared with amitriptyline. The drug is not recommended for use in children.

Dose : Equivalent of 30 to 100 mg of nortriptyline base daily, in divided doses.

Nortriptyline is available in 10, 25 mg capsules and 10 mg/5 ml in injectable form.

Preparations : Nortriptyline capsules, B.P. Nortriptyline tablets, I.P., B.P.

Brand Names : Primox®, Secmin-25®, Sensival®

Monoamine Oxidase Inhibitors

In 1952, it was observed that tuberculosis patients on treatment with isonicotinic acid hydrazide (INH) were more active and also sometimes more irritable. This observation was attributed to CNS stimulation. This observation also held good for another derivative of INH, called iproniazid. Clinical investigation further revealed that iproniazid was a central stimulant and was useful in the treatment of mental depression. Further biochemical observation led to the conclusion that this class of drugs inhibited an enzyme known as 'mono amino oxidase' (MAO) which was responsible for the destruction of brain amines like norepinephrine and serotonin, with the result, more norepinephrine was in circulation, which naturally gave stimulant effect. Thus, the drugs in this category came to be known as MAO inhibitors and turned out to be CNS stimulants. These drugs are, therefore, used in the treatment of psychotic patients, with mild to severe depression. Patients on treted with these drugs show increased sense of well-being, increased desire and ability to communicate, elevation of mood, increased physical and mental alertness and improved appetite.

1) Phenelzine sulphate

β-phenylethylhydrazine, hydrogen sulphate

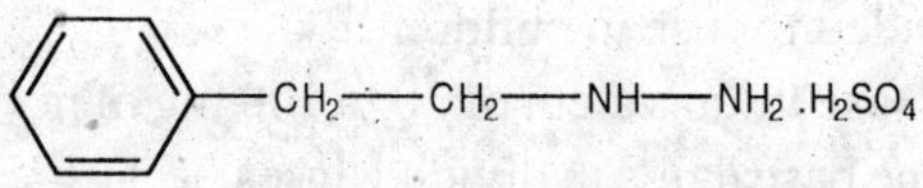

Properties : It occurs as a white powder or pearly platelets with a pungent odour. It is freely soluble in water, very slightly soluble in alcohol.

Storage : It should be stored in airtight containers, protected from light.

Actions and uses : Phenelzine sulphate was introduced in 1959, as a potent MAO inhibitor, used in the treatment of depression. Side effects include postural hypotension, constipation and edema.

Preparations : Phenelzine tablets, B.P.

Dose : 15 mg tablet a day.

2) Tranylcypromine sulphate

(±) trans-2-Phenylcyclopropyl amine sulphate

Properties : It occurs as a white crystalline powder. It is odourless and has an acid like taste. It is soluble in water, very slightly soluble in alcohol and in ether.

Actions and uses : This drug was introduced in 1948 as an amphetamine analog. The drug was retested for MAO inhibitory action and was reintroduced in 1961, as MAO inhibitor, for the treatment of patients with psychoneurotic and psychotic depression. The drug however gave rise to hypertensive crisis and was withdrawn briefly in 1964. But due to its effectiveness in the treatment of depression, it was allowed to be used in hospitals under strict observation. It was prohibited for patients over 60 years of age and with a history of cardiovascular diseases.

Dose : 20 mg a day, in two doses.

Preparations : Tranylcypromine tablets, B.P.

Drugs For Further Study

Tricyclic Antidepressants

1) Doxepin - Doxin®, Spectra®
2) Trimipramine - Surmontil®
3) Dothiepin - Doreme®, Dothip®, Exodep®
4) Clomipramine - Anafranil®, Clofranil®, Clomidac®
5) Nitroxazepine - Sintamil®
6) Amoxapine - Demolox®

Tetracyclic Antidepressants

7) Mianserin - Depnon®, Seridac®
8) Mirtazapine - Mirazep®, Mirnite®, Mirt®, Mirtaz®

MAO Inhibitors

9) Moclobemide - Morex®, Rimarex®

Selective Serotonin Reuptake Inhibitors (SSRIs)

10) Fluoxetine - Fludac®, Fluxal®, Prodac®, Pronil®
11) Sertraline - Daxid®, Serenata®, Serlift®
12) Venlafaxine - Flavix®, Venla®, Venlift®, Vexor®
13) Citalopram - Celica®, Citalop®, Citara®, Feliz®
14) Escitalopram - Articalm®, Citalop-S®, Feliz-S®
15) Paroxetine - Panex®, Pari®, Raxit®, Xet®
16) Reboxetine - Narebox®, Reboxxin®
17) Fluvoxamine - Fluvoxin®, Sorest®, Voxamin®
18) Duloxetine - Delok®

Miscellaneous

19) Trazodone - Tazodac®, Trazalon®, Trazonil®
20) Tianeptine - Stablon®

Exercise

Q1. Define and classify 'Antidepressants'. Give structure and chemical name of imipramine hydrochloride. (Summer 06)

Q2. Explain 'Depression' with suitable example. (May-June 04)

Q3. What are antidepressants? Discuss desirable properties of antidepressant drugs. Classify them and write structure of atleast three drugs from same class. (May 07)

14 Analeptics

Analeptics are agents used to reduce narcosis brought about by excess of depressant drugs. These drugs often stimulate a variety of other centers as well. Many analeptic drugs are also pressor drugs because of their action of stimulation of the vasomotor center. Stimulation of emetic centre, also located in medulla, also gets affected by some of these drugs. Their action as central stimulant also results in decrease in appetite and gives an 'anorexigenic effect'. These drugs are, therefore, used - although not rightfully - to reduce appetite and thereby control obesity. Analeptic drugs have variety of actions such as cortical stimulants (theophylline, caffeine, dextroamphetamine), medullary stimulants (coramine), spinal stimulants (strychnine), central stimulants (nicotine) and respiratory stimulants (picrotoxin, nikethamide, caffeine).

Some of the important drugs in this class are as follows -

1) Nikethamide

N,N-Diethylnicotinamide

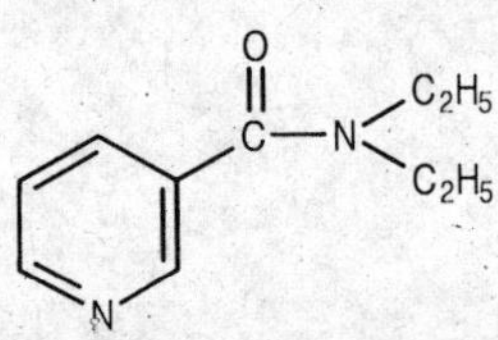

Properties : Nikethamide occurs as a colourless or slightly yellow oily liquid. Freezing point is about 23-25°C or crystalline mass. It has a slight characteristic odour and a slightly bitter, burning taste. It is miscible with water, alcohol and ether.

Actions and uses : Nikethamide is a respiratory stimulant. It has an intermediate central stimulatory effect. Often it is used as an emergency drug for patients in coma or in the state of shock. However, its narrow margin between the analeptic and convulsant dose makes it questionable in the treatment of coma.

Dose : Usual dose is IM or IV 1.25 gm, repeated as needed at 5 minute interval.

Preparations : Nikethamide injection I.P., B.P.

2) Dextroamphetamine phosphate

(Dexamphetamine phosphate)

(+)-α-methylphenethylamine dihydrogen phosphate

Properties : Dextroamphetamine is used as phosphate and sulphate salts. They occur as white, odourless, crystalline powders with a bitter taste. They are soluble in water and slightly soluble in alcohol.

Incompatibility : The salts are incompatible with alkalies and with calcium salts.

Actions and uses : It is a potent central stimulant and is, therefore, used as analeptic in reversing the profound central depression due to anesthetic, narcotic and hypnotic drugs. Narcoleptic patients show considerable relief from attacks of sleep and cataplexy is often improved by this drug. It also has anorexigenic effect and sometimes it is used as adjunct to dietary control in the management of obesity. The drug is also used - although not correctly - to overcome fatigue and as "pep-pills" especially by students during examinations. Although this is a kind of drug abuse, it does not lead to 'true addiction'. Tolerance of larger doses is reported, with without increased effect, and habituation does occur.

Dose : Orally 5 mg, three times a day, IM and IV products also available with same dose.

Preparations : Amphetamine sulphate tablets B.P.

3) Caffeine

1,3,7-Trimethylxanthine

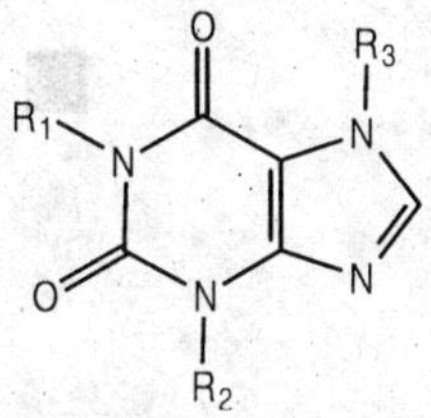

	R_1	R_2	R_3
Caffeine	CH_3	CH_3	CH_3
Theophylline	CH_3	CH_3	H
Theobromine	H	CH_3	CH_3

Properties : Caffeine is a very weak base and does not form salts. It is a white powder with glistening crystals and has a bitter taste. It is soluble in water (1:50) and in hot water (1:60). A cup of coffee or tea contains about 60 mg caffeine.

Stability : Caffeine is a very weak base and is decomposed by strong solutions of caustic alkalies. Its salts are decomposed by water.

Storage : It should be stored in airtight containers.

Actions and uses : The physiologic action of caffeine, theophylline and theobromine are almost alike. The primary effect is a stimulation of CNS. There is also a direct stimulation of all muscles, partly due to central effect and partly due to peripheral effect. It causes diuretic action and vasodilation by direct action on peripheral vessels. The dominant effect on the psychic centre, causes increased flow of thoughts, lessens drowsiness, relieves mental fatigue and headache. All this results in a sense of comfort and well-being, although impairment of these qualities do take place after sometime.

Caffeine is often used in headaches of certain kind like neuralgia, rheumatism, migraine and due to fatigue. For such purposes, it is often given in combination with phenacetin or aspirin or other analgesics. One such example of a popular formulation is 'Anacin®'. Large doses of caffeine, however cause insomnia, restlessness, excitement, mild delirium, tachycardia and diuresis.

Dose : 100 to 300 mg

Preparations : Aspirin and Caffeine tablets, B.P.

Caffeine iodide elixir, B.P.C.

Brand Names (with a combination) : Coldact Plus®, Coldoff®, Dristan®, Novacold®, Nescold®, Paramol-C®, Sinarest®, Snizof®

4) Theophylline

1,3-Dimethylxanthine

Properties : Theophylline occurs as an odourless, white, crystalline powder with a bitter taste. It is slightly soluble in water; sparingly soluble in alcohol; soluble in solutions of alkali hydroxides. It is a weak base and forms salts with acids and soluble derivatives with alkali metals. It combines with ethylene diamine to give the compound aminophylline.

Incompatibility : It is incompatible with tannins. Aminophylline is incompatible with acids with lactose and other sugars.

Actions and uses : Theophylline has actions resembling those of caffeine and theobromine. It is a more powerful relaxant of bronchial smooth muscle. Its soluble derivatives such as aminophylline are used in the treatment of bronchial asthma.

Dose : 60 to 200 mg, 3 to 4 times a day.

Preparations : Aminophylline injection, I.P., B.P.

Aminophylline tablets, I.P.

Mersalyl injection, B.P.

Brand Names :

Theophylline - Broncordil®, Deriphyllin®, Etosalbetol®, Duralyn-CR®, Phylobid®, Theobid®

Aminophylline - Aminophylline® (GSK), Minophyl®

Exercise

Q1. Name the central nervous system stimulant each among the following category. Give the structure of any one of them - i) An amide & ii) A xanthine derivative. (Kachchh Univ. 06, May 05)

Q2. Write the structure and chemical name of Caffeine. (Karnataka Univ., Winter 04, Winter 06)

Q3. Write the structure of - 1,3,7- Trimethyl xanthine. (Summer 03)

Q4. Write the uses of nikethamide. (Summer 03)

Q5. Define 'analeptics'. Write structure, chemical name and uses of coramine. (Summer 06, Winter 04)

■

15 Adrenergic Drugs

The autonomic nervous system is made up of two parts, adrenergic and cholinergic. In adrenergic system, noradrenaline is the neurotransmitter released at the postganglionic synapse.

Adrenergic receptors are of two main types α and β. Effects mediated by α-receptors include vasoconstriction of peripheral arterioles, dilation of pupils, inhibition of motility of stomach, intestine and bladder and liberation of glucose from liver. Important α-agonists are metaraminol, noradrenaline and phenylephrine, α-blockers include tolazoline and phentolamine. Effects mediated by β-receptors are increase of heart rate and force of myocardial contraction and relaxation of uterine and bronchial muscles. Important β-agonists are isoprenaline and orciprenaline. The β-blockers include propranolol and practolol.

Adrenergic Agonists

The adrenergic or sympathomimetic drugs are agents that mimic the responses obtained as a result of stimulation of the sympathetic or adrenergic nerve. (Fig. 15.1)

Majority of these substances contain an intact or a partially substituted amino ($-NH_2$) group. The adrenergic agonists increase the activity of the sympathetic system and are also called as 'sympathomimetic amines'.

Structural Relationship of Adrenergic Drugs

Most of the drugs in this class can be divided into two broad groups.

a) Compounds with OH substitution in 3 and 4 position of phenyl ring termed as catecholamines.

b) Those compounds which lack the hydroxyl groups known as non-catecholamines.

The basic structural moiety to which all these drugs can be related is called phenyl ethyl amine. When the phenyl ring is substituted by -OH groups at 3 and 4 positions, it is called 'catechol'. Thus, in figure 15.2 the basic phenyl ethyl amine moiety is shown with its relationship to the major adrenergic drugs.

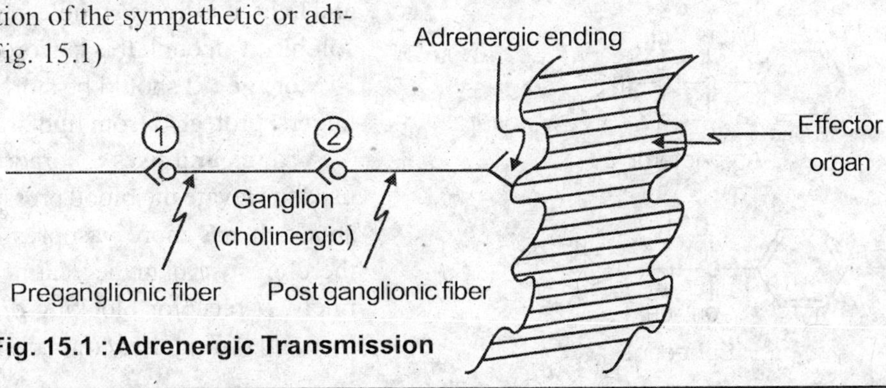

Fig. 15.1 : Adrenergic Transmission

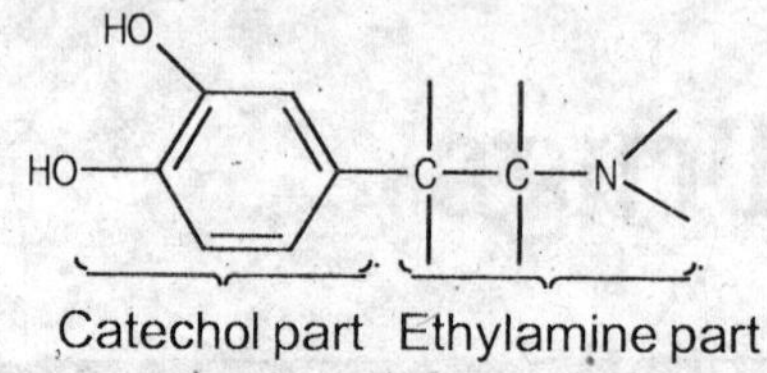

Fig 15.2

a) Catechol Amines

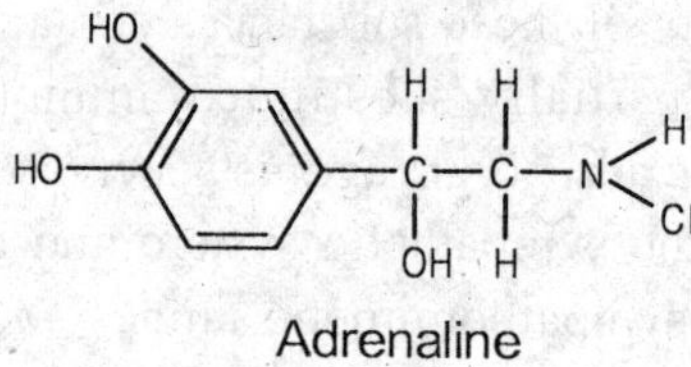

Adrenaline

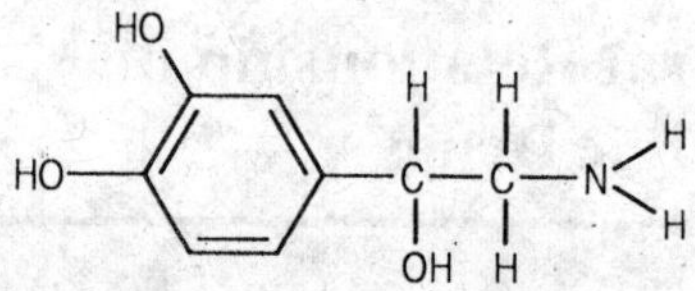

Noradrenaline

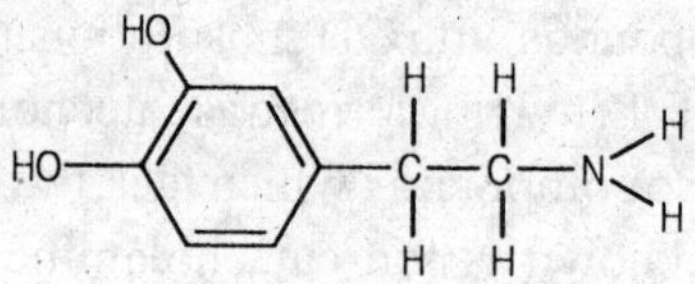

Dopamine

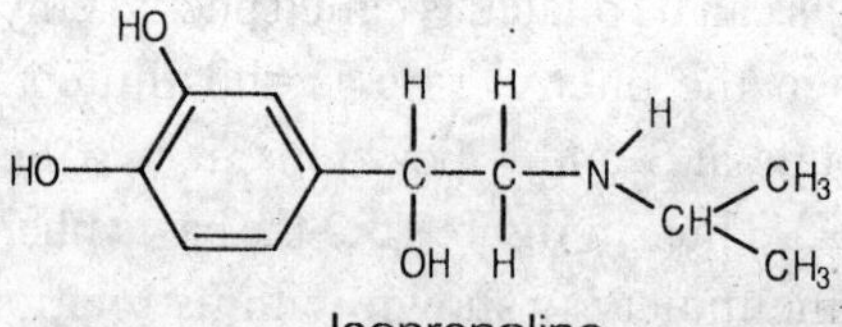

Isoprenaline

b) Non-catechol amines

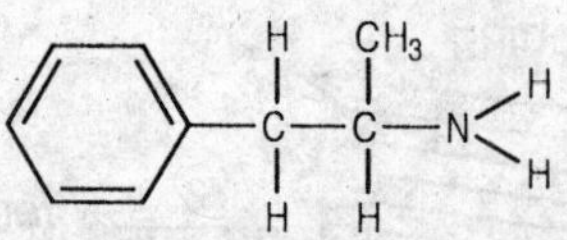

Amphetamine

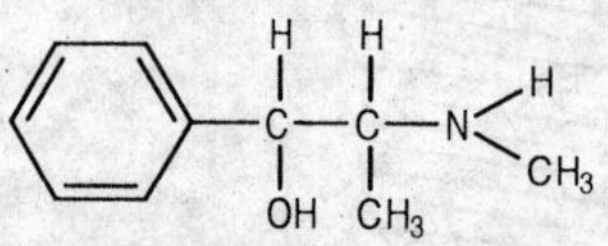

Ephedrine

Classification of Adrenergic Drugs

From the therapeutic point of view these drugs can be classified as follows,

I] Adrenergic drugs used to raise blood pressure (vasoconstrictive) - noradrenaline (norepinephrine).

II] Those drugs used for their inotropic actions on the heart - dopamine, isoprenaline.

III] Those used as central stimulant (CNS stimulant) - amphetamine.

IV] Those used as smooth muscle relaxants - adrenaline, isoprenaline or selective β_2 stimulants like salbutamol.

V] Those used in allergic reactions - ephedrine.

VI] Those used for local vasoconstrictor effect like nasal decongestion effect - phenylephrine, naphazoline, pseudoephedrine.

VII] Those used for suppressing appetite (anorexigenic effect) - amphetamine, phentermine.

I] Adrenergic drugs used to raise blood pressure

1) Noradrenaline

(-)3,4-Dihydroxy-α-(amino methyl) benzyl alcohol

Properties : Noradrenaline is official in I.P. as the acid tartrate salt. This compound occurs as an odourless, white crystalline powder with a bitter taste. It slowly darkens on exposure to air and light. It is freely soluble in water and slightly soluble in alcohol. It is laevorotatory.

Storage : It should be stored in airtight containers, protected from light.

Actions and uses : Noradrenaline is mainly used to elevate the blood pressure of a patient in shock. It has more vasopressor action and is, therefore, useful in the treatment of shock. Routinely, α-receptor blocking drugs are used before and during the removal of pheochromocytoma. If there is a fall in blood pressure after the removal of tumor, noradrenaline is considered to be useful.

Dose : 8 mcg per minute, IV infusion.

Preparations : Noradrenaline injection, B.P.C.

Sterile strong noradrenaline solution, B.P.C.

Noradrenaline bitartrate, I.P.

Brand Names : Adrenor® inj., Norad®, Nordren®, Vescue®

2) Adrenaline (Epinephrine)

(-)3, 4-Dihydroxy-α [(methylamino) methyl] benzyl alcohol.

Adrenaline is official in I.P. as the free base and as bitartrate salt.

Properties : Adrenaline occurs as a white or creamy white, crystalline, odourless powder. It is very slightly soluble in water; practically insoluble in alcohol and ether. It is readily soluble in solutions of mineral acids and of alkali hydroxides. It is laevorotatory. Adrenaline acid tartrate is freely soluble in water.

Stability : Adrenaline and its salt darken slowly on exposure to air and light. Degradation reactions in aqueous solutions include racemisation and conversion to adrenochrome. These reactions are catalysed by hydrogen ions and hydroxide ions. Solutions are most stable at pH 3.2 to 3.6.

Incompatibility : Adrenaline and its salt are incompatible with oxidising agents, alkalis, copper, iron and other metals, gum, tannin and sodium metabisulphite.

Storage : It should be stored in airtight containers, preferably in an atmosphere of nitrogen, protected from light.

Actions and uses : Adrenaline is important historically as the first hormone to be isolated and first to be synthesised. In the body it is biosynthesised from the amino acid, phenylalanine, phenylalamine is hydroxylated to produce tyrosine and then dopa, which is then decarboxylated to give dopamine. This dopamine is then hydroxylated at the β-carbon to give noradrenaline. Initially adrenaline was isolated from the medulla of the adrenal glands of animals and, therefore, the name adrenaline.

The synthetic adrenaline is a racemic mixture of *l* and *d* form. Natural *l* -form is nearly 15 times more active than the racemic mixture. As a free amine, it is available in oil solution for IM injections. Adrenaline is destroyed readily by alkaline solutions weak oxidising agents and oxygen from air.

Adrenaline is used to raise the blood pressure and to accelerate the heart rate. It is used as an emergency drug to relax bronchial muscles in an asthmatic attack and in anaphylactic reactions. It is given intravenously to treat acute circulatory collapse. However, adrenaline has following disadvantages like, it is not active orally, it has short duration of action, it decomposes very readily, its vasoconstrictive action is frequently followed by vasodilation.

Dose : 200-500 mcg IM and 100-250 mcg IV.

Preparations : Neutral adrenaline eye drops, B.P.C

Adrenaline tartrate injection, I.P., B.P.

Compound adrenaline and atropine spray, B.P.C.

Brand Names : Adrenaline tartrate® (P&B), Xylocaine® inj. with Adrenaline, Medicreme® cream, Vasocon®, Brovon® inhalant

II] Antiasthmatic drugs

1) Isoprenaline

(Isoproterenol, Isopropylarterenol)

3,4-Dihydroxy-α-[(isopropyl amino) methyl] - benzyl alcohol hydrochloride

Properties : Isoprenaline is a white, odourless, slightly bitter, crystalline powder. Its salts are soluble in water (1:3) and alcohol (1:50). A 1 per cent solution in water is slightly acidic (pH 4.5 to 5.5). It is official in I.P. as hydrochloride and sulphate salts.

Stability : It gradually darkens on exposure to air and light. Solutions should contain an antioxidant such as sodium metabisulphite. Contact with metals should be avoided as it causes discolouration and loss of activity.

Storage : It should be stored in airtight containers, protected from light.

Actions and uses : Many of the actions of isoprenaline are similar to adrenaline and noradrenaline.

a) It is used in the treatment of acute attack of bronchial asthma. It sometimes works better than adrenaline and theophylline combination in some patients.

b) In Stokes-Adams syndrome, it is preferred to adrenaline because it produces less cardiac arrhythmias.

c) Isoprenaline is sometimes advocated as cardiac stimulant in the treatment of shock. However, the use of this drug must be carefully supervised. The drug should not be given parenterally, because of its stimulation of the heart muscle. It should not be given along with adrenaline, but may be alternated with it.

Dose : IM or SC 200 mcg. Oral inhalation 125-750 mg as a 0.25 to 1 per cent solution.

Preparations : Isoprenaline hydrochloride injection, I.P., B.P.

Isoprenaline tablets, I.P., B.P.

Isoprenaline aerosol inhalation, B.P.C.

Brand Names : Autohaler®, Isolin®, Isoprin®

2) Salbutamol

2-(Tert-Butylamino)-1-(4-hydroxy-3 -hydroxy methyl phenyl) ethanol

Properties : Salbutamol sulphate occurs as an odourless white powder with a slightly bitter taste. It is freely soluble in water, soluble in alcohol and ether.

Storage : It should be protected from light.

Actions and uses : Salbutamol is chemically related to isoprenaline. It has a prominent β-2 receptor action, i.e., bronchodilator action, but poor cardiac stimulant action (β_1). Therefore it is less likely to produce palpitation or rise in blood pressure at therapeutic dose.

It is more effective by inhalation (dose 100 mcg) than orally (dose 2-4 mg). It can also be given by IM or IV injection (dose 0.5 mg every 4 hours). Because of its poor cardiac stimulant action, it is far safer drug than adrenaline or isoprenaline. Therefore, it is a preferred drug in the treatment of asthma. It is a drug of choice in acute precipitation of asthma. It is also useful in the prevention of bronchospasm, precipitated by exercise or other stimuli. Some of its side reactions are tremors, especially of hands. Surprisingly, the drug does not develop clinically significant tolerance to bronchodilator effects, even after regular and continued use by the asthma patients.

Dose : By inhalation 100 mcg by mouth.

Oral dose : 2-4 mg, 2 to 3 times a day.

Preparations : Salbutamol tablets, I.P., B.P.

Salbutamol inhaler, I.P.

Salbutamol injection, I.P.

Salbutamol syrup, I.P.

Salbutamol aerosol inhalation, B.P.C.

Brand Names : Asthalin®, Salbutol®, Salbetol®, Salmodil® syrup, Salbid®

3) Terbutaline sulphate

1-(3,5-Dihydroxyphenyl)-2-tertiary butyl-aminoethanol sulphate.

Properties : It occurs as a white to greyish-white crystalline powder. It is odourless and has a bitter taste. It is freely soluble in water, very slightly soluble in alcohol.

Actions and uses : This drug was introduced with the implication that it acts preferentially at β-2 receptor site, making it useful in the treatment of bronchial asthma and related conditions. However, the common cardiovascular effects that are common with other adrenergic drugs are also seen in the use of terbutaline sulphate.

Dose : Oral - 5 mg, three times a day.

Preparations : Terbutaline injection, I.P.

Terbutaline tablets, I.P.

Brand Names : Bricanyl® inhaler, Bliskof® syrup, Bricarex® expectorant, Terpect®

V] Drugs used in allergic reactions

1) Ephedrine

(-) Erythro-2-methylamino-1-phenylpropanol

Ephedrine is an alkaloid obtained from the stems of various species of Ephedra. The drug 'ma huang', containing ephedrine was known to Chinese in 2000 B.C. The active principle, epherine was isolated in 1885, and was synthesised in 1920.

Properties : Ephedrine has two asymmetric carbon atoms and thus, there are 4 optically active forms. The erythro racemate is called ephedrine and the threo racemate is known as pseudoephedrine. Natural ephedrine is D(-) and is the most active of the 4 isomers as a pressor amine. Ephedrine alkaloid occurs as a waxy solid and as crystals or granules and has a characteristic pronounced odour. It is unstable in light and decomposes gradually and darkens. It is soluble in alcohol and water (5 per cent) and in organic solvents. The free alkaloid is a strong base and an aqueous solution has a pH of 10. The salt form has a pKa of 9.6.

Storage : It should be stored in airtight containers, protected from light.

Actions and uses : Therapeutic uses of ephedrine are,

1) In acute and chronic attack of asthma.

2) Relief from nasal decongestion.

3) Prevention and treatment of hypotension.

4) In Stokes-Adams syndrome (although isoprenaline is preferred drug).

5) Ephedrine eye drops are employed to produce mydriasis without cycloplegia.

6) In narcolepsy because of its central effect (but amphetamine is the preferred drug).

7) Other uses include prevention of nocturnal enuresis (passing urine at night), relief from whopping cough.

Dose : Oral - 50 to 300 mg a day.

Preparations : Ephedrine tablets, I.P., B.P.

Ephedrine elixir, B.P.C.

Paediatric belladonna and ephedrine mixture, B.P.C.

Brand Names : Efipress® amp., Sulfidrin® inj.

VI] Drugs used for local vasoconstrictor effect

1) Phenylephrine hydrochloride

3-Hydroxy-α(methyl aminomethyl) benzyl alcohol

Properties : It is a white, odourless, crystalline, slightly bitter powder. It is freely soluble in water and alcohol. It is relatively stable in alkaline solution and can withstand heat sterilisation.

Stability : In aqueous solution, it is gradually oxidised with the formation of coloured products. Discolouration is retarded by sodium metabisulphite and disodium edetate.

Storage : It should be stored in airtight containers, protected from light.

Actions and uses : It is twice as longer acting than adrenaline. It is a vasoconstrictor and is orally active. Its main use is in the relief of nasal congestion. It is also used as mydriatic agent and also to prolong the action of local anesthetics and to prevent a drop in blood pressure during spinal anesthesia.

Dose : 5 mg by SC or IM injection.

Preparations : Phenylephrine injection, I.P., B.P.

Phenylephrine eye-drops, B.P.C.

Brand Names : Drosyn® eye drops, Penrex® drops, Cool® eye drops, Ocurest® eye drops, Fenox® nasal drops, Tuspress®

2) Pseudoephedrine hydrochloride

(+)-Threo- α-[1-(methylamino)ethyl] benzyl alcohol

Properties : As mentioned above, pseudoephedrine is a threo racemate of ephedrine. It is a white crystalline powder, soluble in water, alcohol and chloroform.

Actions and uses : Like ephedrine, this racemate is also used as bronchodilator, but is much less active in increasing blood pressure. This makes it a little safer to formulate in cough mixture, along with antihistamines. However, it should be used with caution in hypertensive patients.

Dose : 30 - 60 mg three times a day.

Preparations : Pseudoephedrine tablets, I.P.

Pseudoephedrine syrup, I.P.

Brand Names : Alerfri®, Allkof® suspension, Amodex® syrup, Nasoryl®, Recofast®, Sinarest-AF®

Adrenergic Antagonists

The actions produced by stimulation of the adrenergic (sympathetic) nervous system, can be blocked peripherally by drugs called as 'Adrenergic Antagonists'.

Classification of drugs reducing adrenergic activity

I] Drugs that induce depletion of catecholamines from various body tissues, eg. reserpine.

II] Drugs that interfere with the synthesis of adrenergic transmitters (norepinephrine, dopamine) either in the adrenergic neuron or in adrenal medulla eg. α-methyl-p-tyrosine.

III] Drugs that interfere with the transmission of impulses across postganglionic adrenergic ending eg. blocking agents like guanethidine.

IV] Drugs which block the adrenergic receptors,

a) α-receptor blockers - dibenamine, phenoxybenzamine, tolazoline, phentolamine and

b) α-receptor blockers - propranolol, atenolol, metoprolol, practolol. This is the class of adrenergic antagonists. Only three drugs, representative of this class, will be considered here.

Drugs which block the adrenergic receptors :

a) α-receptor blockers

1) Tolazoline hydrochloride

2-Benzyl-2-imidazoline hydrochloride

Properties : This drug is a typical α-adrenergic blocking agent, belonging to the imidazole chemical class. The drug occurs as a white or off-white, bitter, crystalline powder with a slight aromatic odour. It is freely soluble in water or alcohol.

Storage : It should be stored in airtight containers, protected from light.

Actions and uses : The drug has the ability to block circulating adrenaline, it also blocks sympathetic nerve activity. In addition, it also has histamine-like activity which gives it a vasodilating property. For this reason, it finds its chief use in the treatment of peripheral vascular diseases. Tolazoline, because of its predominant cardiac effect, often evokes a mild rise in blood pressure. The salivary, lacrimal, respiratory and pancreatic secretions are also augmented. The compound also exerts a mild anti-serotonin activity.

Dose : Oral 25 to 75 mg. Injection, 25 mg per ml.

Dose 50 mg , 2 to 4 times a day SC or IM

Preparations : Tolazoline tablets, B.P.

b) β-receptor blockers

1) Propranolol hydrochloride

1-(Isopropylamino)-3(-1-naphthoxy)2-propanol hydrochloride

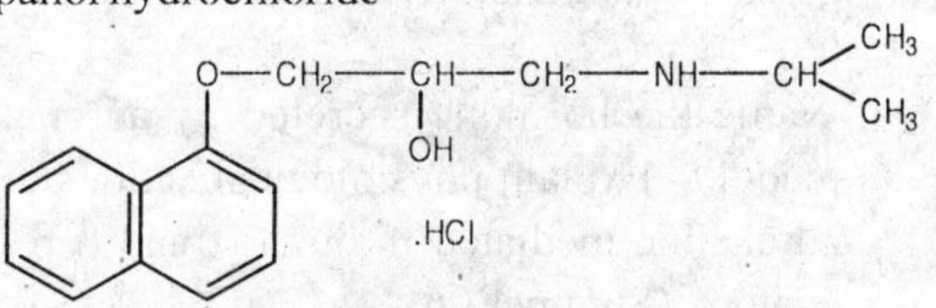

Properties : It occurs as an odourless white powder with a bitter taste. It is soluble in water and alcohol.

Stability : It is affected by light. Oxidation occurs in aqueous solution and causes discolouration. Solutions are most stable at pH 3 and decompose rapidly when alkaline.

Storage : It should be protected from light.

Actions and uses : Propranolol is a typical β-adrenergic blocking agent. There are a variety of β-blockers. Briefly they are (i) specific β - blockers eg. Timolol. (ii) α-blockers with membrane stabilising activity and sympathomimetic activity eg. Oxprenolol, pindolol (iii) β-blockers with only membrane stabilising activity e.g. Propranolol (iv) β-blockers with cardio selective activity eg. Atenolol (v) β-blockers with additional α blocking property eg. Labetalol.

Propranolol has only membrane stabilising effect. But its therapeutic uses are like other β-blockers. It is useful in (a) Angina pectoris (b) Coronary atherosclerosis (c) Cardiac arrhythmias (d) Hypertension (e) Thyrotoxicosis. But it is contraindicated (i.e. not to be used) in bronchial asthma, allergic rhinitis during change of season, sinus, bradycardia, right ventricular failure, patients on CNS stimulant drugs like MAO inhibitors.

Brand Names : Ciplar®, Corbeta®, Betacap TR®, Inderal®

2) Practolol

4'-(2-Hydroxy-3-isopropylaminopropoxy) acetanilide

Properties : Practolol occurs as an odourless, fine white powder with a bitter taste. It is slightly soluble in water and sparingly soluble in alcohol. Aqueous solutions are most stable at pH 6.

Storage : It should be protected from light.

Actions and use : Practolol is another β-blocker and has similar actions as that of propranolol. Practolol is largely excreted unchanged by kidneys while atenolol and acebutolol are excreted by both the routes (liver and kidney). Because of this the relative bioavailability of practolol is better and variations in plasma levels are much less. The plasma half-life of β-blockers which are metabolised mostly by liver (like propranolol) is short (2-3 hours), whereas that of drugs like practolol, which are mainly excreted unchanged by kidneys is longer (8-12 hours). However, plasma half-life does not cor-

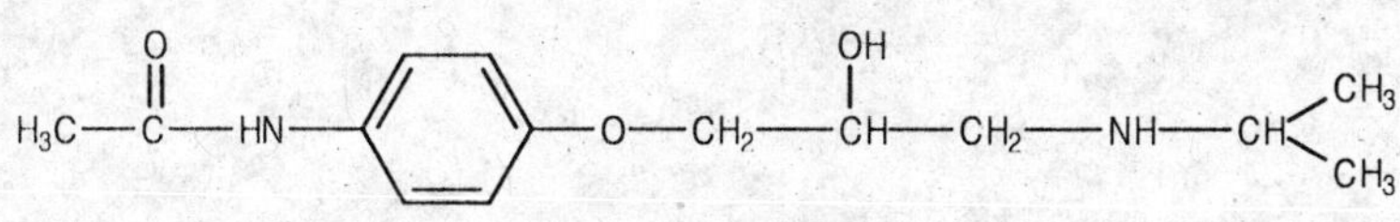

Practolol

relate well with the therapeutic effects, which are relatively long lasting.

Dose : 5 to 20 mg, intravenous injection.

Preparations : Practolol injection, B.P.

Drugs For Further Study

Adrenergic agonists

1) Bambuterol - Abel®, Bambudil®, Bemlo®, Roburol®
2) Orciprenaline - Alupent®
3) Clonidine - Arkamin®, Catapres®, Clothalton®

Adrenergic antagonists - α-blockers

4) Prazosin - Cyber-CR®, Minipress®, XLGITS®, Prazopress®
5) Terazosin - Hytrin®, Teradip®, Terapress®, Teraz®
6) Doxazosin - Alfazosin®, Doxacard®, Duracard®
7) Phenoxybenzomine - Fenoxene®

Adrenergic antagonists - β-blockers

8) Metroprolol - Betaloc®, Lopresor®, Metolar®
9) Atenolol - Altol®, Atecard®, Aten®, Atenova®
10) Pindolol - Visken®
11) Oxprenolol - Trasicor®
12) Bisoprolol - Biselect®, Bisocar®, Concor®
13) Celiprolol - Celipres®
14) Nebivolol - Nebicard®, Nebistar®, Nodon®

Adrenergic antagonists - α & β blockers

15) Labetolol - Lobet®, Normadate®
16) Carvedilol - Carca®, Cardivas®, Carloc®

Also see Cardiovascular Drugs.

Exercise

Q1. What do you know of adrenergic drugs? What are their therapeutic uses? Give an account with suitable examples. (Kachchh Univ. 06, May 05, Nov 06)

Q2. Write a short note on adrenergic blocking agents. (Kachchh Univ. 06, May 05)

Q3. In what dosage form the following drug is given - Salbutanol. (Summer 03, Summer 06)

Q4. Name the hormone secreted by adrenal medulla. Explain physiological actions of adrenaline mediated through α and β receptors. (Summer 06)

Q5. What are adrenergic agents? Classify them with suitable example. Give structural formula of - i) Ephedrine, ii) Propanolol, iii) Adrenaline. (May-June 04, Winter 04, Summer 03, Summer 06)

Q6. Write pharmacological action of adrenalin, what are adrenergic agents, classify them with example. (May 07)

Q7. Write note on β-adrenergic blocking agents. (May 07)

16 Cholinergic Drugs

The autonomic nervous system is composed of two parts, namely, the sympathetic and the parasympathetic. Out of these two, sympathetic nervous system has already been discussed under the chapter of 'Adrenergic Drugs'. (Chapter 15)

Acetylcholine mediates (regulates) the transmission of nerve impulses in the ganglia of the sympathetic system and in both the preganglionic and postganglionic fibres, i.e. at the ganglia and the neuromuscular junctions in the parasympathetic system. (Fig. 16.1)

Acetylcholine acts on muscarinic and nicotinic receptors. Muscarinic stimulation leads to cardiac inhibition, peripheral vasodilation, miosis, increased salivation and other secretions, increased motility of gastrointestinal tract and genitourinary tract. Stimulation of nicotinic receptors cause stimulation of skeletal muscles, autonomic ganglia and adrenal medulla.

Acetycholine, like noradrenaline, is stored in vesicles, and is released at the time of nerve impulse transmission, and is also released (in greater quantities) to many emergency demands. The Acetylcholine System, is composed of

i) Acetylcholine (a neurohumoral agent).

ii) Acetylcholine esterase (an enzyme which hydrolyses excess of acetylcholine).

iii) Choline acetylase (an enzyme which resynthesises acetylcholine from choline and acetic acid, via acetylcoA).

The major sites of activity of acetylcholine are:

i) The postganglionic parasympathetic receptor (as shown in Fig. 16.1)

ii) The autonomic ganglion (See Chapter 15)

iii) Skeletal neuromuscular junction.

Cholinergic Agonists

The postganglionic fibres of parasympathetic nerve system are called 'cholinergic' and the drugs that mimic the action of acetylcholine are called 'cholinergic agonists'. It is now established

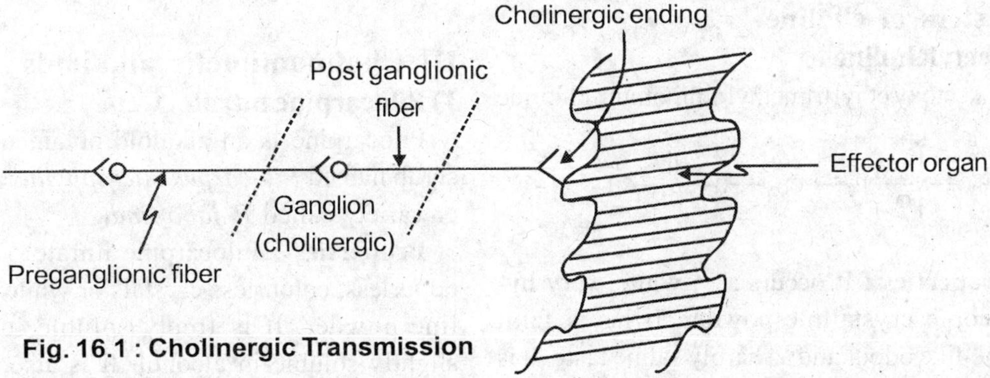

Fig. 16.1 : Cholinergic Transmission

that when a nerve impulse (coming through brain, through autonomic nervous system) reaches a certain synapse (nerve ending), the action potential in the presynaptic nerve causes the release of certain quantum of acetylcholine, which then diffuses across the synaptic gap (and fills it) to allow the impulse to pass further to the postsynaptic acetylcholine receptor and bring about the parasympathetic action. This mode of transmission is sometimes referred to as cholinergic transmission, as it brings about typical cholinergic actions.

The drugs in this class are, therefore, called cholinergic or parasympathomimetic drugs, which stimulate the effect or cells (or organs) innervated by postganglionic parasympathetic cholinergic nerves. In general, their actions are similar to those seen following the stimulation of parasympathetic nervous system.

Classification of Cholinergic Drugs

I) Esters of Choline

eg. Acetylcholine, methacholine

II) Cholinomimetic Alkaloids

eg. Pilocarpine, arecoline,

III) Cholinesterase Inhibitors

(indirectly acting cholinergic agonists)

eg. Neostigmine, insecticides

I] Esters of choline

1) Acetylcholine

2-Acetoxy ethyl trimethyl ammonium chloride

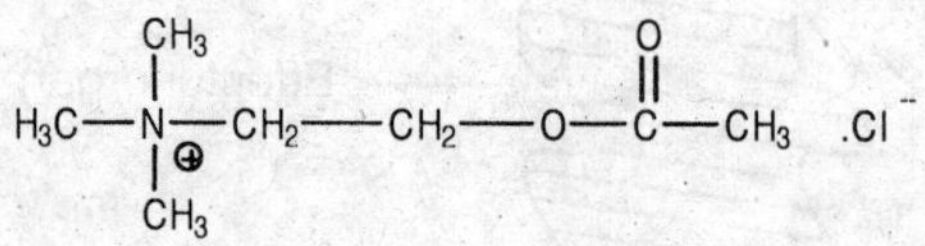

Properties : It occurs as a white, very hygroscopic crystalline powder. It has a faint amine-like odour and a sharply saline taste. It is very soluble in water and in alcohol. Aqueous solutions are unstable.

Incompatibility : It is incompatible with alkalies and acids.

Storage : It should be protected from light.

Actions and uses : The representative drug of this class, it is used as a short acting miotic in eye during cataract surgery.

2) Methacholine

2-Acetoxypropyl trimethyl ammonium chloride

Properties : Methacholine chloride occurs as odourless, deliquescent, colourless or white crystals or white crystalline powder. It is very soluble in water, freely soluble in alcohol.

Storage : It should be stored in airtight containers.

Actions and uses : Unlike acetylcholine, methacholine is stable and not readily hydrolysed by the enzyme acetylcholine esterase. This is because of its β-methyl group, which slows down the hydrolysis. It is, therefore, longer acting than acetylcholine, and gives sustained parasympathetic stimulation. It does not give nicotinic effect. It exerts a depressant action on cardiac auricular mechanisms which is blocked by quinidine, a stimulation of gastrointestinal peristalsis and a general vasodilation followed by fall in blood pressure. All these reactions are blocked or reversed by atropine.

Dose : 20 mg by SC injection.

II] Cholinomimetic alkaloids

1) Pilocarpine nitrate

Pilocarpine is an alkaloid obtained from a shrub named *Pilocarpus microphyllus* and other variety called *P. jaborandi*.

Properties : Pilocarpine nitrate occurs as odourless, colourless crystals or white crystalline powder. It is freely soluble in water; slightly soluble in alcohol. It is also used as hydrochloride. It is dextrorotatory.

Stability : Solutions of pilocarpine salts degrade by hydrolysis and epimerisation. Degradation is catalysed by hydrogen ions and hydroxide ions. Solutions are most stable at pH 4 to 5.

Incompatibility : It is incompatible with chlorhexidine acetate, phenylmercuric salts and benzalkonium chloride.

Storage : It should be protected from light.

Actions and uses : It acts by direct action (stimulation) on the effector organs and produces both cholinergic and nicotinic actions. It exerts miotic effect on eye by reducing the intraocular pressure. It produces increased sweating, salivation and gastric secretion. It also produces secretion in the respiratory tract and is, therefore, sometimes used as expectorant.

Dose : 0.5 to 4 per cent aqueous solutions are used as eye drops to treat glaucoma. It is formulated in a transdermal patch 'Ocusert' (to be worn in the eye) which releases drug for 7 days.

Preparations : Pilocarpine eye drops, B.P.

Physostigmine and pilocarpine eye-drops B.P.C.

Brand Names : Carpine® drops, Pilocar® drops, Locarp® drops

III] Cholinesterase inhibitors

1) Physostigmine

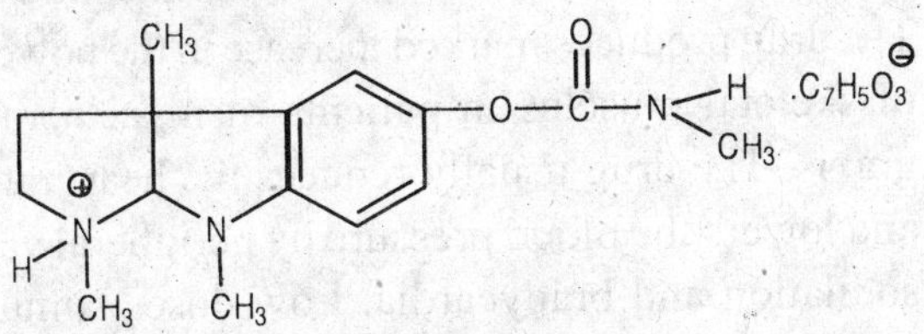

Physostigmine is an alkaloid obtained from the seeds of *Physostigma venenosum*. It is official in I.P. as the salicylate salt.

Properties : Physostigmine salicylate occurs as odourless, colourless or faintly yellow crystals. It is sparingly soluble in water; soluble in alcohol. It is laevorotatory.

Stability : The drug powder becomes pink on exposure to air and light. In aqueous solution, physostigmine is hydrolysed to eseroline, which is oxidised to coloured products. Hydrolysis is catalysed by hydrogen ions and hydroxide ions. Solutions are most stable at pH 3.7.

Storage : It should be stored in airtight containers, protected from light.

Actions and uses : This drug is among those that inhibit the action of the enzyme acetylcholine esterase, reversibly, and thus, conserve the supply of acetylcholine, and thereby bring out the cholinergic action.

The enzyme acetylcholine esterase, as mentioned earlier, hydrolyses the excess of acetylcholine liberated at the postganglionic synapse (junction). It has the following features -

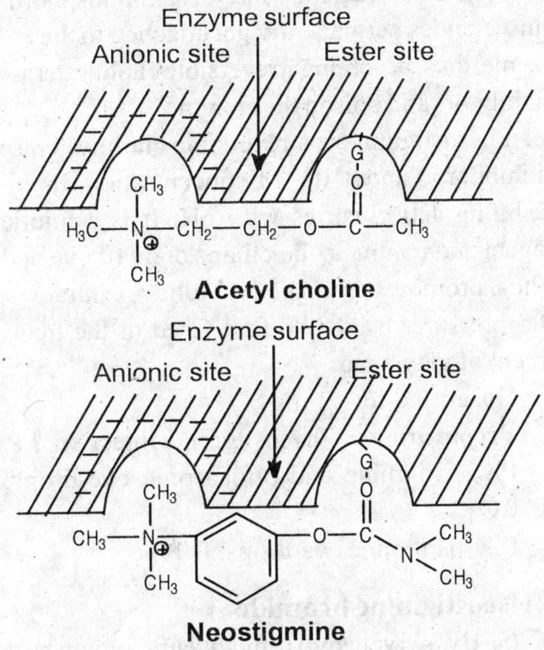

Fig. 16.2 : Interaction of drugs with acetylcholinesterase

i) It has two active sites namely the anionic site and ester site, separated by two methylene

($-CH_2-CH_2-$) groups. The distance between the two active sites is about 7A°.

ii) The positively charged nitrogen and its three methyl groups fit into the anionic site which is largely negatively charged. The acetyl group is attached to the ester site, through a linkage group -G .

iii) Any drug which has a similar spatial arrangement of groups, closer to acetylcholine, will also occupy the same position on the enzyme surface and will thus, compete with the natural acetylcholine liberated at the junction. Neostigmine, whose structure fits into the enzyme sites (as shown in the fig. 16.2), thus, can compete with the natural acetylcholine. The drug neostigmine therefore, becomes a reversible cholinesterase inhibitor and in a way saves or conserves the natural acetylcholine. The drug thus, becomes a cholinergic agent. But some other chemical agents, like organophosphorus insecticides permanently get attached to the enzyme, thus, becoming irreversible cholinesterase inhibitors and poison the enzyme.

Physostigmine is a reversible cholinesterase inhibitor at about 10^{-6} M concentration. Its inhibiting action varies with pH. It is a miotic agent and contracts the ciliary body of eye and thus, promotes drainage and relieves intraocular pressure. It is, therefore, used in the treatment of glaucoma.

Dose : 0.6 to 1.2 mg

Preparations : Physostigmine injection, I.P.

Physostigmine and pilocarpine eye-drops, B.P.C.

Physostigmine eye-drops, B.P.

2) Neostigmine bromide

(*m*-Hydroxyphenyl) trimethylammonium bromide dimethylcarbamate

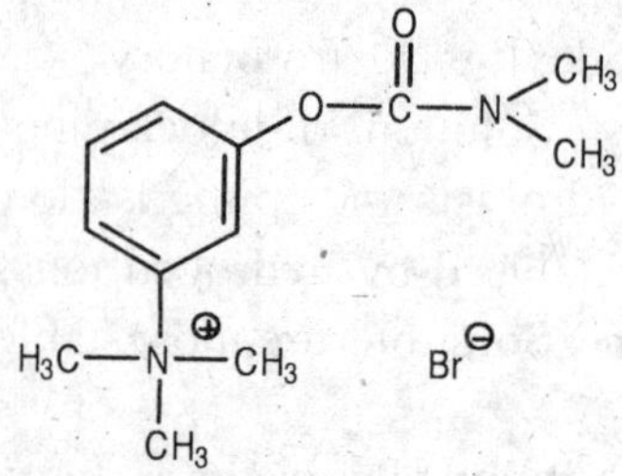

It is official in I.P. as bromide and methylsulphate salts.

Properties : Neostigmine bromide occurs as odourless, colourless crystals or white crystalline powder. It is very soluble in water, freely soluble in alcohol.

Storage : It should be stored in airtight containers, protected from light.

Actions and uses : The structure of physostigmine was modified and the first drug developed was neostigmine. The trimethylamino group was placed meta to dimethyl carbamate group in phenyl ring to obtain neostigmine. A better stability was obtained by this modification and neostigmine was found to be more resistant to hydrolysis.

Neostigmine has action similar to physostigmine. It inhibits cholinesterase at 10^{-6} M concentration. But unlike physostigmine, its activity is independent of pH.

The uses of neostigmine are similar to those of physostigmine. However, its miotic activity is better than that of physostigmine. It finds an important use in the treatment of myasthenia gravis. The drug produces marked increase in the power of skeletal muscles in patients of myasthenia gravis. The drug usually reduces the heart rate and lowers the blood pressure by peripheral vasodilation and bradycardia. Low doses stimulate autonomic ganglia, while large doses block them. Like other cholinergic drugs, it increases various secretions. It produces bronchoconstriction and increased uteral peristalsis.

Dose : 15-30 mg

Preparations : Neostigmine bromide tablets I.P., B.P.

Neostigmine injection I.P., B.P. - contains neostigmine methylsulphate

Brand Names : Myo-pyrolate®, Tilstigmin®, Prostigmin®

3) Pyridostigmine Bromide

3-Hydroxy-1-methylpyridinium bromide dimethylcarbamate

Properties : It occurs as a white deliquescent crystalline powder. It has an agreeable characteristic odour and a bitter taste. It is very soluble in water, alcohol and chloroform.

Storage : It should be stored in airtight containers, protected from light.

Actions and uses : Pyridostigmine is more toxic than neostigmine. Its activity is similar to neostigmine. The drug is used in myasthenia gravis. It has a longer duration of action and has less muscarinic effect on gastrointestinal tract. It is better tolerated by myasthenic patients. However, the drug is less potent than neostigmine. Slow release tablets have duration of 4-10 hours.

Dose : 60 to 240 mg.

Preparations : Pyridostigmine injection, I.P. Pyridostigmine tablets, I.P.

Brand Names : Distinon®, Gravitor®, Myestin®

Antidote for cholinesterase inhibitors : Pralidoxime chloride

2-Pyridine aldoxime methyl chloride (2-PAM)

Properties : It occurs as an odourless, white to pale yellow, crystalline powder. It is freely soluble in water, sparingly soluble in alcohol.

Actions and uses : Pralidoxime is a drug which is used as an antidote for the treatment of poisoning due to parathion and related insecticides. It is also an antagonist for neostigmine and pyridostigmine. In addition, it affects depolarisation at the neuromuscular junction. It is anticholinergic, cholinomimetic and it regenerates cholinesterase. It is effective upto 2 hours, and a concentration of 8 mcg/ml in blood effectively reduces poisoning due to parathion and other organophosphorus insecticides. But it has to be given within 2 hours of poisoning.

Dose : 1 to 2 gm by IM or IV injection.

Brand Names : 2-PAM-I® inj., Aldopam® inj., Clopam® inj., Neopam®, Unipam®

Cholinergic Antagonists

The cholinergic antagonists or the parasympatholytic drugs include atropine and its congeners, synthetic and semisynthetic atropine substitutes, synthetic compounds of aminoalcohols, their esters, ethers, carbamates and amino amides. The main therapeutic actions of this group of drugs are:

i) Dilation of pupil, mydriasis.

ii) Antispasmodic action - to reduce spasms.

iii) Antisecretory action - to dry up secretions.

iv) Bronchodilator action.

v) CNS depressant action.

vi) As preanesthetic medication.

Some of the drugs have all these actions, like atropine; while some in this series, especially those with modified atropine structure have specific one or two of the above actions.

1) Atropine

(($\pm$) Hyoscyamine)

Tropan-3-yl ($\pm$)-tropate; Tropine ester of tropic acid.

Atropine is prepared by racemisation of (-) hyoscyamine, an alkaloid obtained from Hyoscyamus species and other solanaceous plants. Atropine sulphate and atropine methonitrate are official in I.P.

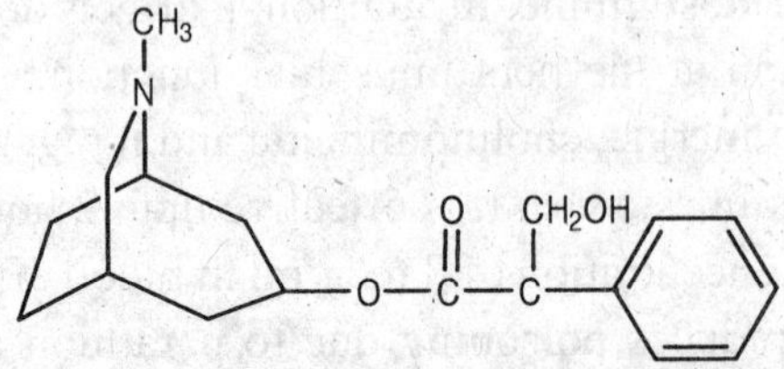

Properties : Atropine is a tropine ester of racemic tropic acid and is optically inactive. It also occurs naturally as Solanaceae alkaloids. Atropine occurs in the form of optically inactive, white odourless crystals having a bitter taste. It is slightly soluble in water (1:460), but freely soluble in alcohol (1:2). Aqueous solutions are alkaline (pH 9.5). Its salt atropine sulphate is freely soluble in water.

Stability : In aqueous solutions, atropine is slowly hydrolysed to tropine and tropic acid. Hydrolysis is catalysed by hydrogen ions and hydroxide ions. The solutions are most stable at pH 3.8.

Incompatibility : Atropine salts are incompatible with bromides, iodides, alkalis, tannic acid, quinine and salts of mercury.

Actions and uses : Atropine is used by ophthalmologists for its mydriatic effect, paralysing the iris and ciliary muscle, Its 0.5 to 1 per cent solution is widely used for fitting glasses. Atropine is also used as preanesthetic medication before administering general anesthesia, to decrease oral and air-passage secretions. It is also useful in decreasing respiratory depression, when morphine is used in surgical operations. Because of its ability to dry up secretions, atropine is sometimes used for symptomatic relief in cold. Its use as antispasmodic agent finds many useful applications like decreasing smooth muscle spasm, acute abdominal pains, appendicitis pain etc. One of the most important emergency use of atropine is as antidote in organophosphorus poisoning - to prevent muscarinic effects of acetylcholine accumulation. Atropine is also somewhat useful in Parkinson's disease, to relieve rigidity and tremors of patients suffering from this disease. This action of atropine is due to its CNS effect.

Dose : 250 mcg 3 times a day.

In organophosphate insecticide poisoning 2-4 mg IV, followed by 2 mg IM every 5 to 10 minutes, till symptoms disappear or signs of atropine toxicity appear.

Preparations : Atropine sulphate eye drops, B.P.

Atropine sulphate injection, I.P.

Atropine sulphate tablets, I.P.,B.P.

Morphine and atropine injection, I.P.

Atropine eye ointment, I.P. - contains atropine methonitrate.

Compound adrenaline and atropine spray, B.P.C. - a spray containing atropine methonitrate, to be inhaled through mouth.

Brand Names : Atro® eye drops, Atrocycline® ointment, Atroren® ointment, Tropine®, Topin®

2) Hyoscine

(Scopolamine)

(-)-,6, 7-Epoxytropan-3-yl tropate

Hyoscine is an alkaloid obtained from species of Datura and other solanaceous plants. It is used as the hydrobromide salt.

Properties : Hyoscine hydrobromide occurs as odourless, slightly efflorescent, colourless crystals of white crystalline powder. It is freely soluble in water; soluble in alcohol. It is laevorotatory.

Storage : It should be stored in airtight containers, in a cool place, protected from light.

Actions and uses : Hyoscine is mainly used to prevent motion sickness during journeys. The greatest advantage of this drug is it produces slight sedation at the oral dose of 0.5 to 1 mg. The action lasts for 4 to 6 hours and is, therefore, suitable for short journeys. It however, does not prevent nausea or vomiting. Hyoscine (scopolamine) has been a subject of drug delivery system and a transdermal patch to be worn behind the ear has been developed to prevent motion sickness.

Hyoscine has peripheral and central actions. Its antimuscarinic properties produce mydriasis and relaxation of accommodation. It depresses the cerebral cortex and is, therefore, used in mania, cerebral excitement and delirium.

Dose : 0.5 to 1 mg

Preparations : Hyoscine hydrobromide tablets, I.P., B.P.

Hyoscine injection, I.P., B.P.

Hyoscine eye drops, B.P.C.

Hyoscine eye ointment, B.P.

Brand Names : Belloid®, Buscopan®, Hyospan®

3) Homatropine

Tropan-3-yl mandelate

Properties : Homatropine hydrobromide occurs as odourless, colourless crystals or white crystalline powder. It is freely soluble in water and sparingly soluble in alcohol.

Stability : In aqueous solution, the drug is hydrolysed into tropine and mandelic acid. Hydrolysis is catalysed by hydrogen ions and hydroxide ions. The solutions are most stable at pH 3.7.

Actions and uses : Homatropine hydrobromide is used in eye as 1-2 per cent solution to produce mydriasis and cycloplegia - but it is not ideal for producing complete cycloplegia as its action persists for 1-3 days. It behaves very much like atropine.

Preparations : Cocaine and homatropine eye-drops, B.P.C.

Homatropine eye drops, B.P.

Homatropine hydrobromide eye drops, I.P.

Brand Names : Homarin Forte®, Homide® drops

4) Propantheline bromide

N,N-Diisopropyl-N-methyl- N-[2-(xanthen-9-yl-carbonyloxy)ethyl] ammonium bromide

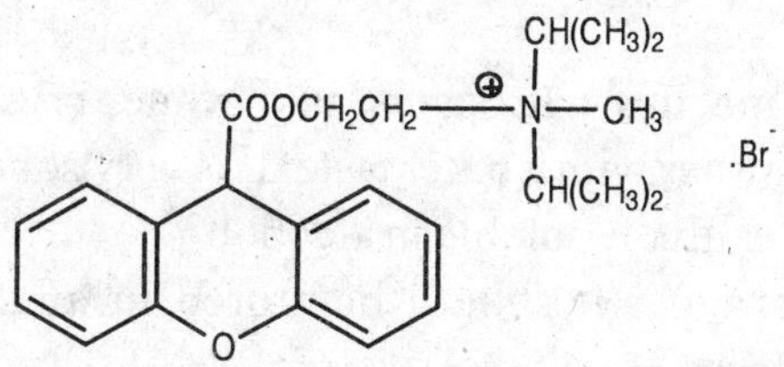

Properties : It occurs as a slightly hygroscopic, white or yellowish white powder. It is odourless and has a very bitter taste. It is soluble in water, alcohol and chloroform.

Storage : It should be stored in airtight containers.

Actions and uses : Propantheline bromide and its congener, methantheline bromiode, belong to the chemical class of quaternary amino alcohol esters where the nitrogen atom is quaternised and bears a positive charge. These drugs produce a high ratio of ganglionic and muscarinic blockage. The GI effects of these drugs are higher than atropine and have longer duration of action of 4-6 hours. Since their primary action is antisecretory, they are used in peptic ulcer. The drugs have many serious side effects. They produce postural hypotension, impotence, urinary retention and neuromuscular blockade. Other side effects are euphoria, restlessness, acute psychosis and dermatitis. Since, new and more effective drugs like cimetidine and ranitidine have come up for peptic ulcer, these drugs have lost ground.

Dose : 15 mg, 3 times a day.

Preparations : Propantheline tablets, I.P., B.P.

Methantheline Bromide : The isopropyl groups on nitrogen are replaced by ethyl groups, the remaining structure is similar to propantheline.

Brand Names : Pro-Banthine®, Spastheline®, Pepler®

5) Benztropine

3-Benzhydryloxytropanium methanesulphonate

Properties : It occurs as a white, crystalline powder with a bitter taste. It is very soluble in water, freely soluble in alcohol.

Storage : It should be stored in airtight containers.

Actions and uses : Benztropine is a synthetic atropine analog and has many features of atropine structure. It is a potent blocker of receptors of dopamine and, therefore, is used in Parkinson's disease. It also has a pronounced CNS effect. It also has peripheral anticholinergic effect, slight antihistaminic, sedative and local anesthetic activity.

Dose : 1.4 to 5 mg per day.

Preparations : Benztropine injection, B.P.C. Benztropine tablets, B.P.

6) Biperiden

α-(5-norbornen-2yl)-α-phenyl-γ-piperidyl propanol

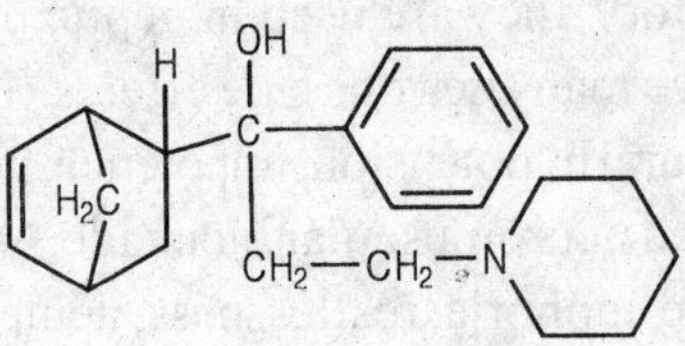

Properties : Biperiden occurs as a white crystalline, odourless powder. It is very slightly soluble in water; sparingly soluble in alcohol; soluble in ether. Biperiden hydrochloride is used orally and lactate salt is used parenterally.

Storage : It should be protected from light.

Actions and uses : This drug which was introduced in 1959, has weak peripheral anticholinergic but strong nicotinic activity. These weak anticholinergic effects, make this drug useful in Parkinson's syndrome.

The drug is used in all kinds of Parkinson's diseases like postencephalitic, idiopathic, arteriosclerotic; and helps to eliminate akinesia, rigidity and tremors. The drug is also used to eliminate drug induced extrapyramidal symptoms and thus enables continued use of tranquilisers. Biperiden is also useful in spastic disorders not related to Parkinsonism such as multiple sclerosis, spinal cord injury and cerebral palsy. It is, however, contraindicated (not to be used) in epilepsy.

Dose : 2 mg IM, to be repeated half-hourly, until relief, but not more than 4 times a day. 5 mg IV to be repeated only once in 24 hours.

Preparations : Biperiden lactate injection, I.P.

7) Tropicamide

N-ethyl-2-phenyl-N(4-pyridylmethyl) hydracrylamide

Properties : The drug belongs to aminoamide class of synthetic anticholinergic drugs. It occurs as a white powder, slightly soluble in water, but freely soluble in alcohol and in chloroform. The pH of ophthalmic solutions is usually between 4 and 5.0.

Actions and uses : The drug is used as anticholinergic in ophthalmic procedures where mydriasis is produced by relaxation of sphincter muscle of the iris. The effect is achieved in 20 to 25 minutes and lasts for about 20 minutes with complete recovery in 6 hours. It is, therefore, more useful in many eye manipulations. However, its use over homatropine to achieve cycloplegia is in question. Its use in glaucoma is contraindicated like other mydriatics.

Dose : Eye drops 0.05 to 0.1 ml of 1 per cent solution repeated in 5 minutes.

Preparations : Tropicamide eye-drops, I.P., B.P.C.

Brand Names : Drosyn-T® drops, Tropicamet® drops, Tricoyl® drops, Itrop Plus®, Picamid®

Drugs For Further Study

Cholinergic agonists

1) Bethanechol - Urotone®

Cholinergic antagonists - Muscarinic blockers

2) Oxyphenonium bromide - Antrenyl®
3) Clidinium bromide - Clidox®, Equirex®, Spasril®
4) Hyoscine - Belloid®, Buscopan®, Hyospas®
5) Pipenzolate methylbromide - Pipen®, Piplar®, Piptal®
6) Dicyclomine - Cataspa®, Centwin®, Clo-act®, Dicomin®, Spasmindon®
7) Cyclopentolate - Cyclogik®, Cyclogyl®, Cyclopent®
8) Trihexyphenidyl - Bexol®, Dystonil®, Pactiane®, Parkitane®
9) Procyclidine - Kemadrin®
10) Orphenadrine - Orphipal®

Cholinergic antagonists - Nicotinic blockers (Neuromuscular blockers)

11) Atracurium - Artacil®, Atrelax®, Tracrium®
12) Pancuronium - Neocuron®, Panuron®, Pavulon®
13) Succinylcholine - Entubate®, Myorelex®, Suxomin®

Exercise

Q1. Define cholinergic agents. Classify it giving suitable examples. Name the drugs used as antidote for anticholinesterase agents. (Kachchh Univ. 06, May 05)

Q2. Classify cholinergic drugs and write the structure of neostigmine. (Karnataka Univ. Winter 06)

Q3. Define Parasympathomimetics. (Winter 04)

Q4. Define and classify anticholinergic drugs giving examples of each class. (Winter 04)

Q6. What are 'Cholinergic antagonists'. Give their examples and name the drug used in 'Parkinson's disease'. (Summer 03)

Q7. Write structures of - i) Biperiden & ii) Propantheline. (Summer 06)

Q8. Define Anticholinesterases. (Summer 06)

Q9. Define and classify cholinergic drugs. Give names and uses of ganglionic blocker. (May-June 04)

Q10. Write category and use of following - i) Physostigmine & ii) Atropine. (May 07, Nov 06)

■

17 Diuretic Drugs

Kidney

The kidney is an important and very vital organ of human body. Its function is to remove the waste from body fluids, convert it into urine and eliminate it from the body. Its functioning is therefore vital and can turn out to be a matter of life and death to a person. The functional unit of kidneys is termed as 'nephron'. There are approximately one million nephrons in each kidney. A simplified diagram of a nephron is given below.

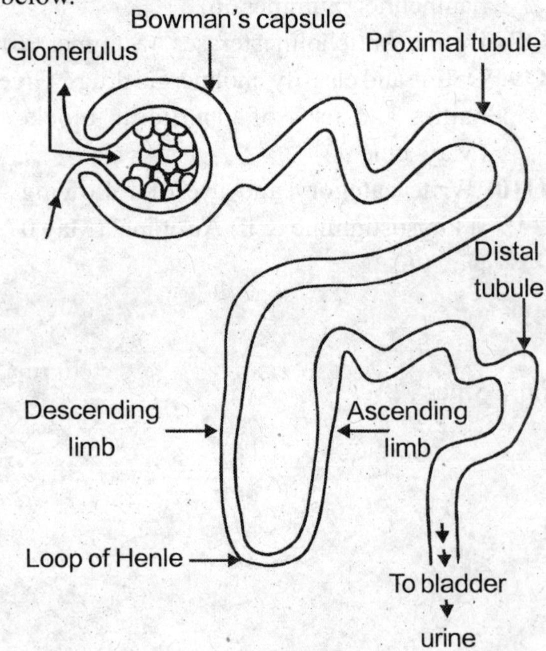

A nephron

Each nephron has three functional parts namely,

1) The renal capsule, consisting of a cluster of capillaries, known as glomerulus, which is enclosed in Bowman's capsule. The blood enters the nephron through the afferent arteriole under high capillary pressure and portions of the dissolved substances are filtered through the walls of the capillaries and the epithelium of Bowman's capsule into the lumen of the capsule.

2) The renal tubule, which has three segments i) the proximal tubule ii) the loop of Henle and iii) the distal tubule.

3) The collecting tubule, which leads to the renal pelvis, the ureter and finally to the larger collecting duct emptying into the bladder where urine is collected for excretion.

The volume and composition of urine are essentially determined by i) Glomerular filtration ii) Tubular reabsorption iii) Active tubular secretion.

The urine formation begins at the glomerular capillaries by the process of ultrafiltration. The glomerular filtrate is a protein-free ultrafiltrate of the plasma. It requires about 100 ml of glomerular filtrate to produce 1 ml of urine. The filtrate then reaches the proximal tubule. Here about 70 per cent of water and sodium ions and essentially all of potassium ions are reabsorbed. The fluid which is isotonic then enters the loop of Henle It becomes increasingly more concentrated as it passes through the descending limb, either by loss of water or concentration of solutes from capillaries. The fluid then comes into ascending limb and becomes increasingly more dilute, as about half of the remaining sodium ions may be reabsorbed by a cation exchange mechanism, which is controlled by a hormone named aldosterone. Sodium ion from renal tubular fluid is exchanged for potassium ion, and to a lesser extent, hydrogen ions from blood. Reabsorption of water from the hypotonic fluid of the distal tubule takes place primarily under the influence of antidiuretic hormone (ADH), vasopressin, from the posterior pituitary gland.

Most of the clinically used diuretics increase the excretion of sodium ion (as chloride or bicarbonate) by decreasing the reabsorption of the ion in the renal tubules. Any compound that interferes with the process of reabsorption of water and solute from glomerular filtrate will give a diuretic action. Since most of the reabsorption takes place in the proximal tubules, the most potent diuretics, like thiazides, act primarily on the proximal tubules. About half of the sodium ion remaining after the passage on the proximal tubule, is reabsorbed on its passage through the loop of Henle. Some of the extremely powerful diuretics like furosemide and ethacrynic acid, block sodium transport in the ascending limb of the loop of the Henle and are, therefore, (sometimes) referred to as loop diuretics. Only a small number of diuretics act primarily on the distal tubules, these are known as weak diuretics (like aldosterone inhibitors and triamterene). This site, i.e., distal tubule governed by aldosterone, is also a site where sodium-potassium exchange occurs, leading to increased potassium secretion. Some of these diuretics which act on distal tubule, reduce potassium excretion and are called potassium sparing diuretics, eg. spironolactone.

Therapeutic Applications

The general therapeutic uses of diuretics can be listed as follows

i) For the treatment of all kinds of oedema. Especially useful in oedema associated with congestive heart failure, premenstrual tension, oedema of pregnancy, renal oedema.

ii) Oedema induced by other drugs like ACTH and corticosteroids.

iii) To relieve intraocular pressure in glaucoma.

iv) In the treatment of mild hypertension.

v) In toxicosis, to excrete toxins out of the body.

Classification of Diuretics

I] Weak diuretics

a) Osmotic Diuretics eg. sodium and potassium salts, urea

b) Non electrolytes eg. mannitol

c) Carbonic Anhydrase Inhibitors eg. acetazolamide

d) Xanthine Derivatives.

II] Moderately potent diuretics

eg. chlorothiazide, benzothiazide

III] Very potent diuretics

eg. furosemide, old-time diuretics eg. mercurial diuretics, ethacrynic acid. These are also known as 'loop diuretics'.

IV] Potassium sparing diuretics

eg. triamterene, aldosterone blocking agents eg. spironolactone.

Sometimes diuretics are also classified according to their chemical structures.

I] Weak diuretics

a) Osmotic diuretics

1) Urea

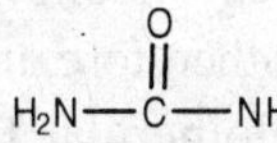

Properties : Urea occurs as colourless, slightly hygroscopic, prismatic crystals. It is odourless and has a cooling and saline taste. It is very soluble in water and soluble in alcohol.

Storage : It should be stored in airtight containers.

Actions and uses : This is a typical osmotic diuretic belonging to the weak diuretics class. When administered in large amounts, electrolytes are excreted and mobilisation of oedema fluid takes place. Oral administration is rarely used for cardiac oedema and nephrosis since it requires large doses upto 20 g, 2 to 5 times a day. Usual dose is IV 1 g to 1.5 g per kg of body weight, as a 20 per cent solution in Dextrose injection. A cream containing 10 per cent of urea is used as keratolytic in hyperkeratosis.

Preparations : Urea cream, I.P., B.P.C.

Urea injection, B.P.

Brand Names : Cotaryl® cream, Moisturex® cream, Skin-KR® cream

b) Non Electrolytes

1) Mannitol

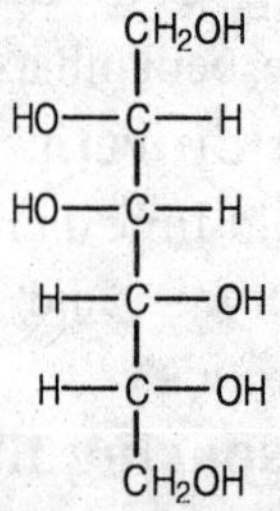

Mannitol is a hexahydric alcohol related to mannose and isomeric with sorbitol.

Properties : It occurs as an odourless white, crystalline powder, with a sweetish taste. It is freely soluble in water and very slightly soluble in alcohol. It is dextrorotatory.

Actions and uses : It is a sugar alcohol (polyhydroxy aliphatic alcohol). It is filtered by the glomerulus, and therefore, used as diagnostic agent to measure glomerular filtration rates. It is a typical osmotic diuretic and is effective in various oedematous states including those which fail to respond to thiazides. It is particularly useful in barbiturate poisoning to increase the urinary elimination of barbiturates. In such cases it is used as a 5-25 per cent solution. Mannitol is used as a 20 to 25 per cent solution for intravenous injection.

Dose : 50 to 100 gm a day IV injection.

Preparations : Mannitol injection I.P., B.P.

Marketed by - Albert David, Cadila Pharma, Core.

II] Moderately potent diuretics

1) Chlorothiazide

6-Chloro-2H-1,2,4-benzothiadiazine-7-sulphonamide-1,1-dioxide

Properties : It occurs as a white crystalline powder with a slightly bitter taste. It is very slightly soluble in water and slightly soluble in alcohol.

Storage : It should be stored in airtight container.

Actions and uses : Chlorothiazide was first introduced in 1958. It gives primarily a saluretic effect, but may produce significant loss of potassium, and therefore potassium supplement like KCl solution has to be given. Chlorothiazide is a potent diuretic and is used for the treatment of all types of oedemas. It is also useful in the management of mild hypertension but is not useful in glaucoma.

Dose : 1 to 2 gm a day.

Preparations : Chlorothiazide tablets, B.P.

2) Hydrochlorothiazide

6-Chloro-3,4-dihydro-2H,1,2,4-benzothiadiazine-7-sulphonamide 1,1-dioxide

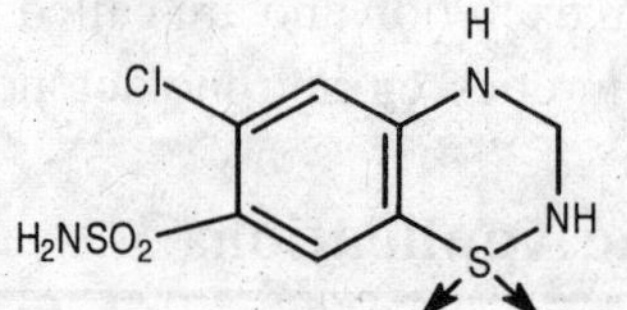

Properties : It occurs as a white crystalline powder. It is practically insoluble in water and soluble in alkali hydroxide solutions.

Actions and uses : Reduction of 3, 4 positions of the thiadiazine ring, increases the activity of the benzothiadiazines by nearly 10 times. Hydrochlorothiazide is the parent compound belonging to the class of reduced benzothiadiazines. Qualitatively, the drug has about the same diuretic activity as chlorothiazide. The dose is smaller and diuresis occurs in 2 hours and the action lasts for about 6-12 hours. The drug is useful in oedema associated with congestive heart failure, hepatic cirrhosis, steroid therapy and renal dysfunction. It is also used in mild hypertension along with other antihypertensive drugs.

Dose : 50 to 200 mg a day.

Preparations : Hydrochlorothiazide tablets, I.P., B.P.

Brand Names : Aquazide®, Hydride®, Esidrex®

3) Benzthiazide

3-[(Benzylthio)methyl]-6-chloro-2H-1,2,4 benzothiadiazine, 7-sulphonamide,1,1,dioxide

Properties : It occurs as a white, crystalline powder. It has a characteristic odour and a bitter taste. It is practically insoluble in water and slightly soluble in alcohol. It is freely soluble in solutions of alkalies.

Storage : It should be stored in airtight containers.

Actions and uses : Benzthiazide is a substituted chlorothiazide, at 3 position, where a benzyl thio methyl group appears. It is significantly more active than its parent compound, chlorothiazide, but about 85 per cent as active as hydrochlorothiazide. It gives similar electrolyte excretion pattern and also has the same problems like excretion of potassium ion, causing hypokalemia.

Dose: 50 to 200 mg a day. For hypertension - 25 to 50 mg, twice a day.

Preparations : Benzthiazide tablets U.S.P.

III] Very potent diuretics

1) Furosemide (Frusemide)

4-Chloro-N-furfuryl-5-sulphamoylanthranilic acid

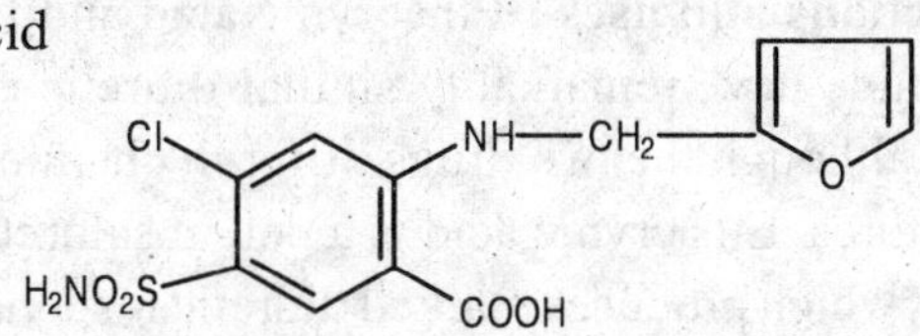

Properties : It occurs as a white, crystalline powder. It is odourless and almost tasteless. It is very slightly soluble in water, sparingly soluble in alcohol. It is soluble in solutions of alkali hydroxides.

Actions and uses : Furosemide is a typical loop diuretic, acting on the entire nephron including the loop of Henle. It is a powerful diuretic, produces rapid diuretic response within an hour and the action lasts for about 4-6 hours. It inhibits the reabsorption of sodium throughout the renal tubules and produces a saluretic action. Like the thiazides, it also produces potassium excretion, and therefore, has to be supplemented with potassium salts like KCl. It also causes disturbances in glucose tolerance and gives rise to blood urea. It is used in mild hypertension, besides all kinds of oedema.

Dose : 20 to 80 mg a day.

Preparations : Frusemide injection, I.P., B.P. Frusemide tablets, I.P., B.P.

Brand Names : Lasix®, Exna-K®, Fru® inj., Frusenex®, Tebemid®

2) Ethacrynic acid

[2,3-Dichloro-4-(2-methylenebutyryl) phenoxy] acetic acid.

Properties : Ethacrynic acid is an odourless, white crystalline powder. It is very slightly soluble in water but freely soluble in alcohol, chloroform and benzene. The solution of sodium salt at pH 7 is stable at room temperature, but stability decreases with increased temperature and pH. Neutral solutions of the sodium salt in 5 per cent dextrose or sodium chloride injection are used to prepare intravenous injections.

Actions and uses : Ethacrynic acid and furosemide have remarkably similar diuretic effects although the two drugs differ in chemical structures. Ethacrynic acid is a potent saluretic agent which produces marked diuretic response in certain cases of refractory oedema. The diuretic action begins within 30 minutes of oral dose and within 5 minutes of intravenous administration. Ethacrynic acid inhibits sodium reabsorption primarily at two sites in the nephron i) in the ascending limb of loop of Henle and ii) in the distal tubule where urinary dilution takes place. Thus, it is also a typical loop diuretic. Ethacrynic acid produces systemic alkalosis, due to chloride excretion. It may also produce hypoalbuminemia, hypochloremia, hyponatremia, hypokalemia and metabolic alkalosis. The drug also has one serious side effect and that is, it sometimes produces transient deafness and sometimes even permanent deafness. The cause of this side effect is not known.

Ethacrynic acid is useful in the treatment of refractory oedema and may be used in combination with potassium sparing diuretic or with potassium supplement.

Dose : 50 to 100 mg oral, once or twice a day. 500 mcg to 1 mg per kg of body weight for IV

Preparations : Ethacrynic acid tablets, I.P., B.P.

Ethacrynic acid injection, B.P.C.

IV] Potassium sparing diuretics

1) Spironolactone

This drug is an aldosterone antagonist. It acts by competitive antagonism of aldosterone in the distal tubule of nephron, thereby preventing the potassium secretion and decreasing the sodium reabsorption. Its diuretic action is weak.

Dose : 100 to 200 mg per day

Brand Names : Aldactone®, Fruselac®, Lasilactone 50®

2) Triamterene

This is another drug of the potassium sparing diuretic class. It also acts on the distal tubule of nephron and has actions similar to spironolactone.

Dose : 100 mg a day.

Brand Names : Ditide®, Frusemene®

Drugs For Further Study

1) Chlorthalidone - Hydrazide®, Hythalton®
2) Xipamide - Xipamid®
3) Clopamide - Brinaldix®
4) Metolazone - Metolaz®
5) Torasemide - Dytor®, Retrolix®, Torsinex®
6) Amiloride - Amifru-40®, Amimide®, Frumil®
7) Acetazolamide - Avva®, Diamox®, Iopar-SR®

Exercise

Q1. Write short notes on - a) Carbonic anhydrase inhibitors, b) Thiazides and hydrothiazides & c) High-ceiling diuretics. (Kachchh Univ. 06, May 05, Nov 06)

Q2. Define and classify diuretics. Write the structure and chemical name of hydrochlorthiazide, frusemide, urea and mannitol. (Karnataka Univ., May-June 04, Winter 06, Nov 06)

Q3. Define Diuretics with suitable examples of drugs. (Summer 03)

Q4. Define diuretics. Classify them and write structure of atleast two drugs from each class. (May 07)

18 Cardiovascular Drugs

Cardiovascular drugs are used for their action on the heart or on other parts of the vascular system. These drugs modify the total output of heart or the distribution of blood to certain part of circulatory system. There are many drugs which can be listed under the title of cardiovascular drugs, but these can be classified according to their specific pharmacological action.

Classification of Cardiovascular Drugs

I] Cardiotonic drugs

These are mainly used for their inotropic effect and for effect on the conducting system of the heart, eg. Digitalis and other cardiac glycosides.

II] Antianginal drugs and vasodilators

These primarily act on the vascular system, like organic nitrates and nitrites, eg. glyceryl trinitrate.

III] Antihypertensive drugs

These cause fall in blood pressure. There are several such hypotensive drugs - Rauwolfia alkaloids (reserpine), guanethidine, alphamethyldopa, α and β adrenergic blocking agents such as phentolamine, atenolol.

IV] Antiarrhythmic drugs

These drugs modify the cardiac rhythm eg. quinidine.

V] Antihyperlipidemic drugs

These lower the cholesterol levels in blood, eg. clofibrate.

VI] Other drugs

These do not necessarily have a direct action on cardiovascular system, but are of considerable value in the treatment of cardiac diseases. These include (a) Diuretics (b) Anticoagulants (c) Hypoglycemic agents (d) Thyroid hormones.

I] Cardiotonic drugs

Cardiac glycosides : Cardiac glycosides have primarily the action of increasing the force of contraction (called as positive inotropic effect) of the heart without increasing its oxygen consumption. They are used to slow down heart rate in the atrial arrhythmias, particularly atrial fibrillation. They are also used in congestive heart failure. Thus, their main therapeutic uses can be listed as follows :

i) In congestive heart failure (low output failure).

ii) In left ventricular failure.

iii) In atrial fibrillation with tachycardia.

iv) In atrial flutter.

v) In atrial and AV nodal paroxysmal atrial tachycardia.

The cardiac stimulating properties of digitalis, strophanthus and squill are due to the cardiac glycosides present in them. On hydrolysis they yield corresponding aglycones and sugars. The cardiac activity resides in the aglycone portion, but the sugar residue provides favourable solubility and distribution characteristics.

Digitalis contains several cardiac glycosides. Lanatoside C is constituted of the aglycone,

Table 18.1

Source	Precursor Glycoside	Glycoside	Aglycone Portion	Sugar
1) Digitalis	Purpurea Glycoside A	Digitoxin	Digitoxigenin	Digitoxose
Purpurea (leaf)	Purpurea Glycoside B	Gitoxin	Gitoxigenin	Digitoxose
2) Digitalis	Lanatoside A	Digitoxin	Digitoxigenin	Digitoxose
lanata (leaf)	Lanatoside B	Gitoxin	Gitoxigenin	Digitoxose
	Lanatoside C	Digoxin	Digoxigenin	Digitoxose

digoxigenin, two molecules of sugar D-digitoxose, one molecule of acetyldigitoxose and one molecule of D-glucose. Digoxin also has the aglycone digoxigenin and its sugar part is composed of three molecules of D-digitoxose. Digitoxin has the sugar part similar to digoxin, but the aglycone portion is digitoxigenin. The aglycone portions of the cardiac glycosides present in digitalis belong to the chemical class of cardenolides which have an α-β-unsaturated five membered lactone ring attached to position 17 of the steroid nucleus. Digitoxigenin has structure similar to digoxigenin differing only in not having hydroxyl group at position 12. Thus important cardiac glycosides, their aglycone portions, sugars, and their sources can be summarised in the above table. (Table 18.1)

The cardiac glycosides differ much in their speed of the onset, duration of action, time to reach maximum concentration Cmax, plasma half-life and binding to proteins. For example, digoxin has 60-85 per cent absorption, 25 per cent binding to plasma, 24-48 hours of plasma half-life, 4 to 6 hours of Cmax, 3 to 6 days of duration of action and requires only 0.5 to 2 ng/ml of concentration for therapeutic effect. While digitoxin has slow onset, has 90-100 per cent absorption, nearly 90 per cent binding to proteins, 5 to 7 days of plasma half-life, 6 to 12 hours of Cmax, 18 days of duration of action and requires 10 to 35 nanogram (ng) per ml of concentration for therapeutic effect. Digitalis therapy has therefore, to be watched very carefully and overdose (over digitalisation) can cause digitalis toxicity.

Dose :

Digoxin : For the first 24 hours, 0.75 - 1.5 mg oral,

0.5 to 1.0 mg IV

For maintenance (oral) 0.12 to 0.5 mg

Digitoxin : For the first 24 hrs., 0.8 - 1.2 mg oral,

0.8 - 1.2 mg IV

For maintenance (oral) 0.05 to 0.2 mg.

Brand Names : Digox®, Dixin®, Lanoxin®, Sangoxin®

II] Antianginal drugs and vasodilators

The drugs in this class include inorganic and organic nitrites and nitrates. All these drugs act by vasodilation by persistent relaxation of vascular smooth muscle, especially that of smaller blood vessels. The reduction in oxygen demand also results due to vasodilation. These drugs therefore, are primarily utilised in the prophylaxis and in the treatment of angina pectoris.

Classification of Antianginal drugs

I) Organic nitrates

Glyceryl trinitrate pentaerythritol tetranitrate, isosorbide dinitrate

II) β-Adrenergic blockers

Propranolol, metoprolol, atenolol

III) Calcium channel blockers

Diltiazem, verapamil, nifedipine

IV) Potassium channel reactivators

Nicorandil

V) Antiplatelet drugs

Dipyridamole, aspirin

VI) Miscellaneous

Oxyfedrine, lidoflazine, dilazep

1) Ethyl Nitrite : CH_3CH_2ONO and
Amyl Nitrite : $(CH_3)_2CH_2.CH_2ONO$
(Isopentyl nitrite)

Properties : These drugs have definite explosion hazards if the source of ignition is present, even at room temperatures. They are nearly insoluble in water but miscible with organic solvents.

Actions and uses : These two drugs belonging to the organic nitrites and nitrates have their primary utility in the prophylaxis and treatment of angina pectoris. The beneficial action of these drugs is due to the coronary vasodilation that they cause. These compounds also decrease the myocardial work and oxygen consumption of the heart at submaximal exercise levels. They however do not increase the maximum aerobic capacity of the heart.

Both these drugs are rapidly absorbed from lungs and from other mucous membranes after inhalation. Ethyl and amyl nitrite, are decomposed by the gastric juice and hence cannot be administered by mouth.

Dose : Dispensed as pearls in 0.2 and 0.3 ml for inhalation. Pearls when broken make a loud noise. Onset of action within 10 seconds, duration 5-10 minutes.

2) Glyceryl Trinitrate (Nitroglycerin)

This is the trinitrate ester of glycerin and is official in USP as tablet form. It is prepared by carefully adding glycerin to mixture of nitric acid the and fuming sulphuric acid as follows,

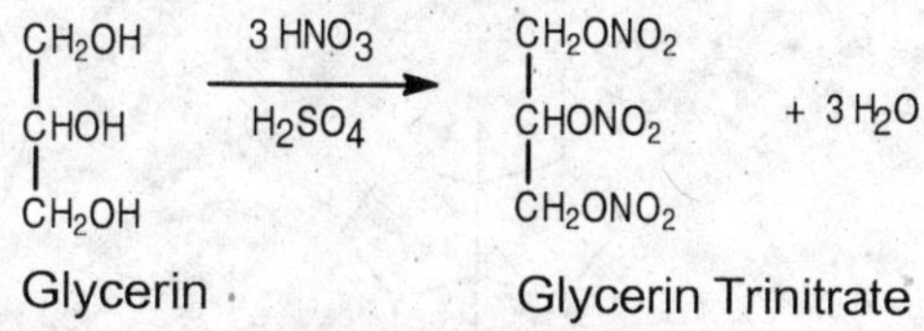

Properties : The ester is colourless oily liquid with a sweet burning taste. It is slightly soluble in water but freely soluble in organic solvents. It is highly explosive.

Actions and uses : It is a strong vasodilating agent and since it is absorbed through skin, it often causes headache. The main therapeutic use is in the treatment of angina pectoris. It also gives dramatic relief in paroxysmal nocturnal dyspnoea of left ventricular failure. It is sometimes used in long term management of chronic heart failure due to ischemic heart disease. The common side effects are headache, transient giddiness, postural hypotension.

Dose : Tablets of 0.3, 0.4 and 0.6 mg. Usual dose 0.2 - 0.6 mg sublingually. Onset 1-2 minutes, duration 15-40 minutes.

Sustained released formulation in 2.6 mg dose for 8-12 hour duration effect.

Preparations : Glyceryl trinitrate tablets, I.P., B.P.

Concentrated glyceryl trinitrate solution, B.P.

Brand Names : Angised®, Myovin®, Nitroject® inj., Nitroderm® TTS (transdermal patch), Nitrolingual® spray.

3) Pentaerythritol tetranitrate

$[C\text{-}(CH_2ONO_2)_4]$

This is also potent and is widely used as prophylactic for angina attacks. The onset of action is about 20 minutes and lasts for 300 minutes.

Dose : 10 mg tablets, 3-4 times a day.

4) Isosorbide Dinitrate and Isosorbide Mononitrate

1,4:3,6 Dianhydro sorbitol 2,5 - dinitrate

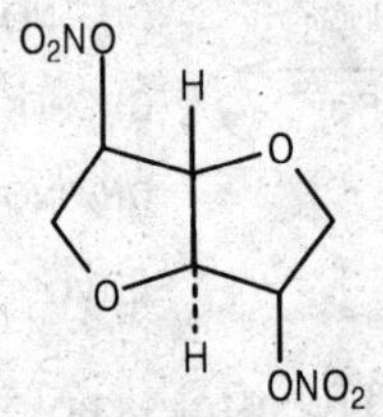

Diluted isosorbide dinitrate is a dry mixture of isosorbide dinitrate with lactose or inert excipient. It is used as oral or sublingual preparation for coronary vasodilation. The onset of action is within 15 minutes and lasts for 4 to 5 hours. Given sublingually, the onset is within 2 minutes. This is a drug that every angina patient is advised to keep with him all the time to meet any emergency situation of angina attack.

Dose : Isosorbide dinitrate 2.5 to 10 mg sublingual.

Isosorbide dinitrate (sustained release) - 40-80 mg orally.

Isosorbide mononitrate (ISMO) 20 mg orally.

Brand Names :

Isosorbide dinitrate - Isordil®, Cardicap-TR®, Dinospray®, Anzidin®

Isosorbide mononitrate - Anginex®, Angitab®, Ismo®, Monicor®, Vasotrate®

III] Antihypertensive Agents

Antihypertensive drugs form a large group of drugs among the cardiovascular agents. These drugs are used in the treatment of hypertension (high blood pressure i.e. diastolic pressure of 100 mmHg or more). These drugs act by reducing the cardiac output and/or reducing the total peripheral resistance. They act on various sites and therefore can be classified according to their site of action as follows,

a) Drugs acting centrally.

This class includes drugs like α-methyldopa and clonidine.

b) Drugs acting on the autonomic ganglia (ganglionic blocking agents).

This class includes drugs such as

i) Quaternary ammonium compounds eg. Hexamethonium, Pentolinium, Chlorisondamine.

ii) Secondary amines eg. Mecamylamine

iii) Tertiary amines eg. Pempidine, Trimethaphan

c) Drugs acting on postganglionic sympathetic nerve endings.

i) Adrenergic neuron blocking agents eg. Guanethidine, Bethanidine

ii) Catecholamine depletors eg. Reserpine

d) Drugs acting on Adrenergic Receptors.

i) α-Adrenergic blocking agents (α-blockers) eg. Phentolamine, Phenoxybenzamine, Prazosin.

ii) β-Adrenergic blocking (β-blockers) eg. Propranolol, Atenolol.

iii) Both α and β-Adrenergic blocking agents eg. Labetalol

e) Drugs acting directly on the vascular smooth muscle.

i) Hydralazine

ii) Calcium Channel Blockers eg. Nifedipine and

iii) Vasodilators eg. Sodium nitroprusside.

f) Drugs acting by reflex action, by stimulating baroreceptors.

(i.e. Receptor sensitive nitroprusside) like Veratrum alkaloids.

g) Drugs which block renin-angiotensin-aldosterone linkage.

i) ACE inhibitors like captopril, enalapril,

lisinopril which block the conversion of angiotensin I to angiotensin II by inhibiting the angiotensin converting enzyme (hence called ACE inhibitors).

ii) Agents which block the action of natural hormone aldosterone called as aldosterone blocking agents, eg. Spironolactone.

h) Miscellaneous Drugs.

Diuretics, MAO inhibitors eg. pargyline etc.

a) Drugs Acting Centrally

1) Methyldopa

(-),3(3,4-Dihydroxy phenyl)-2 methylalanine

Properties : It occurs as a white to yellowish-white fine powder. It is sparingly soluble in water.

Storage : It should be stored in airtight container, protected from light.

Actions and uses : This drug was developed under a research programme to develop an antagonist to inhibit the biochemical synthesis of pressor amines such as adrenaline, serotonin, noradrenaline, etc. Thus, methyldopa was developed and was found to be useful in mild to severe hypertension. Since methyldopa existed in zwitterion form, its ethyl ester, which was more useful for oral administration was used. It is especially useful in patients with compromised renal function. Its hypotensive effect is enhanced by diuretics like thiazides.

Dose : 250 mg, orally three times a day.

Ethyl ester - IV infusion 250 to 500 mg in 100 ml of 5 per cent Dextrose solution over a period of 30-60 minutes, 4 times a day.

Preparation : Methyldopa tablets I.P., B.P.

Methyldopate injection, B.P. - contains the ester form

Brand Names : Aldopam®, Alphadopa®, Emdopa®

2) Clonidine

2-[(2,6-Dichlorophenyl) imino] imidazoline

Properties : This is an imidazoline derivative, and is potent antihypertensive agent. It is a lipid soluble drug and is well absorbed from gut and has a high volume of distribution. It has a half life of 12 hours, therefore, two doses per day are sufficient.

Dose : 0.1 mg tablets

Brand Names : Arkamin®, Catapres®, Clothalton®

b) Ganglionic Blocking Agents

These drugs were popular in the initial period of hypertensive therapy. But due to many adverse reactions, development of tolerance and unpredictable absorption, their use is now not common. Quaternary ammonium compounds like hexamethonium act directly on ganglion, and reduce the cardiac output by reducing the venous return and as a result veins get dilated and blood pressure is lowered. Other agents like mecamylamine and pempidine, which are secondary and tertiary amines, can penetrate into the cell and cross blood- brain barrier, due to less charge on nitrogen (being secondary and tertiary amines). Sometimes these drugs are used in emergency like hypertensive crisis.

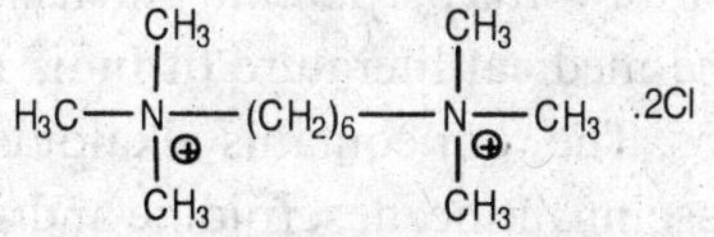

Hexamethonium chloride

c) Drugs acting on the postganglionic sympathetic endings

1) Guanethidine Sulphate

[2-(Hexahydro-1-2H)-azocinyl)ethyl]-guanidine sulphate.

Properties : It occurs as a white or almost white, crystalline powder. It is freely soluble in water.

Storage : It should be stored in airtight container in a cool place.

Actions and uses : This drug is not related chemically to any of the common antihypertensive drugs. It produces a gradual fall in blood pressure, usually after 2 to 7 days of therapy. The peak level effect is maintained for 3-4 days. Because of its slow onset and long duration of action, only a single daily dose is needed. The hypotensive action of guanethidine is attributed to its ability to block adrenergic neurons, by its action on post ganglionic sympathetic nerve ending. It prevents the release of norepinephrine from the nerve terminals. Because of this pharmacological action, the main side effect of the drug is postural hypotension. It usually developes in the morning and is precipitated by physical exercise.

Dose : 10 to 50 mg a day; gradually increased in the increments of 10 to 50 mg a day every 1 to 7 days.

Preparations : Guanethidine tablets, I.P. 1985, B.P.

Guanethidine sulphate has been omitted in I.P. 1996.

2) Reserpine

This drug is obtained from the roots of the plant called *Rauwolfia serpentina* and has been known in the medical literature of India since ancient times. The root contains alkaloids like reserpine, rescinnamine, deserpidine and ajmaline. Reserpine is by far the most potent of all and is in use. Reserpine has also other action (beside antihypertensive action) like sedative, antipsychotic and tranquilising action. Due to other synthetic drugs the use of reserpine is now much less.

Dose : 0.25 mg to 1 mg a day.

Brand Names : Adelphane®, Genophane®, Sarpalzino®, Serpasil®

d) Drugs acting on adrenergic receptors

1) α-Blockers

Drugs like phentolamine and phenoxybenzamine are typical α-adrenergic blocking agents having short duration of action and mainly used in the diagnosis and treatment of pheochromocytoma (tumor of adrenal medulla).

Prazosin is a quinazoline derivative and is a peripheral vasodilator. It is used in the treatment of moderate to severe hypertension frequently in addition to other drugs such as diuretics or β-blocker or methyldopa.

Brand Names :

Prazosin - Cyber-CR®, Minipress®, Prazopress®

Phentolamine - Fentanor®

Phenoxybenzamine - Fenoxene®

ii) β-Blockers

There are relatively new entrants in the treatment of hypertension. These drugs are used to control moderate hypertension. Both systolic and diastolic blood pressure are lowered. All the drugs in this class have about the same activity and clinically there is no single drug which is superior. They have fairly long half life and therefore, are given only once a day. Some drugs are used to reduce intraocular pressure, like timolol (Betim).

Dose : Propanolol - 80-240 mg a day

Atenolol - 50-100 mg a day

Metoprolol - 100-400 mg a day

Timolol - 10-40 mg/12 hour

Acebutolol

Labetalol acts on both α and β receptors 200-800 mg/12 hr.

Brand Names : Propanolol - Inderal®, Ciplar®

Atenolol - Atenol®, Aloten®, Aten®, Atenova®

Metoprolol - Lopressor®, Betaloc®, Metolar®

Timolol - Eymol® drops, Glucomol® drops

Acebutolol - Sectral®

Labetalol - Lobet®, Normadate®

e) Drugs acting directly on vascular smooth muscle

1) Hydralazine/Dihydralazine

Hydralazine was first tested for its antihistaminic activity, but then its hypotensive property was also seen. The drug was almost discarded for its adverse reactions, but again found its usefulness in clinical practice in combination with other agents. The drug lowers blood pressure in both normal subjects as well as in hypertensive patients. Diastolic pressure is reduced more than systolic. Although plasma half life is short, it is still a longer acting agent. Because of the high incidences of adverse reactions and also because of development of other better drugs, use of this drug has now declined.

Dose : 10-50 mg four times a day.

Brand Names : Nepresol®

2) Calcium Channel Blockers

Nifedipine, nitrendipine, nimodipine, verapamil, dilitiazem.

Verapamil, nifedipine and other drugs in this class, block calcium channels in the membranes of smooth and cardiac muscle cells. Both these drugs are useful in the long term treatment of hypertension. Nifedipine has also been used in the management of hypertensive emergencies. It is also a drug of choice in hypertensive patients with impaired renal function and with diabetes. Nimodipine is useful in cerebral haemorrhage. Another drug of recent origin is diltiazem which has its activity in between verapamil and nifedipine.

Dose : Verapamil - 240 to 480 mg/day

Nifedipine - 15 to 60 mg; 6 to 8 hourly

Nifedipine (Retarol) - 20 mg, 12 hourly

Brand Names :

Nifedipine - Angiblock®, Calcigard®, Cardules®, Depicor®, Needin®

Nitrendipine - Nitrepin®, Cardif Beta®

Verapamil - Calaptin®, Vasopten®, Veramil®

Diltiazem - Dilcal®, Dicard®, Angizem®

f) Drugs acting by reflex action by stimulating baroreceptors

The veratrum alkaloids have their primary site of action as afferent receptors predominantly in the heart. As a result of the sensitization of the afferent receptors, the peripheral sympathetic tone is reduced, producing fall in blood pressure. At the same time, the vagal tone is also increased and this induces bradycardia. The drug is now no longer used.

g) Drugs blocking renin-angiotensin linkage (Renin-angiotensin antagonists)

Drugs in this class inhibit conversion of angiotensin I to angiotensin II. This is achieved by inhibiting the enzyme called angiotensin converting enzyme (ACE) which is responsible for the conversion of angiotensin I to angiotensin II. Inhibition of ACE raises the levels of hormone bradykinin, a potent vasodilator. Bradykinin contributes to the cardioprotective effect of these drugs. Thus, captopril, a typical ACE inhibitor lowers systemic arterial resistance and lowers the mean systolic and diastolic pressure. The hypotensive effect is seen in all varieties of hypertension (except primary), but is most marked in patients with renal hypertension. These drugs are also potentiated by diuretics and β-blockers. Enalapril maleate, is a congener of captopril. It is more potent than captopril, produces less side effects and is longer lasting. It is actually a prodrug and gets converted to an active metabolite called enalaprilat.

Lisinopril is another drug in this category and has about the same properties as enalapril.

Dose : Captopril - 25-50 mg twice a day.

Enalapril - 5 to 10 mg once or twice a day.

Lisinopril - 5-20 mg once daily, upto 40 mg/day.

Brand Names :

Captopril : Aceten®, Angiopril®, Capace®, Capotril®

Enalapril - Enace®, Enam®, Enapril®

Lisinopril - Acinopril®, Cipril®, Lipril®, Lisoril®

h) Miscellaneous Drugs

Oral Diuretics : The diuretics of benzothiadiazine series chlorothiazide, hydrochlorothiazide and related phthalimidine compounds : chlorothalidone have proved very valuable in the treatment of mild to moderate hypertension. In addition they enhance the effect of other hypotensive agents like reserpine, vasodilators, adrenergic blocking agents, methyldopa and even ACE inhibitors. Combinations of these drugs with diuretics are now common. The detailed chemistry and pharmacological actions of these compounds have been discussed in the chapter 17.

Other miscellaneous drugs like MAO inhibitors, aldosterone blocking agents like spironolactone have been discussed in chapter 17.

Angiotensin II antagonists :

Drugs which competitively block angiotensin II produce a vasodilatory effect. This class has received a lot of attention since 1990. Losartan was the first drug from this class.

IV] Drugs that modify cardiac rhythm (Antiarrhythmic drugs)

The drugs in this class modify the cardiac rate and rhythm.

Quinidine and procainamide are the most effective drugs for use in the modification of cardiac rate and rhythm. These drugs are therefore used to treat atrial fibrillation and flutter, paroxysmal atrial and nodal tachycardia, to correct atrial and ventricular premature beats and ventricular fibrillation and flutter.

Other drugs which have been found useful in the treatment of arrhythmias are lignocaine (lidocaine), phenytoin (diphenylhydantoin), propranolol and verapamil.

Classification of Antiarrhythmic Drugs :

I] Membrane depressant drugs

Quinidine, procainamide, lignocaine, phenytoin, encainide, flecainide.

II] β-Adrenergic blockers

Propranolol

III] Repolarisation prolongators

Amiodarone, bretylium

IV] Calcium channel blockers

Verapamil, diltiazem.

1) Quinidine sulphate

Quinidine is an isomer of the anti-malarial drug quinine. It is one of the natural alkaloids occurring in the cinchona bark. The beneficial effect of quinine on atrial fibrillation was first noticed by a Dutch colonial doctor, who was treating patients for malaria with quinine and found that in some of the patients, their complaint about the palpitation of the heart, i.e., atrial flutter or fibrillation disappeared after a prolonged treatment of quinine.

Properties : Quinidine sulphate occurs as a white needle like crystals. It is sparingly soluble in water. It darkens on exposure to light. It is dextrorotatory.

Incompatibility : It is incompatible with alkalis, iodides and tannic acid.

Storage : It should be stored in airtight container, protected from light.

Actions and uses : Quinidine has both the cardiac actions and extracardiac actions. Cardiac actions of quinidine include reduced automaticity, depression of excitability, slowing of conduction velocity and prolongation of refractory period. The extracardiac actions include fall in blood pressure due to adrenergic blocking action and action on arteriolar smooth muscle. A typical effect of these two actions is seen on the prolongation of QT interval of the electrocardiogram (ECG).

Dose : 200 to 800 mg repeated at 2 to 3 hour intervals for 5 doses a day. Maintenance dose of 100 to 200 mg; 3 to 6 times a day.

Preparations : Quinidine tablets, I.P., B.P.

Brand Names : Natcardine®

V) Antihyperlipidemic agents

(Antihypercholesterolemic drugs or Cholesterol lowering agents)

It is now well established through several research findings that cholesterol plays an important role in the development of atherosclerosis; the fatty deposits in blood vessels are high in cholesterol, either free or as esters. Further it was observed that those sectors of the population, whose diet was rich in cholesterol, had high incidences of atherosclerosis than those whose diets were low in cholesterol. Since fat is the major source of precursor of cholesterol, control of fat content in the diet, can reduces cholesterol synthesis. This was indeed the case. Use of unsaturated fats from vegetable sources led to the decreased level of serum cholesterol.

In Parallel, efforts were on to find drugs which could lower/control cholesterol levels. One such drug is clofibrate. Gemfibrozil is a congener of clofibrate.

1) Clofibrate

Ethyl,2-(p-chlorophenoxy)-2-methylpropionate.

Properties : Clofibrate is a stable, colourless to pale yellow liquid, soluble in organic solvents, but insoluble in water.

Actions and uses : Clofibrate is absorbed from the GIT and is rapidly hydrolysed by enzymes to free acid, which is then extensively bound to serum proteins. The biological half life is about 12 hours.

It appears that this drug inhibits the cholesterol biosynthesis in the liver at a point prior to mevalonic acid. There is also a considerable evidence that the drug is effective in lowering the serum triglycerides.

Clofibrate is well tolerated and has minor side effects like nausea and gastrointestinal distress. It has drug-drug interaction with anticoagulant drugs and the dose of such drugs has to be adjusted when clofibrate is being used simultaneously.

Dose : 500 mg 4 times a day

Preparations : Clofibrate capsules, I.P. (1985), B.P.

Clofibrate has been omitted in I.P. 1996.

2) HMG - CoA Reductase Inhibitors :

This is a new class of hypolipidemic drugs. These drugs inhibit the enzyme involved in the biosynthesis of cholesterol in the step of the conversion of HMG-CoA to mevalonic acid. The drugs collectively called as statins include lovastatin, simvastatin, pravastain and fluvastatin.

Drugs For Further Study

Cardiotonics

1) Amrinone - Amicor®, Cardiotone®, Indocor®
2) Milrinone - Milicor®, Primacor® IV

Antianginals -

1) Nicorandil - Corflo®, Korandil®, Nikoran®, Zynicor®.
2) Trimetazidine - Cardimax®, Triadin®, Triguard®, Trivedon®.
3) Oxyfedrine - Ildamen®.
4) Dilazep - Cormelian®.

Antihypertensives -

1) Terazosin (α-blocker) - Hytrin®, Teradip®, Terapress®, Teraz®.
2) Doxazosin (α-blocker) - Alfazosin®, Doxacard®, Durocard®.
3) Bisoprolol (β_1-blocker) - Biselect®, Bisocar®, Concor®, Lodoz®.
4) Nebivolol (β_1-blocker) - Nebicard®, Nebistar®, Nodon®, Zinebi®.
5) Carvedilol (α & β-blocker) - Carca®, Carvidas®, Carloc®, Carvedil®.
6) Felodipine (Ca^{++} channel blocker) - Felogard®, Plendil®.
7) Amlodipine (Ca^{++} channel blocker) - Amcard®, Amchek®, Amlocor®, Amlodac®
8) Lercanidipine (Ca^{++} channel blocker) - Landip®-10, Lerez®, Lerka®, Lerva-SC®.
9) Benidipine (Ca^{++} channel blocker) - Caritec®.
10) Ramipril (ACE inhibitor) - Cardace®, Hopace®, Ramipres®.
11) Trandolapril (ACE inhibitor) - Zetpril®.
12) Perindopril (ACE inhibitor) - Coversyl®, Perigard®.
13) Fosinopril (ACE inhibitor) - Fosinace®, Fovas®.
14) Imidapril (ACE inhibitor) - Tanatril®.
15) Losartan (Angiotensin II blockers) - Alsartan®, Losacar®, Losan®, Losartas®, Lostat®.
16) Irbesartan (Angiotensin II blockers) - Irbest®, Irovel®, Xarb®.
17) Candesartan (Angiotensin II blockers) - Candelong®, Candesar®, Candez®.
18) Valsartan (Angiotensin II blockers) - Diovan®, Starval®, Valent®.
19) Telmisartan (Angiotensin II blockers) - Cresar®, Telista®, Telma®, Telpres®.

Antiarrhythmics :

1) Disopyramide - Norpace®, Regubeat®.
2) Adenosine - Adenocor®, Adenoject®, Carnosine®.
3) Amiodarone- Aldarone®, Amiodar®, Cordarone®.
4) Procainamide - Pronestyl®.
5) Lignocaine (lidocaine) - Loxicard 2%®, Xylocard 2%®
6) Mexiletine- Mexitil®.

Antihyperlipidemic agents :

1) Gemfibrozil - Gempar®, Lopid®, Normolip®.
2) Bezafibrate - Bezalip®, Globez®.
3) Lovastatin - Aztatin®, Lostatin®, Lovalip®, Lovatin®.
4) Simvastatin - Simcard®, Simstat®, Simvin®, Starstat®.
5) Atorvastatin - Amat®, Astin®, Atchol®, Atocor®, Atorva®.
6) Pravastatin - Prastatin®, Pravator®.
7) Rosuvastatin - Fortius®, Novostat®, Rovalip®, Rozucor®.

Exercise

Q1. Write short notes on - a) Lipid lowering agents, b) Vasodilators & c) Digitalis glycosides. (Kachchh Univ. 06, May 05, Nov 06)

Q2. Write a note on glyceryl trinitrate and methyl dopa. (Karnataka Univ.)

Q3. Define lipid lowering agents. Give properties, uses and official preparations of clofibrate. (Winter 04)

Q4. Write official preparations, properties and structure of 'nitroglycerin'. (Summer 03)

Q5. Classify the cardiovascular agents with examples of drugs from each class. (Summer 03)

Q6. In what dosage form following drug is adminsitered - Clofibrate. (Summer 06)

Q7. What are cardiac glycosides? Give hydrolysis products of digitalis glycosides. (Summer 06)

Q8. Classify Cardiovascular drugs. Name drugs used in - i) Anginal pain, ii) Irregular beating of heart, iii) High cholesterol in blood & iv) Enlargement of heart. (May-June 04)

Q9. Classify cardiovascular agents, write atleast one structure from each class and write note on cardiotonic or Lipid lowering agents. (May 07)

Q10. Write the brand name of nifedipine. (Nov 06)

Q11. Name a cardiovascular drug having imidazoline derivative. (Nov 06)

Q12. Classify drugs acting on the cardiovascular system with examples. Write the structure, chemical name and uses of propranalol. Add a note on Lipid lowering agents. (Karnataka Univ.)

■

(19) Hypoglycaemic Agents

Diabetes Mellitus

Hypoglycaemic drugs are used in the treatment of diabetes mellitus. Diabetes mellitus is a disease characterised by persistent hyperglycaemia usually with glycosuria. It is caused by a deficiency or diminished effectiveness of insulin. The treatment of diabetes should abolish the disease symptoms, reduce blood glucose levels to normal and maintain suitable body weight. Restriction of carbohydrate intake is essential for all diabetics. Classical symptoms of the disease include thirst, polyuria, dehydration and loss of energy and weight.

The discovery that certain organic compounds lower the blood sugar level dates back to 1918 when guanidine was shown to lower the blood sugar level. Then the discovery that certain trypanosomes need glucose in the medium and will die in its absence, was followed by the observation that galegine, a guanidine derivative, which was trypanocidal in activity also lowered the blood sugar level. This led to the development of a number of very active trypanocidal agents such as bisamidines, di-isothioureas and bisguanidines. Out of which, synthalin and pentamidine were very active trypanocidal agents and also lowered blood sugar levels. In 1942, an antibacterial thiadiazole sulphonamide known as IPTD was found to produce hypoglycaemia. This led to the synthesis and screening of several synthetic hypoglycaemic agents.

There are two main groups among the synthetic hypoglycaemic agents namely, (i) Sulphonylureas and (ii) Biguanides. Following are some of the commonly used drugs.

Classification of Hypoglycaemic Agents

I] Insulins

a) Short acting - Neutral insulin

b) Intermediate acting - Isophane (NPH)-insulin, Lente insulin

c) Long acting - Ultralente insulin

II] Oral hypoglycaemics

a) Sulphonylureas - Tolbutamide, chlorpropamide, glibenclamide, glipizide

b) Biguanides - Phenformin, metformin

c) Miscellaneous - Acarbose, miglitol, repaglinide

I] Insulin

Insulin is the hormone secreted by the beta cells of the Islets of Langerhans and derives its name from the Latin word *'insula'*, which means an island. One of the major strides in medicine in the last century was the extraction of insulin from dog pancreas by Banting and Best in 1922. It was isolated in crystalline form in 1930.

Properties : Insulin is a polypeptide with a molecular weight of about 6000 It consists of two amino acid chains called as A and B, linked by two disulphide bridges. Each chain contains 21 to 30 amino acids, respectively and all are in a known sequence. The active centers of insulin are not exactly known but disulphide bridges are essential for biological activity.

Insulin has been traditionally obtained from bovine and porcine pancreas. Insulin for human use is obtained by chemical conversion of porcine insulin. Recently, 'human insulin' has been biotechnologically processed through cultures of *E.coli* bacteria, and is known as 'Humalin'. Cattle and pig insulin are structurally similar to human insulin in all except for a few amino acid residues.

Insulin is soluble in water, but undergoes molecular aggregation at extreme pH 3.2 and 10. In presence of zinc, aggregation is further encouraged, as it brings about crystallisation of insulin. It is relatively insoluble at pH 4 to 7. It can combine with proteins like protamine and with zinc, which helps preservation of its activity and prolongation of its duration of action.

Actions and uses : Insulin is inactivated *in vivo* by (i) immunochemical system (ii) reduction of the disulphide bonds and (iii) an enzyme called insulinase. Enzymes in the digestive fluids, such as pepsin and chymotrypsin, also inactivate insulin. Therefore, insulin cannot be given orally and is effective only through injection. Insulin has many effects on metabolic processes. These actions can be direct or indirect. Insulin affects skeletal and heart muscle, adipose tissues, the liver, the lens of the eye and leucocytes.

Therapeutic uses : The main use of insulin is in idiopathic diabetes and in secondary diabetes, i.e., diabetes caused by pancreatic disease or Cushing's syndrome. It is also useful in hyperkalemia and in schizophrenia.

Products : Plain insulin is usually injected about half an hour before a major meal. The intermediate and long acting preparations are injected once a day before breakfast. The actions of short acting insulins is so short that several injections per day are required to control diabetes. The action of long acting insulin starts too late to cover the first meal of day, i.e., breakfast. Hence appropriate mixtures have fairly rapid onset and act for about 24 hours. They are usually given before breakfast. Some of the commonly used mixtures are:

1) Protamine zinc insuline (PZI) + plain insulin (1:2 or 3 parts) - PZI contains free protamine which combines with added plain insulin. Hence 2 parts of plain insulin must be added to 1 part PZI otherwise the mixture behaves like PZI only.

2) NPH insulin which is a modified protamine - zinc insulin. It contains just enough protamine to combine with insulin. It behaves like a 1:3 mixture of PZI and plain insulin.

3) Lente insulin is a readymade mixture of amorphous (semi lente) and crystalline (ultralente) insulin zinc suspension in the proportion 3 to 7.

The activities of all these types of insulin are

Table 19.1 : Activities of various types of insulin

Insulin	pH	Type	Protamine	Activity in Hours		
				Onset	Peak	Duration
1) Plain Insulin ZH (semilente)	3.2 clear	Short acting	Nil	1	4	8
2) NPH - insulin ZH (Lente)	7.2 cloudy	Intermediate	Protamine	2	12	24
3) PZI Insulin Zinc suspension (ultralente)	7.2 cloudy	Long acting	Protamine	7	26	36

summarised below.

Dose : Usual dose is 20 to 80 units a day. It should be adjusted according to patient's response.

Preparations : Insulin injection, I.P., B.P.

Globin zinc insulin injection, I.P., B.P.

Isophane insulin injection, I.P., E.P.

Protamine zinc insulin injection, I.P., E.P.

Insulin zinc suspension, I.P., E.P. - It is of two types - amorphous and crystalline.

Insulin injection, Biphasic, B.P.

Neutral insulin injection, B.P.

Brand Names : Human Rapidica® inj., Huminsulin® 30:70 inj., A-traphane HM Penfill® inj.

II] Oral hypoglycaemics

a) Sulphonylureas

1) Tolbutamide

1-Butyl-3-(p-tolylsulphonyl) urea

Tolbutamide belongs to the class of sulphonylurea which has the following general structure

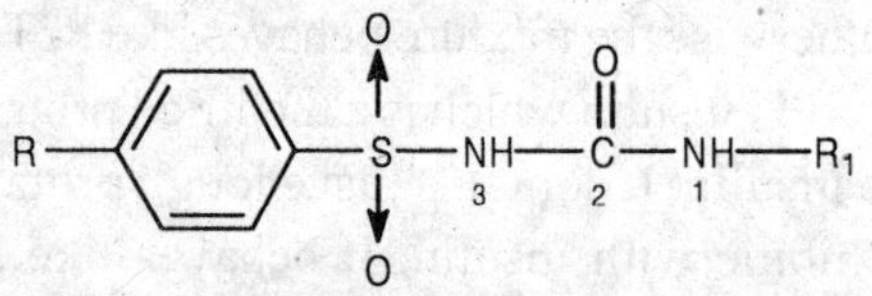

Thus tolbutamide has the following structure

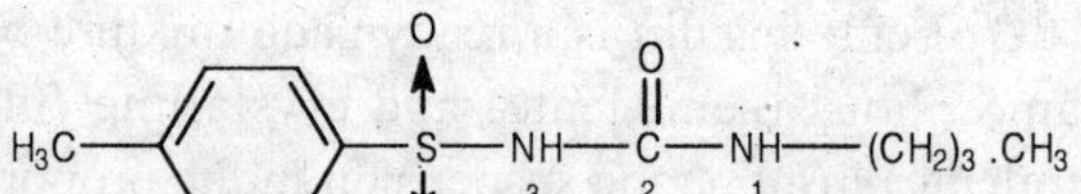

Properties : Tolbutamide is an odourless white crystalline powder, insoluble in water, but soluble in alcohol, alkali and dilute mineral acids.

Actions and uses : It is absorbed rapidly in diabetic patients. This drug should be used only in adult diabetic patients, i.e., only when maturity onset is established. Dietary restrictions have to be continued with the use of this drug.

Dose : Initial, 500 mg twice a day, later on to be adjusted to patient's response.

- Sodium salt : IV equivalent to 1 gm of tolbutamide over a 2-3 minute period.

Preparations : Tolbutamide tablets, I.P., B.P.

Brand Names : Rastinon®

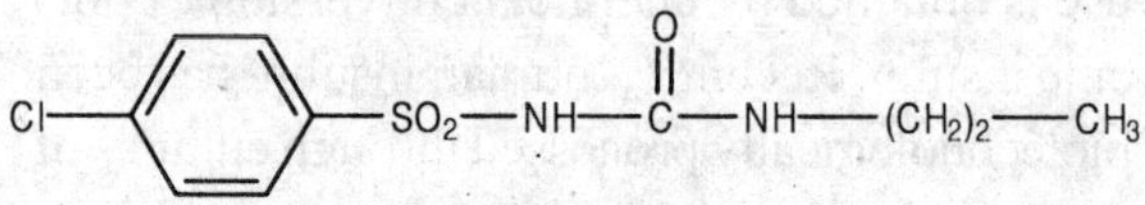

2) Chlorpropamide

1-[(*p*-Chlorophenyl) sulphonyl]-3-propylurea

Properties : It occurs as white, crystalline, powder. It is odourless and tasteless. It is practically insoluble in water; soluble in alcohol and in solutions of alkali hydroxides.

Actions and uses : Because of the chlorine group, the drug is more resistant to oxidation, and thereby resistant to conversion to an inactive metabolite, than is tolbutamide. As a result, the drug is much longer acting. Therefore, after a proper control of sugar in blood is achieved, the drug is required only once-a-day.

Dose : 100 to 200 mg, once or twice a day.

Preparations : Chlorpropamide tablets, I.P., B.P.

Brand Names : Copamide®

3) Glibenclamide

1-{4-[2-(5-Chloro-2-methoxy benzamido) ethyl]-benzene sulphonyl}-3-cyclohexyl urea

Properties : It occurs as white, crystalline, odourless powder. It is very slightly soluble in water and in ether; slightly soluble in alcohol.

Actions and uses : Glibenclamide is effective in a single daily dose and is effective in patients who are not controlled by maximum doses of chlorpropamide. The incidence of hypoglycemic reactions, however, are likely to be more with this drug than with other sulphonylureas. The tolerated dose also varies over a wide range from 2.5 to 200 mg per day. The drug must, therefore be used extremely carefully and in divided doses when more than 5 mg per day is recommended.

Dose : 5 to 20 mg a day.

Preparations : Glibenclamide tablets, I.P., B.P.

Brand Names : Euglucon®, Daonil®, Codica®, Glucosafe®

b) Biguanides

1) Phenformin hydrochloride

General Structure-

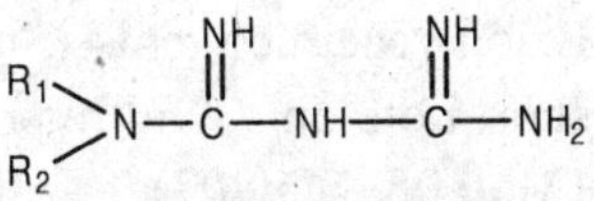

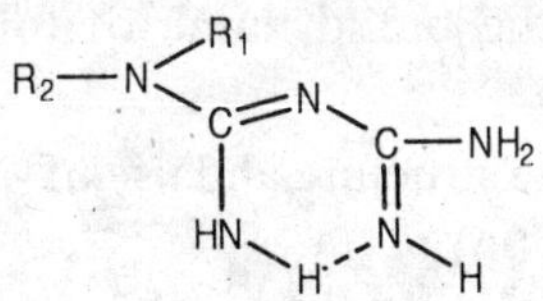

Cyclic form

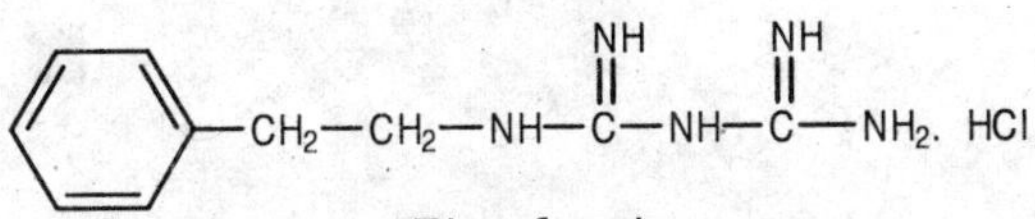

Phenformin

Phenformin and metformin belong to the biguanide group which has a general structure as above.

Properties : Phenformin hydrochloride occurs as an odourless, white, crystalline powder with a bitter taste. It is freely soluble in water and soluble in alcohol.

Actions and uses : These two drugs do not lower the blood sugar in normal subjects, but they do so in all types of diabetes mellitus. They potentiate the hypoglycaemic action of insulin and sulfonylureas, but they themselves do not produce clinical hypoglycaemia in diabetics. Both these biguanides, act extrahepatically and decrease the glycogen content of liver. Unlike insulin they inhibit lipogenesis, but not lipolysis in the adipose tissue. However, they do not stimulate insulin release from the pancrease. Phenformin is not used in the U.K. and U.S.A. It is likely to cause lactic acidosis.

Dose : 25 to 100 mg a day.

Preparations : Phenformin tablets, I.P.

Brand Names : DBI®

2) Metformin hydrochloride

1,1-Dimethylbiguanide hydrochloride

Properties : It occurs as a hygroscopic, white, crystalline powder. It is odourless and has a bitter taste. It is freely soluble in water and sparingly soluble in alcohol.

Storage : It should be stored in airtight containers.

Actions and uses : Metformin is an oral hypoglycaemic agent belonging to the class of biguanides. Its actions and uses are similar to those of phenformin. These drugs control the blood glucose level by increasing its peripheral utilisation and inhibiting gluconeogenesis in diabetic patients. Like phenformin, it may be given in conjunction with a sulphonylurea. It is better tolerated than phenformin and is preferred to it.

Dose : 0.5 to 1.5 gm a day.

Preparations : Metformin tablets I.P., B.P.

Brand Names : Dibeta SR®, Formin®, Forminal®, Metchek®

Drugs For Further Study

1) Glipizide (Sulfonylurea) - Glide®, Glipy-5®, Glucolip®, Glyzip®
2) Gliclazide (Sulfonylurea) - Azukon®, Comzid®, Gliclaz®, Glizid®
3) Glimepiride (Sulfonylurea) - Amaryl®, Azulix®, Euglim®, Glador®
4) Acarbose - Asucrose®, Glucar®, Rebose®, Recarb®
5) Miglitol - Diamig®, Misobit®
6) Repaglinide - Eurepa®, Rapilin®, Repide®
7) Nateglinide - Glinate®, Natelide®, Natiz®, NDS®
8) Rosiglitazone (Thiazolidinedione) - Enselin®, Reglit®, Rezult®, Rosizon®, Rozon®
9) Pioglitazone - Glizone®, Oglo®, Pioglar®, Pioglu®, Piolet®
10) Guargum - Nosulin®

Exercise

Q1. Write a note on insulin. (Karnataka Univ.)

Q2. What are hypoglycemic agents? Give official preparations of insulin. (Winter 04, Summer 06)

Q3. Enumerate the synthetic hypoglycemic agents with their classification. Draw structure of any one. (Summer 03)

Q4. In what dosage form is the following drug given - Insulin. (Summer 03, May-June 04)

Q6. Give uses of glibenclamide. (Summer 06)

Q7. Give stability and storage conditions of insulin. (Summer 06)

Q8. Define Hypoglycaemic agents. (Summer 06)

Q10. Write short note on - Oral hypoglycemic agents. (May 05, May 07)

Q11. Write the brand name of tolbutamide. (Nov 06)

Q12. Write the structure and use of - phenformin. (Nov. 06)

20 Coagulants and Anticoagulants

Anticoagulants

Drugs are used therapeutically to modify the processes of coagulation and thrombus formation. Prevention of clotting is important during blood transfusions, to avoid thrombosis after operation or from other causes, to prevent recurrent thrombosis in pulmonary embolism and to reduce propagation of clots in coronary arteries. Anticoagulant drugs act at various stages of processes of coagulation viz. (i) At platelet aggregation stage (ii) At clot or fibrin formation stage and (iii) at fibrinolysis stage. The mechanism of blood coagulation can be simplified as follows,

1) Platelets + Damaged tissue $\longrightarrow$ Thromboplastin (Lipoprotein)

2) Thromboplastin + Prothrombin $\xrightarrow{Ca^{++}}$ Thrombin

3) Thrombin + Fibrinogen (Globin protein) $\longrightarrow$ Fibrin (Monomer)

$\downarrow$

Fibrin (Polymer)

$\downarrow$

Clot

The drugs in this category are thought to act by interfering with the formation of prothrombin in liver and thus prolonging the prothrombin time and thereby prolonging the formation of blood clot.

Classification of the anticoagulants

a) Parenteral anticoagulants

Heparin, low molecular weight heparins.

b) Oral anticoagulants

Dicumarol, warfarin, phenindione.

Some of the drugs in this category are as follows,

a) Parental anticoagulants

1) Heparin

Heparin is a polysaccharide composed of an unknown number of sulphated D-glucosamine and D-glucuronic acid units linked through an oxygen bridge. It may be obtained from ox lung or from the intestinal mucosa of oxen, pigs or sheep.

Properties : Heparin sodium occurs as a white or creamy-white, hygroscopic powder. It is freely soluble in water. Aqueous solutions at 25°C and pH 7 to 8 are stable.

Storage : It should be stored in airtight containers.

Mode of action : Its anticoagulant activity is attributed to its strong electronegative charge forming complexes with positively charged sites on proteins. Heparin prevents the clotting of blood *in vivo* and *in vitro,* by acting on all the three stages. Prevention of thrombin formation seems to be its prime mechanism, thus preventing the formation of fibrin monomer and further inhibiting its polymerisation which results into clot.

Actions and uses : Heparin administration in therapeutic doses prolongs the clotting time by 2 to $2^1/_2$ times than normal time. However, anticoagulation response (i.e., prolongation of clotting time) is not related to dose and the dose-response relation is not linear. A major disadvantage of heparin is that it is effective only through parenteral route.

Dose : Heparin is available as sodium or calcium salt. The potency of commercial preparations is in the range of 120-190 units/mg.

- IV infusion dose is 5000 units, followed by 20,000 to 30,000 units a day at the rate of 0.5 unit/kg/minute in isotonic saline.

- Low dose (sub G) prophylactic is 5000 units given every 8-12 hours, starting 1-2 hours before surgery and continued till patient is discharged.

- Heparin should not be used intramuscularly.

Preparations : Heparin sodium injection I.P., B.P.

Brand Names : Beparine® gel, Thrombophob® oint., Hepgel® gel

b) Oral anticoagulants :

1) Dicumarol (Bishydroxycoumarin)

3,3`-Methylene bis (4-hydroxy coumarin)

The first coumarin compound was isolated from natural source - a spoilt sweet clover in 1943-44 and was proved to be the cause in a cattle disease called 'Sweet Clover Disease', which caused severe haemorrhagic tendency. Many chemically related compounds were studied, but only a few were clinically useful. One of them was dicumarol.

Mechanism of action : Unlike heparin, dicumarol has no anticoagulant action *in vitro*. Its action depends on its ability to prolong the prothrombin time by suppressing the synthesis of prothrombin and factors VII, IX and X by liver, by competitive inhibition of carboxylation of the glutamic acid residue by Vitamin K in the liver. Dicumarol increases the plasma anti- thrombin levels.

Uses : It is used alone or along with heparin in the prophylaxis and treatment of intravascular clotting. It is used in postoperative thrombophlebitis, pulmonary embolus and thrombotic occlusion of peripheral arteries and recurrent thrombophlebitis. However, it has no effect on already formed clots, but may prevent further intravascular clotting.

Dose : The dose of dicumarol is determined after the determination of prothrombin clotting time. The dose is usually 200-300 mg initially, then 25-200 mg, once a day, depending on prothrombin time. In contrast to heparin, the onset of action of dicumarol is slow and there is a considerable lag time (24-48 hours) between the time of peak plasma level of coumarins and its therapeutic response as measured by prothrombin time. This is because the coumarins act by preventing the formation of essential clotting factors in liver and do not destroy the already circulating ones.

2) Warfarin sodium

3-(α-Acetonyl benzyl)-4-hydroxy-coumarin sodium.

Properties : Warfarin sodium occurs as an odourless, white crystalline powder, with a slightly bitter taste. It is very soluble in water and in alcohol.

Storage : It should be stored in airtight container, protected from light.

Actions and uses : This compound was first used as rodent poison, especially against rats. Then it became widely used coumarin derivative as anticoagulant and many consider it as drug of choice.

After oral administration, absorption is essentially complete and maximal plasma concentrations are reached in 2 to 12 hours. After an initial dose of 40-50 mg, a good prothrombin time is reached in 36 hours and lasts for another 36 hours. When employed in long term therapy, it takes about 3 days for the prothrombin time to return to normal after the drug is discontinued. Unlike dicumarol, warfarin levels are more steady during therapy.

Warfarin is water soluble and it can be administered by intramuscular or intravenous routes.

Warfarin sodium has been made official in I.P. 1996.

Dose : 5 mg tablet once a day.

- Injections 50 mg of sterile drug powder in vials.

- The drug has cumulative action and the maintenance dose has to be gradually decreased after the first week or so.

Preparations : Warfarin tablets, B.P.

Warfarin sodium tablets, I.P.

Brand Names : Uniwarfin®, Sofarin®, Warf®

Coagulants

1) Menadione

2-Methyl-1, 4-naphthoquinone

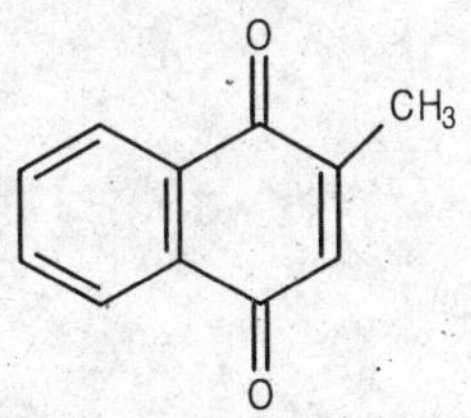

Properties : Menadione is a bright yellow, crystalline powder, nearly odourless. It is greatly affected by light. It is practically insoluble in water, but soluble in oil. Its sodium and diphosphate salts are soluble in water.

Actions and uses : On a mole to mole basis, menadione is equal to vitamin K_1 in activity and can be used as a complete substitute for the vitamin. It is effective orally and also by the IV and IM routes. It is given to patients with biliary obstruction but bile salts or their equivalents have to be given for better absorption. In pre and postoperative jaundice patients, menadione brings about and maintains a normal prothrombin level in the blood.

The activity of dicumarol and related compounds can be reversed by the proper amounts of menadione, and this drug can be used in overdose or toxicity of anticoagulants. Thus in such cases, menadione acts as a coagulant agent.

Dose : Oral and IM 2 to 10 mg a day

Sodium and diphosphate salts - IV and SC 2 mg upto 6 mg a day.

Brand Names : Styptocid®, Styptomet®, Styptorit®, Stypindon®

2) Thrombin

Thrombin is an enzyme which converts human fibrinogen into fibrin. Thrombin is obtained from human plasma. The prothrombin in plasma is converted into thrombin by adding calcium ions and human thromboplastin. The solution is filtered and freeze dried.

Properties : Dried human thrombin occurs as a cream-coloured powder. It is readily soluble in saline solution, forming a cloudy, pale yellow solution. It contains not less than 10 clotting doses per mg.

Storage : It should be stored in an atmosphere of nitrogen, at a temperature below 25°C, protected from light.

Actions and uses : Thrombin is an enzyme with an important role in the clotting process. It is used topically for its haemostatic effect. It is applied as a powder or solution to cuts or injury.

Drugs For Further Study

Anticoagulants

1) Low Molecular Weight Heparin (LMWH) - Clexane®, Clivarine®, Fragmin®
2) Acenocoumarol - Acitrom®
3) Phenindione - Dindevan®

Coagulants

4) Menapthone -Kapilin®
5) Ethamsylate - Alstat®, Clote®, Ethasyl®, Themisylate®
6) Adenochrome monosemicarbazone - Cadisper C®, Styptochrome®
7) Feracrylum -Hemolok®, Sepgard®
8) Aprotinin - Aprotin®, Haemoport®
9) Tranexamic acid - Capitra X®, Dubatran®, Menogia®, Pause®

Exercise

Q1. Explain the phenomenon of blood coagulation. What different drugs are used as coagulants. (Kachchh Univ. 06, Nov 06)

Q2. What are coagulants and anticoagulants? Give suitable examples of each. Draw structure of menadione. (Winter 04, Summer 03)

Q3. In what dosage forms is 'warfarin' administered? (Summer 06)

Q4. Give stability and storage conditions of - thrombin. (Summer 06)

Q5. Explain the phenomenon of blood coagulation. What different drugs are used as coagulants. (May 05)

Q6. Write short note on coagulants and anticoagulants. (May-June 04, May 07, Summer 06)

Q7. Write the structure and use of menadione. (Nov 06)

■

21 Local Anesthetics

Introduction

Local anesthetics are drugs which when applied directly to peripheral nervous tissues, block nerve conduction and abolish all sensations in the part supplied by the nerve. They are generally applied to somatic nerves and are capable of acting on axons, cellbody and synapses.

General Properties

Synthetic local anesthetic drugs have many properties in common. They possess various degrees of water and lipoidal solubility. Since the nervous tissue is rich in lipid, lipoidal solubilities are essential for drug penetration in the neuronal fibre, while water solubility helps to get the drug to the site of action. An effective local anesthetic, therefore, must contain hydrophilic amino group, an intermediate chain and a lipophilic aromatic group.

Thus, a generalised structure would be as follows

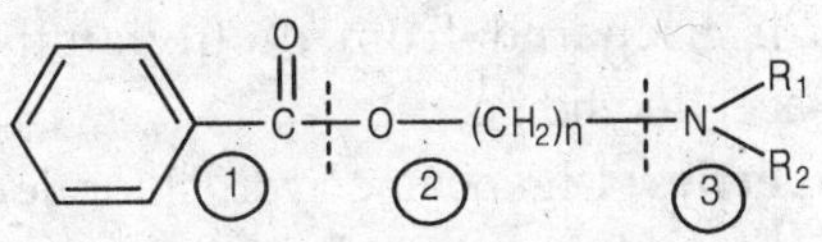

1 - Lipophilic part, 2 - Intermediate chain, 3 - Hydrophilic part

Majority of the clinically useful local anesthetic drugs fall in the above class.

A few drugs of this class will be discussed in this chapter.

Classification of Local Anesthetics

Local anesthetic drugs can be classified as follows,

I] Natural products

eg. cocaine

II] Synthetic compounds

i) Benzoic acid derivatives : eg. hexylcaine, isobucaine

ii) Para-amino benzoic acid derivatives : eg. benzocaine, procaine

iii) Meta-amino benzoic acid derivatives : eg. orthoform

iv) Amides : eg. lidocaine, dibucaine

v) Urethanes : eg. diperodon

vi) Miscellaneous compounds : eg. pramoxin, cincocaine, benzyl alcohol, propanediol.

III] Miscellaneous drugs with local action

eg. clove oil, phenol

1) Benzocaine

Ethyl p-aminobenzoate.

Benzocaine belongs to the p-aminobenzoic acid class.

Properties : It is a white, odourless, crystalline powder with a bitter taste. It is very slightly soluble in water; freely soluble in alcohol, ether and chloroform.

Storage : It should be stored in airtight containers, protected from light.

Actions and uses : Benzocaine is used for its local anesthetic action in powders, upto

20 per cent in ointment and upto 20 per cent in suppositories for various types of surface pain and itching. It is used in throat lozenges and in ulcerative conditions of digestive tract. Often it is used orally to prevent nausea and vomiting alongwith compounds such as aminophylline.

Dose : Benzocaine cream/ointment of -1 to 20 per cent in ointment or cream base.

Preparations : Benzocaine lozenges, B.P.C. Compound benzocaine lozenges, B.P.C.

Brand Names : Chloromycetin® ear drops, Zoken® gel

2) Procaine hydrochloride

2-(Diethyl amino ethyl)-p-amino benzoate hydrochloride.

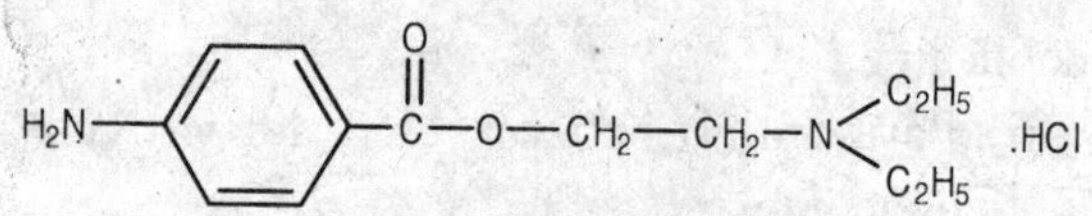

Procaine is one of the oldest and most widely used local anesthetic agents, developed in 1906.

Properties : It occurs as odourless, colourless, crystals or white crystalline powder with salty, bitter taste. It is very soluble in water and soluble in alcohol.

Stability : Procaine is most stable at pH 3.6 and gradually becomes less stable with increase in pH. It was found that slightly alkaline solutions of procaine had some advantage over acidic solutions. However, alkaline solutions were not stable and could not be sterilised. Procaine molecule is subject to hydrolytic decomposition, further the products may be readily oxidised. To overcome this weakness of the molecule an amide-procainamide was made which was much more resistant to hydrolysis and proved to be longer acting.

Storage : It should be protected from light.

Actions and uses : Procaine is not absorbed through intact skin or mucous membrane. It was first used intravenously in 1940, and since then it is being administred by that route for puritis associated with jaundice, for pain due to burns, arthritis and many other conditions. To prolong its activity, adrenaline may be added to constrict blood vessels. When used with penicillin, it forms a procaine-penicillin salt, which helps penicillin to act for a longer time. Procaine is also used to form a sparingly soluble salt of heparin.

Dose : Procaine hydrochloride injection, 25 ml of 1.5 per cent solution upto 200 ml of 0.25 to 0.5 per cent solution. For peripheral nerve block upto 2 ml of 2 per cent solution. For spinal block 1 to 3 ml of 3.3 to 5 per cent solution.

- Procaine + propoxycaine - for Dental use
- Procaine + tetracaine - for Dental use

Preparations : Procaine and adrenaline injection I.P., B.P.

3) Lignocaine (Lidocaine)

2-Diethylamino-2`,6'-acetoxylidide hydrochloride

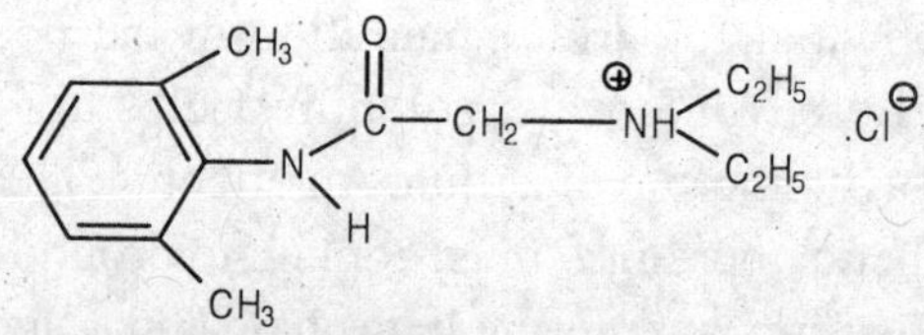

Lignocaine belongs to the amide class of local anesthetics. This is an anilide of 2,6-Dimethylaniline and N,N-diethylglycine. This amide is prepared from diethylamine and chloro-acetyl-xylidide.

Properties : Lignocaine hydrochloride occurs as a white, crystalline powder. It is odourless and has a slightly bitter taste followed by numbing. It is very soluble in water, freely soluble in alcohol and insoluble in ether. It has a pKa of 7.9.

Stability : The free base, an amide is a stable solid, it is most stable among all other local anesthetics. Because of this stability, it can also be autoclaved and therefore lidocaine is the most frequently used local anesthetic. This unusual stability of lidocaine is due to its two methyl groups and ortho to amide linkage. It does not degrade by oxidation.

Incompatibility : Lignocaine base may be precipitated by alkaline solutions.

Actions and uses : It has a quick onset, and high degree of penetration and is twice as potent as procaine. It is also an excellent surface anesthetic. Following an infiltration of 0.25 to 0.5 per cent solution, the duration of action varies from 30 to 60 minutes. Addition of adrenaline prolongs the action for about 2 hours. It is also widely used in dentistry, at 5 per cent concentration in ointment, with polyethylene glycol as base. The drug is recommended for topical use, nerve blocks, infiltration and epidural injection and dental anesthesia.

Dose : Lidocaine ointment for topical use 2.5 to 5 per cent.

- Lidocaine HCl, injection for epidural anesthesia, 10 to 30 ml of 1 per cent solution.

- For infiltration 2 to 60 ml of 0.5 per cent solution.

- For peripheral nerve block 1 to 20 ml of 1 per cent solution.

Preparations : Lignocaine hydrochloride injection, I.P., B.P.

Lignocaine and adrenaline injection, I.P., B.P.

Lignocaine gel, B.P.C.

Brand Names : Xylocaine® oint., Gesicain® inj., Ressocaine® inj, Lignox®

Drugs For Further Study

Bupivacaine - Anawin®, Bupivan®, Sensorcaine®.

Exercise

Q1. Define and classify local anaesthetics with examples. (Karnataka Univ.)

Q2. Give uses of benzocaine. (Winter 04)

Q3. Mention the local anaesthetic drug from "Ester derivatives" with its structure, chemical name and official preparations. (Summer 03)

Q4. Define the following term - Local anaesthetics. (Summer 06)

Q5. Write structure of procaine and state how lignocaine is superior to procaine. (Summer 06)

Q6. What is 'anaesthesia'? Distinguish between general anaesthetics and local anaesthetics. Give stability and storage conditions of diethyl ether. (Summer 06, Nov. 06)

Q7. Explain the following term - IV anaesthetics. (Summer 06)

Q8. Write note on - General anaesthetics. (May-June 04)

Q9. Define anaesthesia, classify general anaesthetics, write atleast one structure from each class. (May 07)

Q10. Write note on - Local anaesthetics. (May 07)

Q11. Answer the following - Name one local anesthetic having an anilide structure. (Nov. 06)

Q12. Write the structure and use of the following - lignocaine. (Nov. 06)

22 Histamine and Antihistaminic Agents

Histamine

Histamine (β-imidazolylethylamine) was discovered in 1907, and was found to be wide spread in nature. It is found in ergot and many other plants. It is also present in many organs and tissues of the human body. Histidine, a naturally occurring amino acid, when decarboxylated, forms histamine and thus may be the source of histamine in the body.

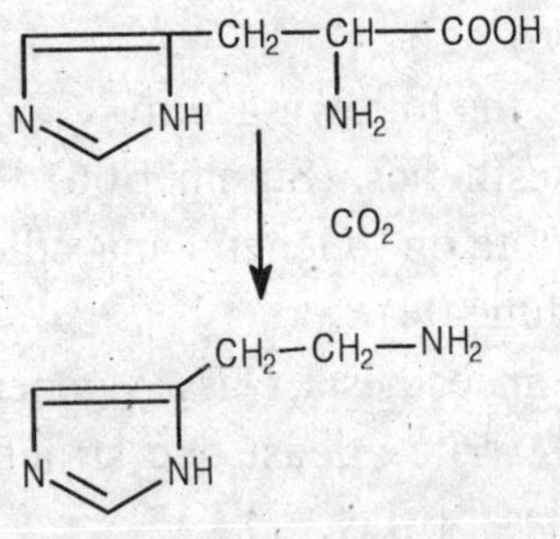

The actions of histamine are mediated by two types of receptors H_1 and H_2. Histamine causes a wide variety of physiological responses, almost every tissue is affected by it. Some of the important physiological reactions are as follows :

i) It produces a strong vasodilation of capillaries.

ii) High doses may even affect permeability, leading to oedema.

iii) It acts on smooth muscles in lungs, producing bronchial constriction.

iv) It has a stimulatory action on certain excretory glands such as lacrimal and nasal, causing increased secretions.

v) Allergic responses : It has been established that histamine plays an important part in human allergy. There are many substances in food and in nature (eg. pollens) which cause symptoms of allergy similar to histamine. These substances are often called as 'histamine - like substances' and their response is similar to many allergic manifestations.

The above effects are mediated by H_1 receptors. H_2 receptor stimulation leads to increased acid secretion in the stomach.

Histamine has little use as remedial agent. The main use of histamine is to diagnose impairment of acid producing cells of the stomach. Normally, histamine is a powerful stimulant, thus if acid is absent even after the injection of histamine, it is considered as proof that acid producing glands are not functioning. Another use of histamine is in what is called "wheal test", which is a diagnostic test for local circulation in which histamine is injected intradermally. In normal subjects a reddish spot "wheal", appears on the skin within about 2.5 minutes, a delay is considered to be a sign of vascular disease.

Preparations and doses

i) Histamine phosphate - Dose 10-40 mcg per kg, SC or IM. Histamine acid phosphate injection, I.P.

ii) Betazole hydrochloride (Histalog) - Dose 40-60 mg, IM or SC.

Brand Names : Algipan®, Histaglobulin®

Antihistaminic Agents

An obvious approach to counter histamine-caused reactions is to develop an antihistamine substance. The origin of antihistamine research dates back to 1937, when sympathomimetic and sympatholytic substances were tried, to block the actions of histamine. Some of the alkyl aromatic amines (sympathomimetic) showed good promise, especially a series of phenylethylenediamines had good activity. Many antihistaminics were then developed and more active antihistaminics had the following general structure

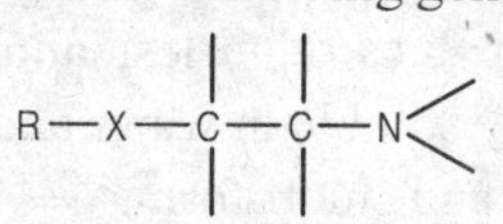

and they all fall in three chemical categories

when X = 0, it was Ethanolamine group (eg. diphenhydramine)

when X = N, it was Ethylenediamine group (eg. mepyramine) and,

when X = C, it was Propylamine (alkylamine) group (eg. chlorpheniramine)

The main therapeutic uses of antihistaminic drugs are,

i) To suppress allergic disorders like pollinosis and urticaria.

ii) In the treatment of seasonal hay fever, to reduce sneezing and rhinorrhoea.

iii) To counteract pruritis and urticaria in atopic and contact dermatitis and that induced by other drugs and chemicals.

iv) In the treatment of Parkinsonism (eg. Diphenhydramine).

v) In the treatment of motion sickness (only a few drugs like Avomine).

The classical antihistamines are H_1 antagonists while H_2 receptor blockers are used as antiulcer drugs eg. cimetidine.

Classification of Antihistaminic Drugs

I] Ethanolamines (aminoalkyl ethers) - Diphenhydramine, doxylamine

II] Ethylenediamines - Tripelennamine, pyrilamine

III] Propylamines - Pheniramine, chlorpheniramine

IV] Piperazines (cyclizines) - Cyclizine, chlorcyclizine

V] Phenothiazines - Promethazine, trimeprazine

VI] Dibenzocycloheptenes - Cyproheptadine, azatadine

VII] Miscellaneous (second generation antihistaminics) - Fexofenadine, loratadine, cetirizine, acrivastine

I] Ethanolamine derivatives

1) Diphenhydramine hydrochloride

2-(Diphenylmethoxy)-N,N-dimethylethanamine hydrochloride

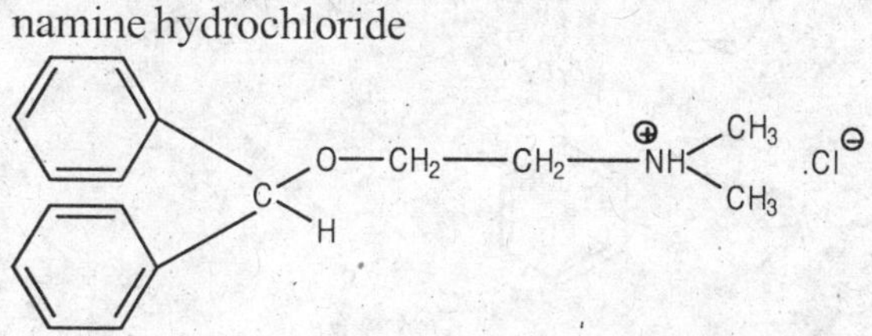

Properties : It is an odourless white, crystalline powder, soluble in water (1:1) or alcohol (1:2), having a bitter taste. The drug has a pKa of 9, and 1 per cent aqueous solution has a pH of 5.

Storage : It should be stored in airtight containers, protected from light.

Actions and uses : Diphenhydramine is recommended in various allergic conditions. It is also of some help in parkinsonism. It is used orally or intravenously in the treatment of urticaria, hay fever, bronchial asthma. The most common side effect is drowsiness. It is found to be useful in the treatment of common cold as a constituent of cough mixtures.

Dose : 50 to 200 mg a day, in divided doses.

Preparations : Diphenhydramine capsules, I.P., B.P.

Diphenhydramine elixir B.P.C.

Brand Names : Benadryl® syrup, Bronolax® syrup, Abcof® syrup.

II] Ethylenediamine derivatives

The first compound of ethylenediamine series was N'-phenyl-N'ethyl, N,N-dimethylethylenediamine.

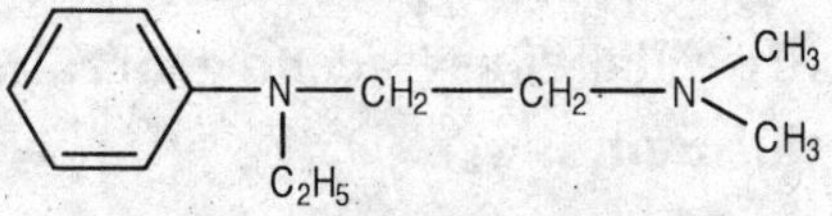

This was found to be toxic and could not be used clinically. Later on N- ethyl group was replaced by benzyl group, which gave the first drug of this series namely, Antergan

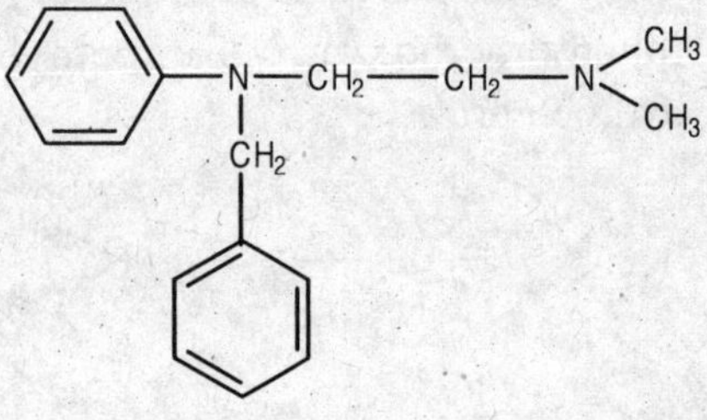

Later on the phenyl ring was replaced by pyridine ring and Tripelennamine was born.

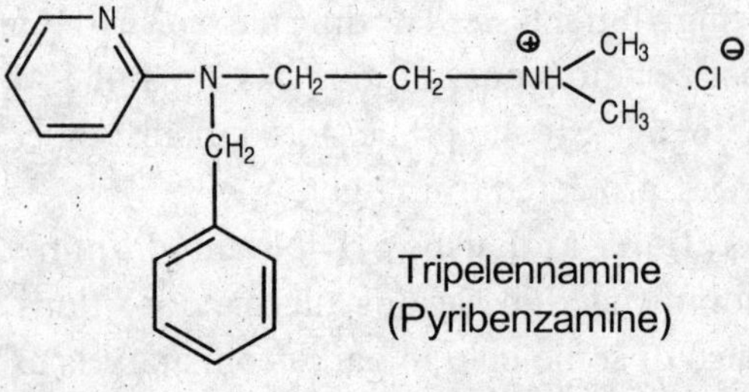

Tripelennamine (Pyribenzamine)

1) Mepyramine maleate

(Pyrilamine maleate)

2-(N-p-anisyl-N-2-pyridylamino) ethyldimethylamine hydrogen maleate

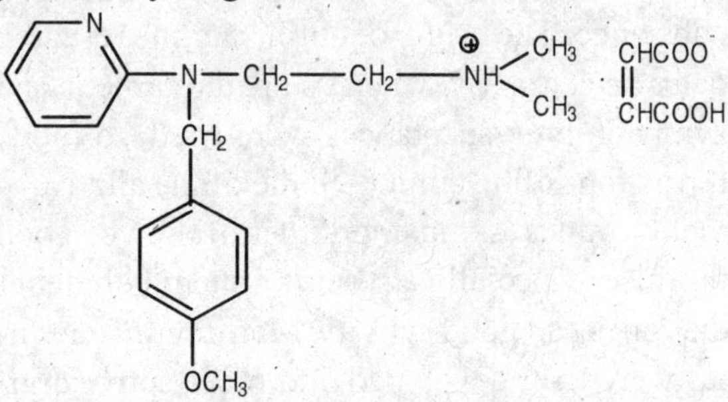

Properties : It occurs as a white or creamy white powder. It is odourless and has a bitter taste. It is very soluble in water and freely soluble in alcohol and chloroform.

Actions and uses : Mepyramine is a similar drug of the same series having similar actions as tripelennamine or methapyrilene. Drugs in this series are clinically better than diphenhydramine and have less side effects. They are also well absorbed orally in a dose of 50 mg per day. It is useful in treating hay fever, but not asthma, atopic dermatitis or eczema.

Dose : 50 mg, 4 times a day

Preparations : Mepyramine tablets, I.P., B.P.

Mepyramine elixir, B.P.C.

Mepyramine injection, B.P.

Brand Names : Histadyl®, Benadryl®

III] Propylamine (alkylamine) derivatives

1) Pheniramine maleate and Chlorpheniramine maleate

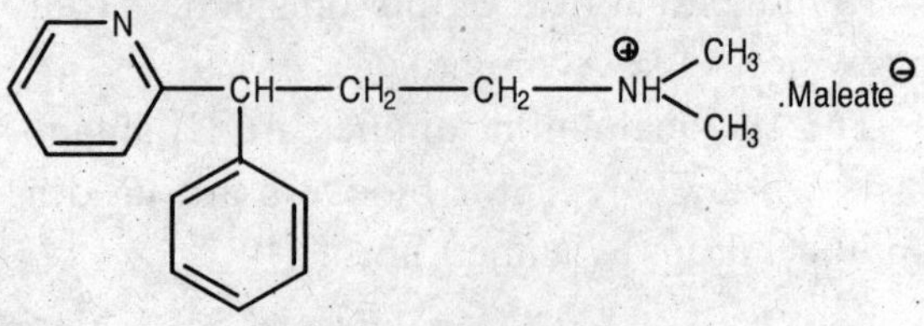

Pheniramine maleate

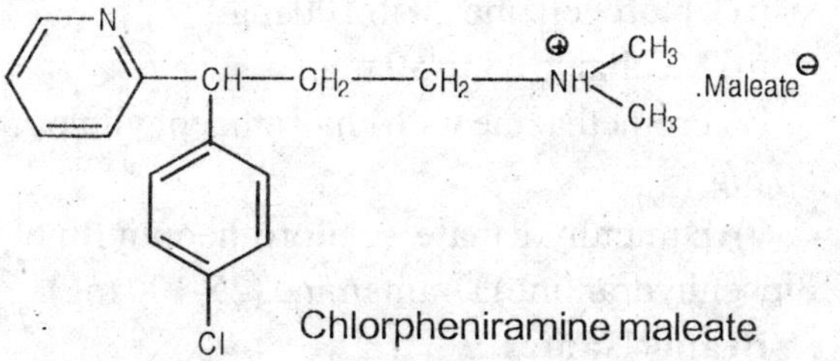

Chlorpheniramine maleate

Properties : Pheniramine maleate occurs as a white crystalline powder with a faint amine-like odour. It is freely soluble in water, very soluble in alcohol. Chlorpheniramine maleate occurs as a white crystalline odourless powder with a bitter taste. It is freely soluble in water and in alcohol.

Actions and uses : In general, compounds of this series are not as potent as those of ethylenediamine series, but they have low toxicity and lower degree of side effects. In chlorpheniramine, activity is increased 20 times because of the chlorine group but there is no lowering of toxicity. Chlorpheniramine has a therapeutic index of 50, as compared to 1 for tripelennamine and 4 for pheniramine.

Dose : Pheniramine - 20-40 mg, 3 times a day.

Chlorpheniramine - 12-40 mg a day, Parenteral 10-20 mg

Preparations : Pheniramine tablets, I.P.

Pheniramine maleate injection, I.P.

Chlorpheniramine tablets, I.P., B.P.

Chlorpheniramine injection, B.P.

Brand Names : Pheniramine - Avil®

Chlorpheniramine - Febrex plus®, Fendyl® Lintus, Cadistin®, Polaramine®

2) Promethazine

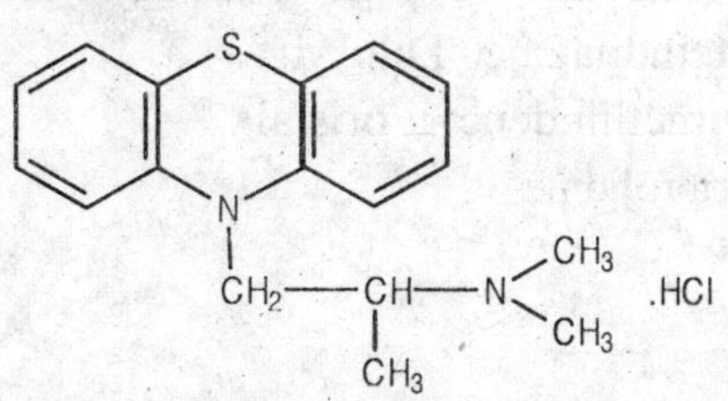

Promethazine is official in I.P. as the hydrochloride and theoclate salts.

Properties : Promethazine hydrochloride occurs as a white or faintly yellow, crystalline powder. It is odourless and has a bitter taste. It is very soluble in water; freely soluble in alcohol.

Stability : The drug is degraded in aqueous solution by heat and light. Degradation is more rapid in the presence of air. Micelle formation decreases the degradation rate.

Storage : It should be stored in airtight containers, protected from light.

Actions and uses : Promethazine is a phenothiazine derivative. When the distance between the two nitrogens is reduced to two carbon atoms, the phenothiazine molecule loses its tranquilising properties and its antihistaminic properties begin to appear. This drug is such an example, where slight modification of this side chain led to an antihistaminic compound. In addition to antihistaminic properties, it also has antiemetic effect, a tranquilising action and a potentiating action on analgesic and sedative drugs. It is 7 times more potent than other antihistaminic drugs and has approximately 3 times the duration of action. One single dose given at night is enough to control symptoms in the majority of cases. It has the usual side effect of drowsiness, but this actually becomes an advantage, when the drug is taken at bedtime.

Dose : 20 to 50 mg a day.

Other drugs of the phenothiazine series having antihistaminic properties are pyrathiazine, trimeprazine and methdilazine.

Preparations : Promethazine tablets, I.P., B.P.

Promethazine syrup, I.P.

Promethazine elixir, B.P.C.

Promethazine hydrochloride injection, B.P.

Brand Names : Phenergan®, Avomine®, Phensedyl® expectorants

3) Cyproheptadine hydrochloride

(Periactin)

4(5H-dibenzo(a,d)cyclohepten-5-ylidene)-1-methylpiperidine hydrochloride.

Properties : It occurs as a white to slightly yellow, crystalline powder. It is almost odourless and has a slightly bitter taste. It is slightly soluble in water, sparingly soluble in alcohol and freely soluble in methanol.

Storage : It should be stored in airtight containers.

Actions and uses : This compound possesses both antihistaminic and antiserotonin activities. Its antihistaminic activity is comparable to chlorpheniramine in potency and duration. This drug, although an antihistaminic, has been used to stimulate appetite in children.

Dose : 4 mg, 3 to 4 times a day; syrup or tablets.

Preparations : Cyproheptadine hydrochloride syrup I.P,

Cyproheptadine tablets, I.P., B.P.

Brand Names : Apitol®, Cedel® syrup, Ciplatin®

4) Antiemetic Drugs (for motion sickness)

Some of the antihistaminic drugs, especially those of the piperazine derivatives series, have in addition to antihistaminic property, antiemetic activity, for which these drugs are used as remedy for motion sickness during long journeys by train, bus or plane.

Dose : Some of the common drugs used for motion sickness and their daily doses are

i) Cyclizine 50 to 200 mg.

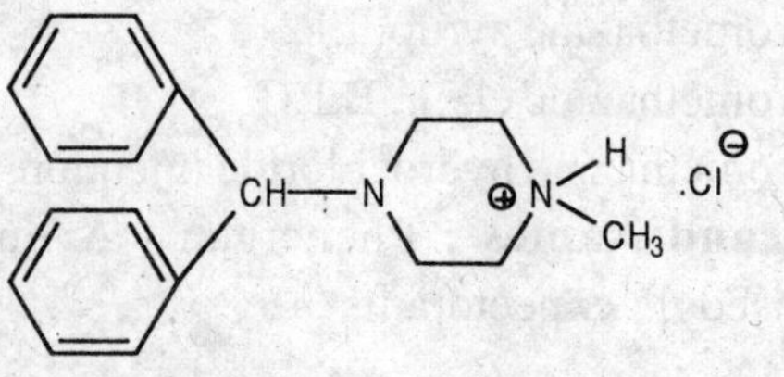

ii) Chlorcyclizine 20 to 100 mg.

iii) Meclizine 25 to 50 mg.

iv) Promethazine with chlorotheophylline 25-50 mg.

v) Dimenhydrinate (Chlorotheophylline + diphenhydramine) Dramamine (25-100 mg).

Brand Names :

Meclizine - Diligan®, PNV®, Pregnidoxin®

Promethazine with chlorotheophylline - Avomine®

Dimenhydrinate - Draminate®, Gravol®

Drugs For Further Study

Non-sedative antihistaminics -

1) Astemizole - Acipax®, Histalong®, Minastem®, Stemiz®
2) Cetirizine - Alday®, Alerid®, Cetiriz®, Cetrine®
3) Levocetirizine - Alertriz®, Histachek®, Levocet®, Levorid®
4) Loratadine - Loridin®, Lormeg®, Roletra®, Tirlor®
5) Desloratadine - Delorta®, Deslor®, Loreta®, Neoloridin®
6) Terfenadine - Terdane®, Terfed®, Trexyl®, Zenad®
7) Fexofenadine - Alernex®, Allegix®, Altiva®, Fexo®
8) Ebastine - Ebast®, Erostin®
9) Mizolastine - Zehist®

Sedative antihistaminics -

10) Azatadine - Zadine®
11) Hydroxyzine - Atarax®, Hydil®, PRV®
12) Clemastine - Clamist®, Tavegyl®
13) Methdilazine - Dilosyn®
14) Dimethindene - Foristal®
15) Triprolidine

Exercise

Q1. Define and classify antihistaminic agents with suitable examples. Give any one structure of drug from each class. (Kachchh Univ. 06, May 05)

Q2. Classify antihistaminic drugs with examples. Write the structure and chemical name of diphenhydramine and chlorpheniramine. Add a note on histamine. (Karnataka Univ.)

Q3. What are antihistamines? Give properties, structure and uses of an aminoalkylether type of antihistamines. (Winter 04)

Q4. Define antihistamines with suitable examples of drugs. (Summer 03)

Q5. Define the term 'Allergy'. Give structure, chemical name and physiological actions of histamine. (Summer 06)

Q6. Explain 'Allergy' with suitable examples. (May-June 04)

Q7. What is allergy? Write physiological action of histamine and classify antihistaminic agents with example. (May 07)

Q8. Write short note on - H_1-receptor antagonists. (Nov 06)

■

23 Narcotic Analgesics

Introduction

Struggle of mankind to relieve pain is as old as mankind itself. Ancient literature and writings are full of serious and fanciful remedies to relieve pain. The pain itself is an unpleasant sensation only the individual who is suffering from it can experience. As a symptom, pain demands instant relief; and in practice, dramatic relief of pain by drugs is highly impressive.

An analgesic may be defined as a drug bringing about insensibility to pain without loss of consciousness. The search for pain-killers, was going on from very early times. Thus, the analgesic activity of morphine was discovered as early as in 1806. Then other man-made analgesic drugs followed, such as acetanilide (1886), phenacetin (1887) and aspirin (1899). The analgesics can be considered in two groups, viz.

1) Morphine and related compounds such as codeine, pethidine and methadone. These are the narcotic analgesics.

2) Antipyretic analgesics such as aspirin, paracetamol, analgin etc. (discussed in chapter 24)

1) Morphine

Morphine is the most important alkaloid of opium and is used as sulphate or hydrochloride. Opium itself is the dried milky exudate obtained by incising the unripe capsule of the poppy plant *Papaver somniferum*. The poppy seeds, however have no pharmacological properties. On drying in the air, the exudate forms a gummy brownish mass. Morphine occurs in opium to the extent of 9 to 14 per cent. It is isolated by various methods, of which the final step is usually the precipitation of morphine from an acid solution by using excess of ammonia. The precipitated morphine is then recrystallised from alcohol.

Properties : The free alkaloid occurs as a laevorotatory, odourless, white, needle-like crystals possessing a bitter taste. It is almost insoluble in water, ether or chloroform. But is somewhat soluble in ethyl alcohol (1:210) at boiling point. Because of its phenolic hydroxy group, it is readily soluble in alkalis. Morphine is a monoacidic base and readily forms water-soluble salts with most acids. Because morphine is poorly soluble in water, its salts are used in clinical

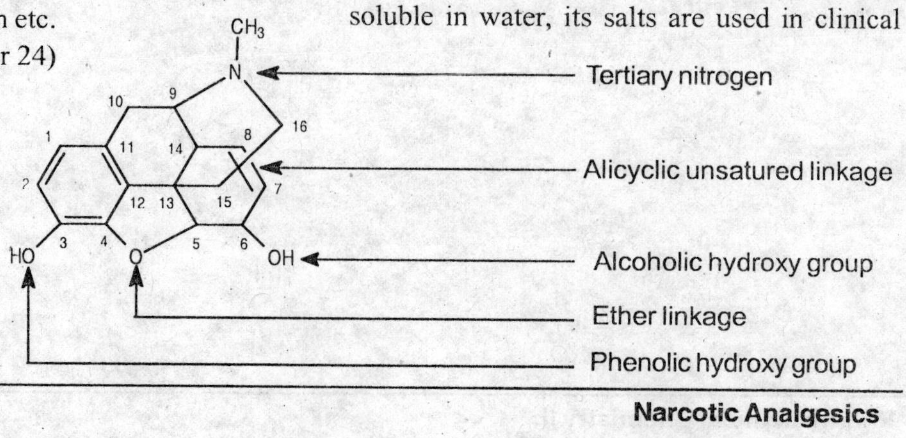

practice. The most preferred salt forms are the sulphate and sometimes hydrochloride and rarely as acetate for some special use (like liquid antitussive formulations).

Therapeutic uses and actions :

1) For relief of pain : Morphine is one of the most powerful analgesics and is able to relieve pain of the highest order, like acute myocardial infarction, fractures of longer bones, amputation of limbs during accidents, pain in renal and biliary cells.

2) For sedation and sleep : Morphine is a valuable sedative in the presence of pain.

3) As preanesthetic medication especially in major surgery.

4) In acute left ventricular failure : Morphine is valuable in the treatment of acute ventricular failure and pulmonary edema.

5) To produce constipation : Tincture opium (0.5 to 1 ml) and paregoric are now rarely used for symptomatic relief of severe diarrhoea, other derivatives of morphine especially diphenoxylate hydrochloride, are more useful and other side effects of morphine are avoided.

6) To suppress cough of the intense order : Although morphine is not recommended for suppressing cough of the intense order, because of its many disadvantages; in the doses of 1 to 3 mg per kg, it is very effective. In the good old days, oil of poppy seeds roasted on fire, was given in small doses along with a spoonful of honey to depress 'whooping cough'.

Adverse reactions of morphine and precautions :

1) Drug dependence : Morphine produces addiction very quickly, which results mainly from its euphoric effects. Morphine addiction is now a world wide problem and many organisations, including W.H.O., are vigorously engaged to resolve this problem. The withdrawal symptoms appear after 6 to 12 hours of abstinence and are so severe that an addict is unable to withstand it without a further dose. This physical dependence has perpetrated the problem of addiction liability of morphine.

2) Tolerance : Repeated administration of morphine results in the development of tolerance.

3) Respiratory depression : Morphine poisoning is characterised by respiratory depression which ultimately results in death.

4) Hypotension : Morphine occasionally produces hypotension as a result of peripheral vasodilation.

5) Other side effects : pinpoint pupils, reduced body temperature, urinary retention, dryness of mouth, mental disorientation, vertigo and tremors.

Dose : As analgesic, 15 to 20 mg.

Preparations : Morphine injection, I.P., B.P.

Morphine and atropine injection, I.P., B.P.C.

Ammonium chloride and morphine mixture, B.P.C.

Chloroform and morphine tincture, B.P.

Kaolin and morphine mixture, B.P.C.

Morphine suppositories, B.P.C.

Brand Names : M-Eslon®, Morcontin®, Duramor®

Morphine antagonists : To counteract acute morphine poisoning and its very serious side effects (sometime fatal), some semi-synthetic congeners of morphine, which have a very close similarity to the morphine structure have been developed. One such morphine antagonist is Nalorphine (N-allyl normorphine), in which N-methyl group of morphine, has been replaced by an allyl group as follows :

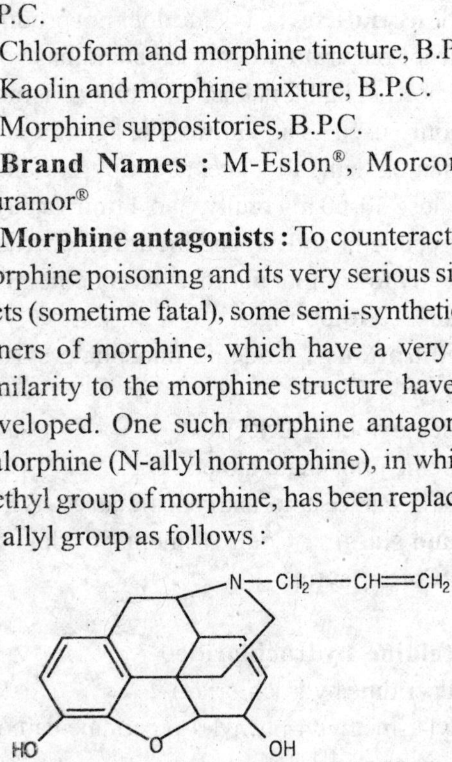

Other morphine antagonists are Naloxone,

Levallorphan, Cyclazocine and Naltrexone.

2) Codeine

3-O-methyl morphine.

Codeine is an alkaloid which occurs naturally in opium, but the amount is so small (0.5 to 2 per cent) that it is of no commercial value. Most of the codeine is, therefore, produced by methylating the phenolic hydroxy group of morphine. This small change in structure makes morphine lose its analgesic activity and codeine is only one tenth as active as morphine in analgesic power.

Properties : Codeine phosphate occurs as small colourless crystals or white crystalline powder. It is odourless and has a bitter taste. It is laevorotatory. It is freely soluble in water while the free base is slightly soluble in water.

Storage : It should be stored in airtight containers, protected from light.

Actions and uses : Codeine does not produce significant respiratory depression and has very low (almost negligible) addiction liability. It is most commonly used as an antitussive agent and in combination with salicylates as antipyretic analgesic (dose 30-60 mg orally, 3 to 4 times a day). Dihydrocodeine and oxycodone are other drugs, used orally for similar purposes as codeine.

Dose : 10 to 60 mg.

Preparations : Codeine phosphate syrup, I.P., B.P.C.

Codeine linctus, B.P.C.

Codeine phosphate tablets, B.P.

Aspirin, Paracetamol and codeine tablets, B.P.C.

Brand Names : Codin® Linctus, Codokuff® syrup, Corex® syrup

3) Pethidine hydrochloride

(Meperidine hydrochloride)

Ethyl-1-methyl-4-phenyl-4-piperidine-carboxylate hydrochloride

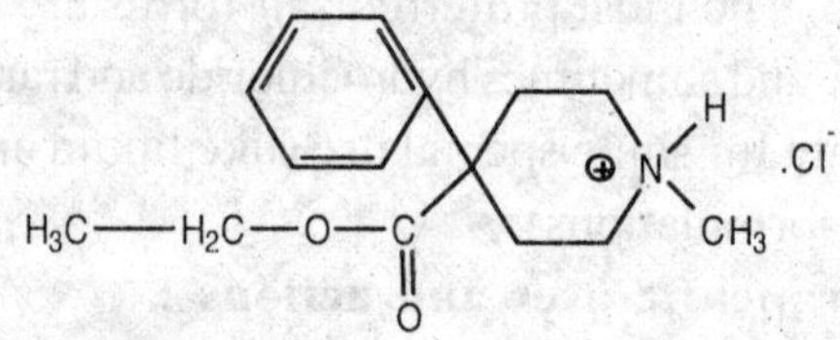

Other pethidine derivatives are piminodine, phenoperidine, fentanyl, anileridine, alphaprodine etc.

In 1938, two scientists named Eisleb and Schaumann reported that a simple piperidine derivative, which came to be known as meperidine, possessed analgesic activity. The compound showed a peculiar erection of tail of mice called as Straub reaction which was characteristic of morphine. The compound was then tested for analgesic properties and was found to be about one fifth as active as morphine. This discovery not only opened a new era of synthetic analgesic drugs, but stimulated research activity in the area of analgesic compounds.

Properties : Pethidine hydrochloride occurs as an odourless, white, crystalline powder with a slightly acidic and bitter taste. It is soluble in water and alcohol.

Therapeutic uses and actions : Pethidine has analgesic, sedative, spasmolytic and local anesthetic actions.

1) Pethidine is about 1/5th as potent as morphine and is useful as analgesic in the majority of cases for which morphine and other opium alkaloids are indicated. But it is especially of value where the pain is due to spasms of intenstine, uterus, bladder and bronchi. It was first discovered as antispasmodic. It is also useful in pains of myocardial infarction, burns and in obsterical gynaecology operations.

2) As a preanesthetic medication in all major surgeries.

3) However, like morphine, pethidine also has addiction liability.

4) Pethidine also affects respiration rate and can cause respiratory depression.

5) It also causes hypotension due to peripherial vasodilation.

6) Pethidine however, is devoid of antitussive activity. but like morphine reduces urinary output.

Dose : 50 to 100 mg by mouth or by SC or IM injection

Preparations : Pethidine injection, I.P., B.P., Pethidine tablets, I.P., B.P.

4) Methadone hydrochloride

6-(Dimethylamino)-4, 4-diphenyl-3-heptanone hydrochloride

Properties : It occurs as odourless, colourless crystals or white crystalline powder with a bitter taste. It is soluble in water and chloroform and freely soluble in alcohol.

Actions and uses : Synthesis of methadone and its analgesic activity proved yet another departure from pethidine structure. It proved that piperidine ring was after all not necessary for the analgesic activity and as long as (even) the aliphatic chain takes the conformation of a cyclic ring (piperidine), the activity will be retained. This is what exactly happened with methadone, which had analgesic activity twice that of morphine and nearly 10 times that of meperidine.

Methadone is a very effective analgesic used to alleviate many types of pains. It produces less sedation and narcosis than morphine and is therefore useful in chronic pains. It has recently found use in the treatment of addiction. It is used as a substitute for morphine and pethidine in the treatment of opioid withdrawal symptoms. However, it has all the drawbacks of morphine and pethidine, like tolerance, addiction liability, dry mouth, dizziness, constipation and mental clouding. Its antitussive property is comparable to morphine, but codeine is preferred for this use.

Dose : IM and SC 2.5 to 10 mg, 6 to 8 times a day, upto 15-50 mg a day for analgesic action.

Oral : 5 to 10 mg, every 4 hours.

Preparations : Methadone injection, I.P., B.P.
Methadone tablets, I.P., B.P.
Methadone linctus, B.P.C.

5) Dextropropoxyphene hydrochloride

(+)-4-Dimethylamino-3-methyl-1,2-diphenylbut-2-yl propionate hydrochloride.

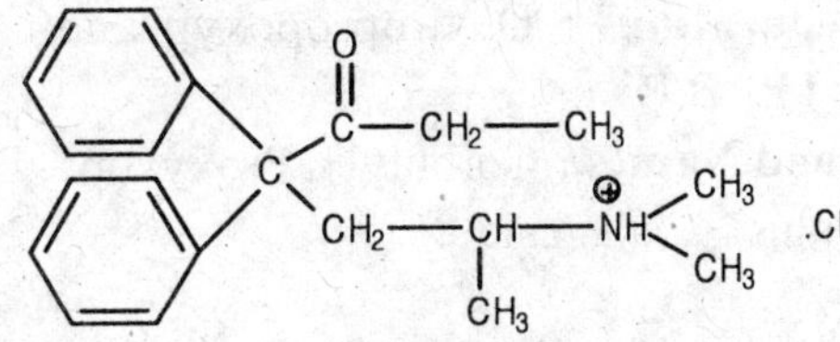

Methadone HCl

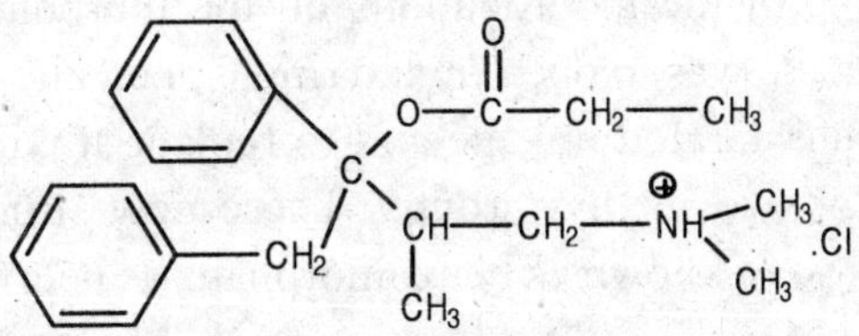

Dextropropoxyphene HCl

Properties : Dextropropoxyphene hydrochloride occurs as a white or slightly yellow, odourless powder with a bitter taste. It is very soluble in water, freely soluble in alcohol and practically insoluble in ether. It is dextrorotatory. The napsylate salt is very slightly soluble in water.

Storage : It should be stored in airtight containers.

Actions and uses : Success of methadone led to further modifications of its structure, but all the modifications did not yield active compounds. One such compound is dextropropoxyphene (d-propoxyphene), which had negligible analgesic properties, almost equal to codeine. The similarity of the structures between methadone and d-propoxyphene can be seen above.

Dextropropoxyphene is orally active in a dose of 30 to 60 mg upto 65 mg. As an analgesic, it is only half as active as codeine and is almost comparable to aspirin (65 mg of d-propoxyphene

- 650 mg of aspirin). It is, therefore, often combined with aspirin for treatment of simple pains like headache, bodyache, etc. It cannot produce euphoria, but has a low degree of addiction liability. It has no antitussive property. It produces mild sedation, but has less other side effects associated with other narcotic analgesics.

Dose : 30 to 60 mg.

Preparations : Dextropropoxyphene capsules, I.P., B.P.

Brand Names : Corbutyl®, Proxyvon®, Dolopar plus®, Walagesic®

6) Pentazocine

One of the modifications on the morphine molecule was to open up the ring C, i.e., alicyclic unsaturated linkage and to replace it with one or two methyl groups. These new structures were known as benzomorphans as below,

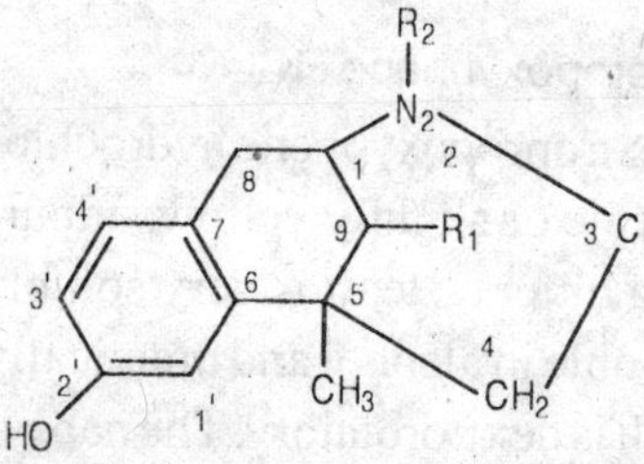

Benzomorphan

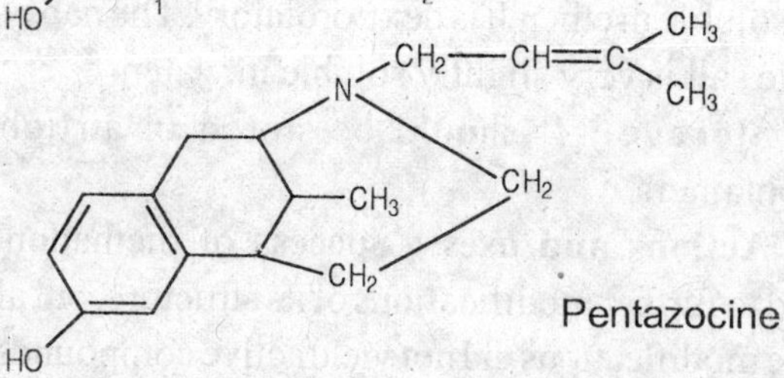

Pentazocine

Properties : It occurs as an odourless, white or creamy-white powder. It is very slightly soluble in water while the hydrochloride salt is soluble in water and in alcohol.

Storage : It should be protected from light.

Actions and uses : Pentazocine is a drug of benzomorphan type. It is a narcotic antagonist. Pentazocine in a parenteral dose of 30 mg or an oral dose of 50 mg is about as effective as 10 mg of morphine. It is believed that (-) isomer is more active as analgesic agent. At a lower dose, the drug seems to be well tolerated with some degree of sedation. The incidence of morphine-like side effects are as high as with morphine for pentazocine also. Pentazocine gives same or slightly greater respiratory depression than morphine, but has less addiction liability and causes almost no euphoria. It, however, precipitates the action of other narcotic analgesics. Unlike morphine, it raises the systemic and pulmonary arterial blood pressure resulting in cardiac load. It is, therefore, not recommended in myocardial infarction. Classical morphine antagonists like nalorphine or levallorphan cannot reverse the action of pentazocine but naloxone can.

It is used as lactate, 30 mg of base per ml, buffered to pH 4 to 5.

Dose : 25 to 100 mg, repeated every 4 hours as required.

Preparations : Pentazocine injection, I.P. Pentazocine tablets, I.P., B.P.

Brand Names : Fortwin®, Pentawin®, Susevin®

Drugs For Further Study

1) Buprenorphine - Bunogesic®, Buprigesic®, Norphin®
2) Butorphanol - Butrum®
3) Tramadol - Adamon®, Dolotram®, Tradol®, Tramazac®
4) Fentanyl - Fendrop®, Fenstud®, Fent®
5) Sufentanyl - Sufentil®

Exercise

Q1. What are opioid analgesics? Classify it giving suitable examples. Write a note on a narcotic antagonist. (Kachchh Univ. 06)

Q2. Define analgesics. Classify narcotic analgesics with examples. Write the structure and chemical name of pethidine & indomethacine. (Karnataka Univ.)

Q3. Define narcotic Analgesics. Give its examples. Draw the structure of pethidine. (Winter 04)

Q4. Define 'narcotic analgesics', give their examples. Draw the structure of 'piperidine derivative' with its chemical name. (Summer 03)

Q5. Write structure, properties, uses and does of acetaminophen. (Summer 06)

Q6. Name the narcotic analgesic containing piperidine heterocycle. Give it's structure and uses. (Summer 06)

Q7. Explain - Antipyretic and analgesics. (Summer 06)

Q8. Give popular brand name of formulation with drug - PethidineHCl. (May-June 04)

Q9. Discuss in detail narcotic analgesics. (May 07)

Q10. Name one analgesic having piperidine derivative. (Nov 06)

■

24 Antipyretic Analgesics and Non-steroidal Anti-inflammatory Agents

Antipyretic Analgesics

1) Aspirin

(Acetylsalicylic acid)

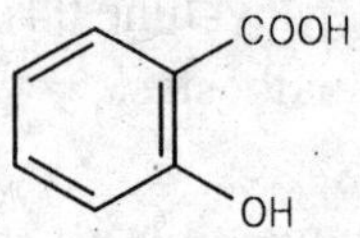

Salicyclic acid

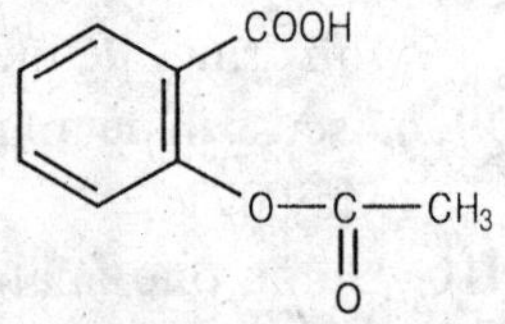

Aspirin (acetyl salicyclic acid)

Aspirin was first introduced in medicine in 1899, although it was synthesised from salicyclic acid by the famous Kolbe's synthesis in 1874 using acetic anhydride. The hydrogen atom of the hydroxyl group in salicylic acid has been replaced by acetyl group.

Properties : Aspirin occurs as white crystals or as white crystalline powder. It is slightly soluble in water (1:300), soluble in alcohol (1:5), chloroform (1:17) and ether (1:15). It dissolves easily in glycerin. Solubility in water can be increased by using acetates or citrates of alkali metals.

Stability : Aspirin is stable in dry air, but in the presence of moisture, it slowly hydrolyses into acetic acid and salicylic acid. Aspirin itself is sufficiently acidic to produce effervescence with carbonates and liberate iodine from iodides. The gastric mucosal irritation produced by aspirin is attributed to the formation of salicylic acid. Dry dosage forms of aspirin (tablets or capsules) should be used. Aspirin in aqueous medium will hydrolyse almost completely in less than a week. However, solutions made with alcohol or glycerin do not decompose as quickly. Citrates retard hydrolysis only slightly. Aspirin lends itself readily to combine with many other substances but tends to soften and become damp with methanamine, aminopyrine, salol, antipyrine, phenol and acetanilide. Aqueous solutions are most stable at pH 2 to 3.

Therapeutic actions and uses :

1) As analgesic antipyretic : Aspirin is useful in variety of minor pains such as neuralgia, toothache and headache. It is also useful in symptomatic treatment of fever.

2) As anti-inflammatory agent : Aspirin is commonly used to treat inflammatory conditions such as arthritis. It modifies and reduces the inflammation, but does not arrest inflammatory response.

3) As antirheumatic : Aspirin administered in sufficiently large dose produces dramatic relief of signs and symptoms of inflammation in acute rheumatic fever. There is considerable and often complete relief of pain with a significant reduction in swelling and immobility of joints.

4) As antiplatelet agent : Aspirin is used to prevent the formation of platelet-fibrin thrombus. Recently, aspirin in lower doses has been recommended as prophylactic for the prevention of heart attacks.

5) Other uses :

i) Prophylactic doses of aspirin have been found useful for prevention of symptoms of food intolerance in patients who show acute GI symptoms after eating specific foodstuff.

ii) Aspirin has been shown to exert beneficial effect in radiation induced diarrhoeas.

iii) Taken orally or applied locally, aspirin has been found useful in reducing erythema due to sun burn.

iv) In local application, aspirin and other salicylates have shown mild antiseptic and antifungal properties.

Dose : 300 mg tablets, 4 to 6 times a day, not to exceed 4 gm/day.

- For rheumatism 4-8 gm, a day in divided doses.
- Soluble aspirin containing citric acid or carbonate are available.
- Buffered aspirin tablets are useful to avoid GI. irritation.
- Methyl salicylate is used for local application as 2.5 per cent in ointment base. Most of the analgesic balms contain this form of salicylic acid.

Brand Names : Anacin®, Disprin®, Colsprin®, Micropyrin®

2) Paracetamol

p- Hydroxy acetanilide.

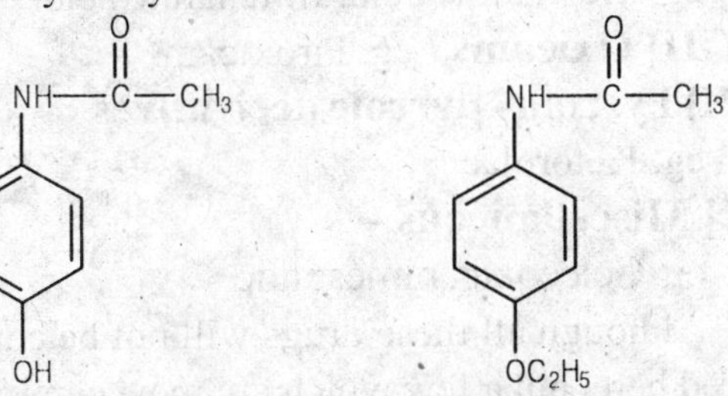

Paracetamol is a paraaminophenol derivative, in which one of the hydrogens of amino group is replaced by an acetyl group. Earlier, acetanilide, and phenacetin (p-Ethoxy acetanilide) were used as antipyretic analgesics, but are no longer used.

Properties : It occurs as an odourless, white crystalline powder with a bitter taste. It is sparingly soluble in water and freely soluble in alcohol.

Storage : It should be stored in airtight containers, protected from light.

Actions and uses : Paracetamol has analgesic and antipyretic action like aspirin, but does not have anti-inflammatory and antiplatelet effect. Unlike salicylates, this drug does not produce acid-base imbalance, electrolyte imbalance or GI irritation. However, paracetamol causes skin reactions and anemia as a result of haemolysis. Its serious side effect is damage to liver which is probably due to its toxic metabolite.

Dose : 250 to 500 mg tablet, not to exceed 2.5 gm in a day for adults.

- Liquid preparations (syrup) are available for children.

Preparations : Paracetamol tablets, I.P., B.P. Paracetamol syrup, I.P.

Aspirin, Paracetamol and Codeine tablets, B.P.C.

Paediatric paracetamol elixir B.P.C.

Brand Names : Crocin®, Metacin®, Calpol®, Pacimol®

3) Analgin (Aminopyrine)

2,3-Dimethyl-4-dimethylamino-1-phenyl-3-pyrazoline-5-one.

Analgin is the sulphate ester of aminopyrine, which is a derivative of 5-pyrazolone.

Analgin is employed as antipyretic analgesic. It is somewhat slower in action, but its effect lasts longer. But it has no uricosuric or antirheumatic effect. It does not have any distinct advantage over aspirin, except that it can be injected.

Some of the side effects of this drug are quite serious, almost toxic, like agranulocytosis. The symptoms of agranulocytosis are, fall in leucocytes, absence of granulocytes in the blood, fever, sore throat and ulceration of mucous surfaces. Many countries have forbidden or greatly restricted the sale of this drug because of this serious side effect.

Dose : Usual dose is 300 mg for headaches, neuralgia and bodyaches.

Preparations : Analgin tablets, I.P.

Brand Names : Novalgin®, Baralgan-M®, Analgin®, Zimalgin®

NSAIDs

Non-steroidal anti-inflammatory drugs commonly known by abbreviation as NSAID, are now drugs of choice to reduce inflammation caused due to various reasons. Inflammation often results into erythema, edema and pain. Rheumatic fever and rheumatoid arthritis are further manifestations of inflammation of the chronic nature.

There are many complicated theories of mechanism of action of NSAIDs, but by and large the following concepts are accepted, as follows,

i) During inflammatory process, arachidonic acid (a fatty acid) is liberated from phospholipid fraction of cell membrane. This arachidonic acid is then converted into another chemical substance called prostaglandins (PG), which are believed to cause edema, erythema and pain. PG does not affect this process of inflammation directly, but through a number of biological processes and mediators such as bradykinin, 5-hydroxytryptamine (5-HT) etc.

ii) NSAIDs have been shown to inhibit release or synthesis of PGs and thus produce beneficial effects.

iii) Arachidonic acid besides getting converted to PGs also gets converted to another chemical known as leukotrienes through an enzyme called lipooxygenase. These leukotrienes activate T-lymphocytes which release lymphokines, which actually play a role in the process of inflammation. Some of the NSAIDs like aspirin inhibit T-lymphocyte activation and their ability to release lymphokines, thus reducing inflammation.

iv) NSAIDs also unmask T-cell suppressing activity, thus decreasing the production of factors (or chemicals) which cause rheumatoid arthiritis or fever.

Classification of NSAIDs

Most of the non-steroidal anti-inflammatory drugs fall into the following chemical group.

I] Salicylates and their derivatives

eg. Aspirin. (discussed earlier)

II] Para-aminophenol derivatives

eg. Phenacetin, paracetamol (discussed earlier) (although both these two drugs have little anti-inflammatory action).

III] Pyrazolone derivatives

eg. Phenylbutazone, oxyphenbutazone.

IV] Indole acetic acid derivatives

eg. Indomethacin, sulindac.

V] Phenylacetic acid derivatives

eg. Diclofenac sodium.

VI] Propionic acid derivatives

eg. Ibuprofen, ketoprofen, naproxen etc.

VII] N-Arylanthranilic acid derivatives (Fenamates)

eg. Mefenamic acid, flufenamic acid.

VIII] Oxicams - eg. Piroxicam.

IX] Pyrrolo - pyrrole derivatives

eg. Ketorolac

X] Miscellaneous -

eg. Celecoxib, nimesulide

Although all these drugs will not be considered here, but a few which are most commonly used are as follows,

1) Phenylbutazone (Butazolidin) and Oxyphenbutazone

Both these drugs are prazolone derivatives.

Phenylbutazone
1,2-Diphenyl-4-butyl-3,
5-pyrazolidine dione

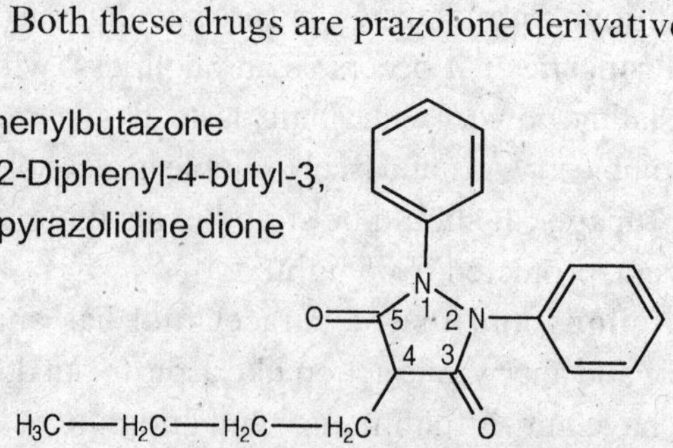

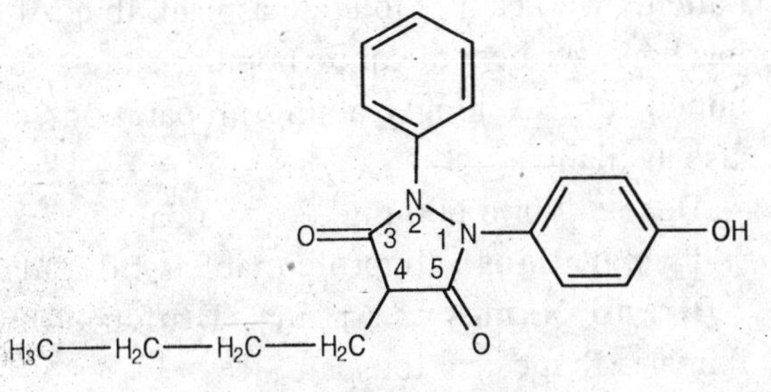

Oxyphenbutazone
4-Butyl-1-(p-hydroxy phenyl)-2-phenyl-3,
5-pyrazolidine dione

Properties : Phenylbutazone occurs as an odourless, white crystalline powder having a bitter after taste. It is very slightly soluble in water, soluble in alcohol and in solutions of alkali hydroxides. Oxyphenbutazone also shows the above characteristics.

Stability : Aqueous solutions of phenylbutazone containing alkali hydroxides are slowly hydrolysed and oxidised by atmospheric oxygen.

Actions and uses : The principal use of phenylbutazone is in the treatment of painful symptoms of gout, rheumatoid arthritis, spondylitis and acute arthritis of joints. However, due to its many serious side effects like agranulocytosis, aplastic and megaloblastic anemia, nephritis, aggravation of peptic ulcer, skin rashes and even, blurred vision, the drug is no longer a drug of choice in therapy.

Phenylbutazone is extensively bound to plasma proteins (98 per cent), hence increasing the dose only increases the side effects. Because of this high protein-binding, it displaces oral anticoagulants, hypoglycemic agents and sulphonamides, causing increased toxicity of these drugs (as they appear in plasma at a much higher concentration).

Phenylbutazone is completely metabolised in liver. One of the major metabolites of the drug is oxyphenbutazone, which also has anti-inflammatory properties. Oxyphenbutazone also shares all the toxic effects of phenylbutazone and does not seem to have any significant advantage over phenylbutazone. Only advantage is it seems to have less gastric irritation.

Dose : Phenylbutazone

Tablets 100 mg, 200 to 400 mg a day in divided doses.

- IM injections (150 mg per ml) 600 mg every 2 to 3 days.

- For oxyphenbutazone 400 mg a day, in divided doses.

Preparations : Phenylbutazone tablets, I.P., B.P.

Phenylbutazone suppositories, B.P.

Oxyphenbutazone tablets, I.P., B.P.

Oxyphenbutazone eye ointment, B.P.C.

Brand Names : Phenylbutazone - Aristopyrin®

Oxyphenbutazone - Sioril®, Oxy-Triactin®

2) Indomethacin

1-(p-Chlorobenzoyl)-5-methoxy 2-methylindole-3-acetic acid

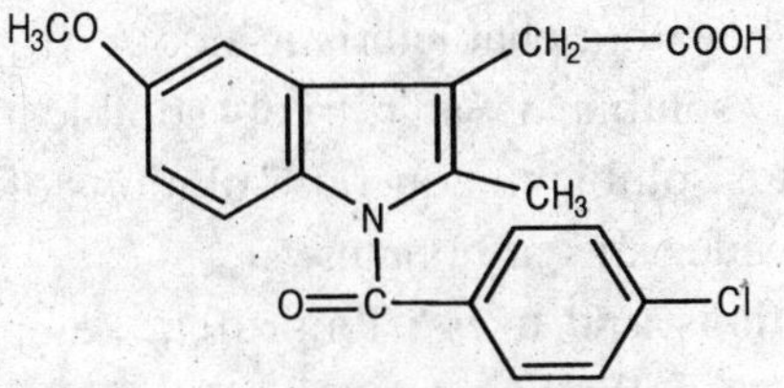

Properties : It occurs as a pale yellow to brownish-yellow powder. It is odourless and almost tasteless. It is very slightly soluble in water and sparingly soluble in alcohol.

Storage : It should be protected from light.

Actions and uses : Introduced in 1965, indomethacin is a typical indole acetic acid derivative. The drug has both analgesic and anti-inflammatory properties. It is useful in rheumatoid arthritis, spondylitis and osteoarthritis. It is however, not much effective in treating gout.

Some of its side effects are gastric distress, headache, blood disorders and aggravation of peptic ulcer. It is, therefore, not recommended for children. It may be preferred in the treatment of acute gout and in ankylosing spondylitis. However, much of the evidence from clinical practice suggests that this drug is neither superior nor has any special advantage over the well established drugs like aspirin.

Sulindac is a derivative of indomethacin, with a fluorine group, instead of chlorine, in the structure and has similar actions.

Dose : 50 to 150 mg a day in divided doses, after food.

Preparations : Indomethacin capsules, I.P., B.P.

Indomethacin mixture, B.P.C.

Indomethacin supporitories, B.P.

Brand Names : Artisid®, Clinoril®, Indoflam®, Inocin-TR®, Indocap®

3) Ibuprofen

2-(4-Isobutylphenyl)propionic acid.

Properties : It occurs as a white powder or crystals with a characteristic odour. It is very slightly soluble in water; freely soluble in alcohol. It is soluble in aqueous solutions of alkali hydroxides and carbonates.

Actions and uses : Ibuprofen, ketoprofen, fenoprofen, flurbiprofen and naproxen are typical propionic acid derivatives among the NSAIDs. Ibuprofen has analgesic, antipyretic and anti-inflammatory properties and is tolerated better than salicylates and other NSAIDs.

Ibuprofen and other propionic acid derivatives, are useful in rheumathoid arthritis, osteoarthritis and ankylosing spondylitis, especially in patients who cannot tolerate aspirin. Ibuprofen has however become quite popular and its sustained release, longer acting preparations are also available.

Dose : 400 to 600 mg, thrice a day.

Preparations : Ibuprofen tablets I.P., B.P.

Brand Names : Arflur®, Brufen®, Ibuflamar®, Ibugesic®, Ibuspan SR®

Drugs For Further Study

1) Flurbiprofen - Froben®
2) Ketoprofen - Ketofen®, Ketonal-D®, Rhofenid®
3) Naproxen - Artagen®, Naprosyn®, Xenobid®
4) Diclofenac - Argesic®, Dicloact®, Diclomol®, Voveran®
5) Aceclofenac - Acefen®, Acota®, Movon®, Zerodol®
6) Piroxicam - Brexic®, Dolonex®, Pirox®, Pyrodex®
7) Tenoxicam - Novotil®, Tobitil®
8) Meloxicam - Ecwin®, M-Cam®, Melflam®, Melogesic®
9) Celecoxib - Celact®, Celcib®, Celcox®, Coxib®, Zycel®
10) Valdecoxib - Revaldo®, Valcox®, Valdez®, Valdone®
11) Parecoxib - Paroxib®, Bioval-P®, Praxis-40®
12) Etoricoxib - Eteron®, Etoshine®, Etoxib®, Etrobax®
13) Nimesulide - Emsulide®, Genlide®, Neosaid®, Nimbid®
14) Nabumetone - Nabuflam®, Niltis®

Drugs acting by mechanisms other than inhibiting PG synthesis

15) Gold (Auranofin) - Goldar®, Ridaura®
16) Penicillamine - Cilamin-250®
17) Etanercept - Enbrel®
18) Lefulnomide - Arava®, Cleft®, Lefra®, Lefumide®
19) Glucosamine - Artica®, Cartigen®, Cartilamine®
20) Hyaluronic acid - Halonix®, LG Hyruan®

Exercise

Q1. What are anti-inflammatory agents. Give an account of anti-inflammatory agents with suitable examples. (Kachchh Univ. 06)

Q2. Write structure and uses of the following - a) Aspirin, b) Methyl salicylate & c) Paracetamol. (Kachchh Univ. 06)

Q3. Write structures of oxyphenbutazone. (Winter 04)

Q4. What are anti-inflammatory agents? Give chemical name and structure of ibuprofen. Explain its action mechanism. (Winter 04)

Q5. Give structure, chemical name, properties, uses and trade names of paracetamol. (Winter 04)

Q6. Give structure, chemical name and uses of indomethacin. Mention its brand names. (Winter 04)

Q7. Define "Non-steroidal Anti-inflammatory agents". Enumerate examples from pyrazole derivatives, with the structure of phenylbutazone. (Summer 03)

Q8. Give uses of ibuprofen. (Summer 06)

Q9. Define NSAID. (Summer 06, May-June 04)

Q10. Define and classify analgesics, giving suitable example. Give structural formula and specific uses of - i) Paracetamol and ii) Aspirin. (May-June 04, 2005)

Q11. What are opioid analgesics? Classify it giving suitable examples. Write a note on narcotic antagonists. (2005)

Q12. What are anti-inflammatory agents. Give an account of anti-inflammatory agents with suitable examples. (2005)

Q13. Define antipyretics and anti-inflmmatory agents. Classify antipyretics and draw the structure of any four - i) Paracetamol, ii) Aspirin, iii) Analgin, iv) Indomethacin, v) Ibuprofen & vi) Mefenamic acid. (May 07, Nov 06)

25 Thyroxine and Antithyroid Drugs

Thyroid Hormones

The thyroid gland synthesises two important hormones namely thyroxine and triiodothyronine.

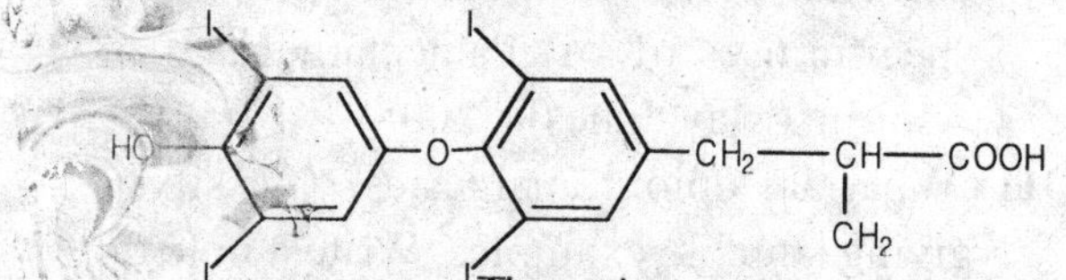

Thyroxine

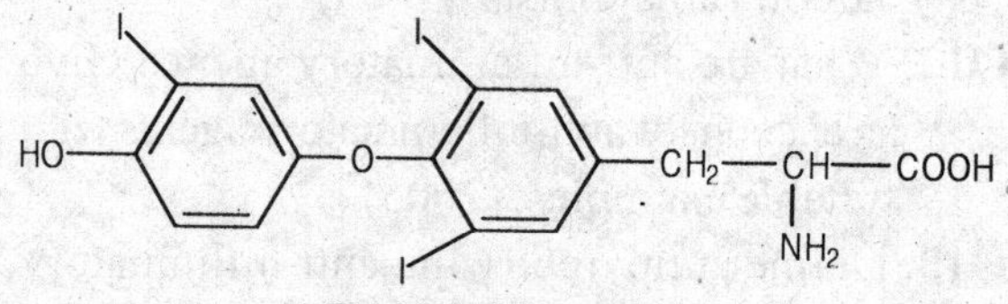

Tri-iodothyronine

Thyroxine

It is now established that thyroxine may be storage form of the hormone while triiodothyronine is the circulating form. In blood, thyroxine is more firmly bound to the globulin fraction, than triiodo thyronine form, which can then enter the tissue cells. Thyroxine was first obtained in crystalline form in 1915 and later on was synthesised in 1927.

Actions and uses : Thyroxine is used in therapy, as replacement therapy, especially in adult hypothyroidism (deficiency of natural thyroxine), in non-toxic goitres, in the treatment of obesity (with caution), in post-surgical treatment of thyroid carcinoma, as diagnostic test for hyperthyroidism, during pregnancy to avoid hypothyroidism and as serum cholesterol lowering agent.

Properties : Thyroxine exists in optically active forms. Levo isomer of thyroxine is active physiologically and is known as levothyroxine which is available in sodium salt form. The salt is a light yellow, tasteless, odourless powder. It is hygroscopic but stable in dry air at room temperature.

Thyroxine sodium is slightly soluble in water and in alcohol. It is soluble in solutions of alkali hydroxides.

Storage : It should be stored in airtight containers, protected from light.

Uses : Levothyroxine sodium is used in replacement therapy of decreased thyroid function. In general 100 mg of levothyroxine sodium is clinically equivalent to 30 to 60 mg of thyroid. Triiodothyronine or leothyronine is more active than thyroxine. It has similar applications, viz.- treatment of metabolic insufficiency, male infertility and some gynaecological disorders.

Dose : 25 to 400 mcg once a day.

- usual dose range is 25 mcg to 1 mg a day.
- pediatric dose, 6 mcg per kg of body weight.

Preparations : Thyroxine tablets, I.P., B.P.

Brand Names : Eltroxine®, Roxin®, Thyrox®

Antithyroid Drugs

Hyperthyroidism (excessive production of thyroid hormone), usually requires surgery. But prior to that, the patient is prepared by treatment of antithyroid drugs to reduce or control hyperthyroidism. Some of the drugs used as antithyroid drugs for this purpose are as follows,

1) Methimazole

1-Methylimidazole-2-thiol

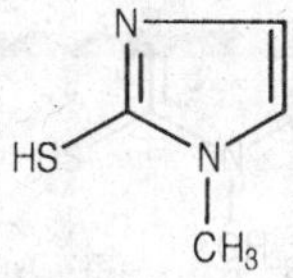

Properties : It occurs as a white to pale buff crystalline powder. It has a faint characteristic odour and a slightly bitter taste. It is freely soluble in water and alcohol.

Storage : It should be stored in airtight containers, protected from light.

Actions and uses : This drug is used in the treatment of hyperthyroidism. It is more potent than propylthiouracil (see below). The side effects are similar to that of propylthiouracil. The patients have to be kept under strict medical observation.

Dose : 5-20 mg, three times a day not to exceed 60 mg.

Preparations : Methimazole tablets, U.S.P.

2) Propylthiouracil

6-Propyl-2-thiouracil

Properties : It occurs as white or pale cream coloured crystals or crystalline powder. It is odourless and has a bitter taste. It is very slightly soluble in water, alcohol and ether. It is soluble in solutions of alkali hydroxides.

Actions and uses : The drug is a derivative of thiouracil, which was formerly used for treatment of hyperthyroidism. Thiouracil was discontinued because of its side effect causing agranulocytosis.

The drug has a slow onset, but has the advantage of not interfering with natural thyroid hormones stored in the thyroid gland.

Dose : 100 to 300 mg, three times a day, not to exceed 900 mg a day. Maintenance dose is 50 mg, 2 to 3 times a day.

Preparations : Propylthiouracil tablets, I.P., B.P.

Brand Names : PTU®

3) Methylthiouracil

6-Methyl-2-thiouracil

Properties : It is a white, odourless crystalline powder. It is very slightly soluble in water and slightly soluble in alcohol.

Storage : It has to be stored in tightly closed, light resistant containers.

Uses : It is used for the treatment of hyperthyroidism. Its actions are similar to propylthiouracil.

Dose : 50 mg, four times a day.

Preparations : Methylthiouracil tablets, B.P.

Drugs For Further Study

1) Carbimazole - Anti-thyrox®, Neo-mercazole®, Thyrozole®
2) Iodine - Collosol iodine® oral

Exercise

Q1. Write short note on - Antithyroid drugs. (Kachchh Univ. 2006)

Q2. What are thyroidal hormones? Give their examples and write structure of Thyroxine. (Winter 04, Summer 03)

Q3. Give uses of Propyl thiouracil. (Winter 04)

Q4. Explain Thyroid and Antithyroid drugs. (Summer 06, 2005)

Q5. Specify dosage forms (tablet, capsule etc..) for Thyroxine. (May-June 04)

Q6. Write the structure and use of Thyroxine. (Nov 06)

26 Diagnostic Agents

Introduction

Diagnostic agents are used to detect impaired function of the body organs or to recognise abnormalities in tissue structure. These agents, usually, have no therapeutic use. The usefulness of a diagnostic agent depends on its solubility, mode and rate of excretion, metabolism, chemical configuration, colour and chemical functional groups (like iodine, sulpha groups).

Classification of Diagnostic Agents

These agents fall into three categories,

I) Radio-opaque agents

a) Water soluble contrast media.
b) Water insoluble contrast media.

II) Compounds for testing functional capacity

a) Agents for kidney function test.
b) Agents for liver function test.
c) Agents used for miscellaneous tests.

III) Compounds modifying a physiologic function

a) Gastrointestinal agents.
b) Gold compounds.
c) Alcohol deterrent agents.
d) Sun-screen agents.
e) Uricosuric agents.

In this chapter, only the radio-opaque agents and compounds for testing functional capacity will be considered. These agents are marketed by generic names by manufacturers such as Qualigens, Loba and BDH.

I) Radio-opaque agents

An ideal radio-opaque substance should have adequate radio-opacity (about 50 per cent), the agent should be able to concentrate in desired parts of body like kidney, gall bladder, etc., should be able to remain in the desired area of the organ for sometime, should have high solubility and absolutely low toxicity.

a) Water soluble contrast media

All these compounds contain iodine, as a functional group to the extent of 50 to 65 per cent. These agents are used to cast shadows (of the organ) on x-ray films. This water soluble group is used mainly for urography and also in angiography, cholangiography and cerebral angiography. These agents are usually injected intravenously before taking the x-ray picture. Therefore, sterile solutions meeting all the specifications of a sterile product according to I.P., are a strict requirement. Some of the common agents in this class are,

i) Sodium iodohippurate ii) Acetrizoate sodium, iii) Diatrizoic acid and its sodium salt, iv) Iodipamide, v) Ipodate sodium and calcium salt, vi) Sodium iothalamate.

b) Water insoluble contrast media

This group is mainly used for cholecystography, bronchography and myelography. Unlike the water soluble group, these compounds are usually taken orally, after a fat-free meal and then some hours later, (nearly 12 hours later) or on the next day, X-ray is taken, on an empty stomach. A general formula of most of these agents can be represented as follows,

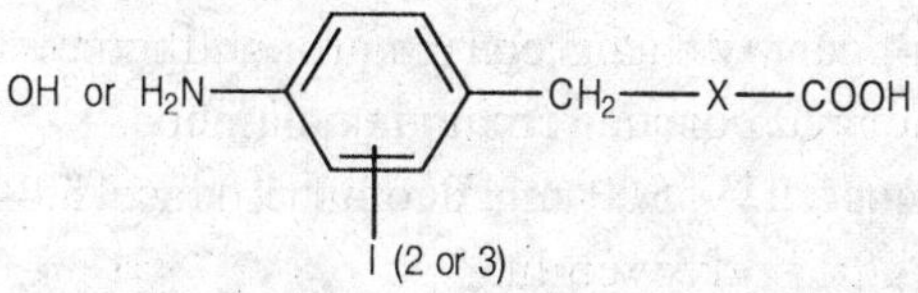

X = a group separating CH_2 and COOH

Some of the agents in this class are -

1) Iopanoic acid

2-(3-Amino-2,4,6-triiodobenzyl) butyric acid

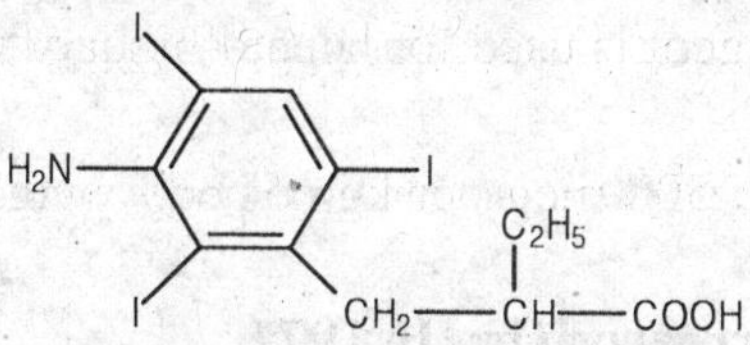

Properties : Iopanoic acid occurs as a white to cream-coloured, odourless, almost tasteless powder. It is practically insoluble in water, soluble in alcohol and in solutions of alkali hydroxides.

Storage : It should be protected from light.

Uses : Iopanoic acid is a radio-opaque compound which is absorbed from the gastrointestinal tract and excreted in the bile. It is used as a contrast medium in radiography of the gall bladder.

Dose : 3 gm

Preparations : Iopanoic acid tablets. B.P.

2) Propyliodone

Propyl-1,4-dihydro-3,5-diodo-4-oxo-1-pyridylacetate.

Properties : It occurs as an odourless, white crystalline powder. It is very slightly soluble in water and in ether.

Storage : It should be protected from light.

Actions and uses : This agent is used as a sterile aqueous or oil suspension for installation into trachea, prior to bronchography.

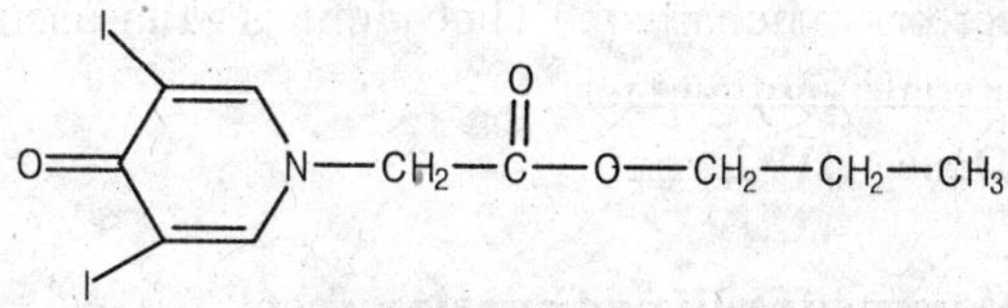

Dose : 0.75 to 1 ml of 60 per cent suspension; introduced by cannula or catheter.

Preparations : Propyliodone injection B.P.
Propyliodone oily injection B.P.

3) Tyropanoate sodium

This compound is used for cholecystography and cholangiography.

4) Iocetamic acid

It is used for gall bladder shadow and for biliary tract observations.

II) Agents for testing functional capacity of organs

a) Agents for kidney function test

1) Indigotindisulphonate sodium (Indigo carmine)

This dye is used as a colouring agent, stain and reagent to determine renal function and to locate the ureteral orifice. Normally it appears in urine in 10 minutes and about 10 per cent of the solution is eliminated in one hour.

Dose : IV 40 mg.

2) Aminohippuric acid

p-Amino hippuric acid

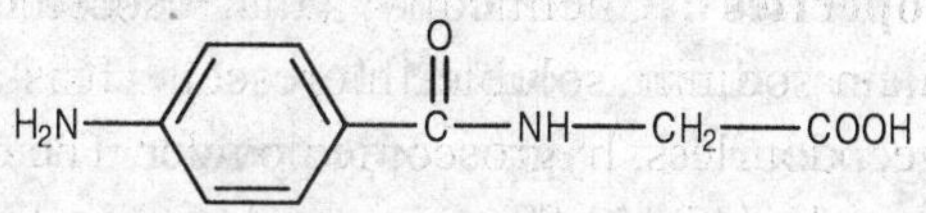

This compound is used as sodium salt, which is excreted by the tubular epithelium of the kidney and by glomerulus. Thus, it serves as a means for measuring the effective renal plasma flow and for determining the tubular excretory mechanism. The agent is thus used for renal function test.

Dose : IV 2 gm.

b) Agents for liver function test

1) Rose bengal

Chemically this is tetraiodo, tetrachloro, fluorescein. It is used for liver function test. The liver almost exclusively removes this dye from blood stream. A normally functioning liver will remove 50 per cent of the dye in 2 minutes from a dose of 100-150 mg of the dye injected intravenously. The dye is also available in radioactive form (I^{131}) and the measurement of radioactivity becomes much easier and accurate.

c) Agents for miscellaneous diagnostic tests

1) Evans blue

Evans blue is a complex azo dye, existing as blue crystals, soluble in water. Evans blue when injected into the blood stream, attaches firmly to the plasma proteins, especially albumin. The colour developed is directly proportional to the concentration. By means of colour intensity, the total blood volume is measured. The test is useful as a guide in the replacement therapy, in shock and in haemorrhage.

Dose : IV equivalent of 22.6 mg of dry Evans Blue.

2) Fluorescein sodium

Properties : Chemically, it is resorcinol-phthalein sodium, soluble fluorescein. It is an orange, odourless, hygroscopic powder. The disodium salt is highly fluorescent when dissolved in water. The acidic solution has practically no fluorescence.

Storage : It should be stored in airtight containers.

Uses : Fluorescein sodium is used as an ophthalmologic diagnostic agent. Diseased or abraded areas of the cornea, such as corneal ulcers, are stained green by the solution. Foreign bodies appear with a green ring around them, while the normal cornea remains unstained.

Dose : IV 500 mg Paediatric dose 15.4 mg per kg of body weight.

Preparations : Fluorescein eye drops, B.P.C. Fluorescein sodium eye drops, I.P.

3) Indocyanine green

This agent is used for hepato-biliary function test.

Dose : 500 mcg per kg of body weight.

4) Chlormerodrin Hg 197

This agent is used for locating lesions of brain and for anatomic or functional defects of kidneys.

5) Azuresin

This agent is used for the diagnosis of achlorhydria. The dye is released in gastric acidic conditions and is absorbed from upper intestine and then promptly excreted in urine where it can be measured quantitatively by colourimetric methods.

Dose : 2 gm preceded by 500 mg of caffeine and sodium benzoate.

6) Sulphobromophthalein sodium

Properties : It occurs as an odourless, hygroscopic, white, crystalline powder with a bitter taste. It is soluble in water; practically insoluble in alcohol.

Storage : It should be stored in airtight containers.

Uses : It is used for testing the functional capacity of the liver, particularly of its reticuloendothelial cells. After intravenous injection, the dye is rapidly removed from the blood and excreted in the bile.

Dose : 5 mg per kg of body weight, by slow IV injection.

Preparations : Sulphobromophthalein sodium injection I.P.

7) Congo red

Properties : It is reddish-brown powder. It is soluble in water and sparingly soluble in alcohol.

Storage : It should be stored in airtight container, protected from light.

Uses : Congo red is used for the diagnosis of amyloid disease. It is given by slow intravenous injection and the per cent decrease of dye content of serum within one hour is determined by colourimetry. In normal patients, 10 to 30 per cent of the dye disappears while in patients with amyloid disease, 30 to 100 per cent of the dye disappears.

Dose : 1.25 to 3.75 mg per kg of body weight, IV injection.

Exercise

Q1. Give a detailed account of diagnostic agents. (Kachchh Univ. 06, Winter 04, May 05)

Q2. Give uses of congo red. (Winter 04)

Q3. Write the uses of fluorescein sodium. (Summer 03, Summer 06)

Q4. Explain the term 'diagnostic agents' with its classification; write uses of - i) Evan's Blue, ii) Congo Red & iii) Indigo carmine. (Summer 06)

Q5. Write note on diagnostic agents. (May-June 04, May 07)

(27) Steroidal Drugs

Structures and General Chemistry of Steroids

Steroids have a common tetracylic nucleus as shown below. The rings A, B and C are six membered and ring D is a five membered ring. The sequence of numbering the various carbon atoms is also shown. A group attached to any position and shown by continuous thick line is taken to be above the plane of the nucleus and is designated as 'beta' (β), and a group shown by dotted line is below the plane and is termed as 'alpha' (α).

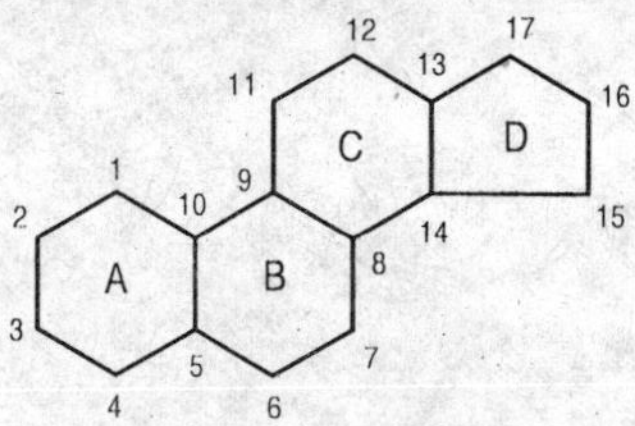

Steroid Nucleus

There are three main groups from which most of the steroidal drugs are evolved and also the nomenclature is derived. They are as follows,

1) Androstane

It is a parent steroid containing 19 carbon atoms, so they are sometimes referred to as C-19 steroid. The most common steroid of this class is the male sex hormone, testosterone.

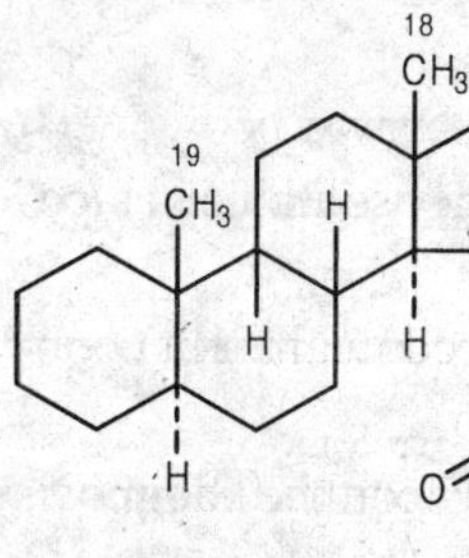

5-α-Androstane

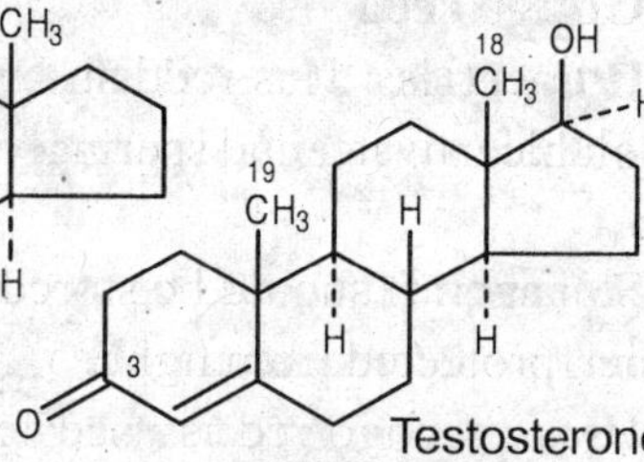

Testosterone

17-β-Hydroxy-4-androsten-3-one

2) Estrane

It is the parent steroid of group two. It has 18 carbon atoms and there is no methyl group attached to the position 10. The common steroidal drug of this class is estradiol (oestradiol).

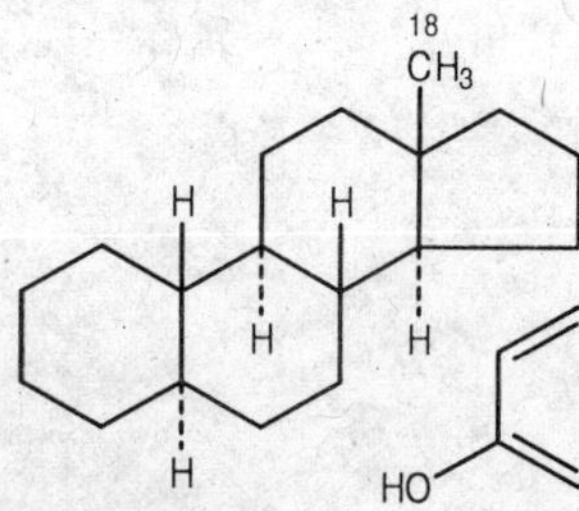

5-α-Estrane

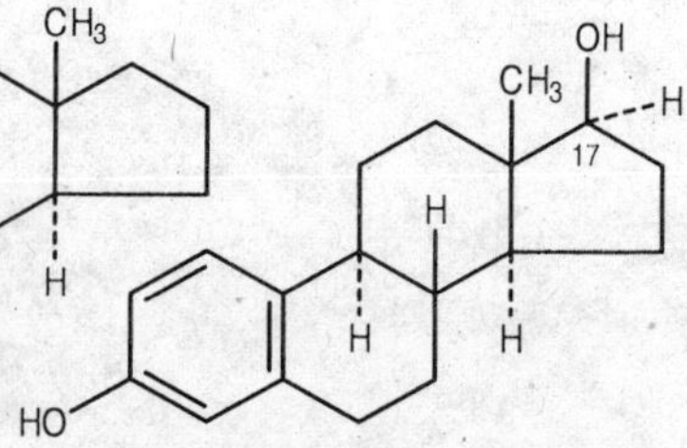

Estradiol (17-β-estradiol)

3) Pregnane

This is a parent steroid of the third group. It has 21 carbon atoms. There is a 2-carbon side chain attached to the 17th position. The most common steroidal drugs belonging to this group are progesterone and adrenocortical hormones.

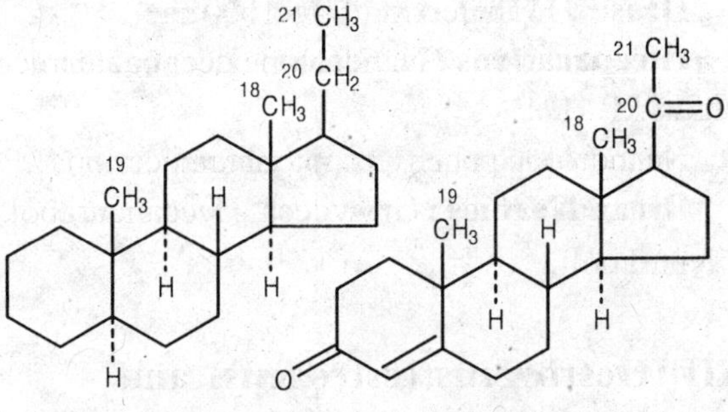

5-α-Pregnane Progesterone

Sex Hormones and Related Steroidal Drugs

Steroidal sex hormones are produced in gonads, ovaries or testes. They are also produced in varying quantities by adrenal cortex and placenta. They influence the development and maintenance of various biological processes which are directly or indirectly associated with reproduction.

Number of synthetic and semi-synthetic steroids have biological activity similar to progesterone and are called 'progestins'. Similarly several non-steroidal compounds have activity similar to estrogens. Although estrogens and progestins have good applications as chemical contraceptive agents for females, they also have a wide range of therapeutic activity for both males and females. Testosterones have two major activities, viz., androgenic, i.e., male physical characteristic activity and anabolic, i.e., muscle building activity. A great deal of interest is on anabolic activity of these steroids, especially its use in disabling and failing conditions of body (especially after a long illness or surgery). Androgenic activity has applications in therapy.

I] Androgens and anabolic agents

a) Testosterone

17 β-Hydroxy-4-androsten-3-one.

Properties : Testosterone occurs as an odourless white crystalline powder. It is very slightly soluble in water and freely soluble in alcohol. It is dextrorotatory. Testosterone propionate has similar properties; it is soluble in ethyl oleate and in arachis oil.

Storage : It should be protected from light.

Actions and uses : Testosterone is the main androgen formed in test and as stated above, it has both androgenic and anabolic activities. Its primary use, therefore, is as androgen replacement therapy in men at maturity age in case of testosterone deficiency. It is useful in certain anemias, osteoporosis and to stimulate growth in undergrown boys. Its anabolic activity has limited use because of side effects. It is believed to improve athletic performance and maintain muscle tone, but this activity has no conclusive evidence. Among its side effects, are hirsutism in females, deepening of voice, increased serum lipids, hypertension and edema. The normal testosterone levels in men are 4 to 12 mg per day and women 0.5 to 2.9 mg per day.

Chemically, testosterone is a derivative of androsterone. It has a hydroxy group at C-17, a double bond between 4 and 5 positions (4-ene) and a ketone group at 3 position (3-one). It is therefore named chemically as 17β-hydroxy-4-androsten-3-one and has the structure as shown in the earlier part of this chapter. Testosterone is usually formulated as 17-β-esters, such as testosterone propionate, or cyclopentyl propionate.

Dose : IM 10 to 50 mg, 2 or 3 times a week, in males.

IM 100 to 300 mg weekly in divided doses, in breast cancer.

Preparations : Testosterone propionate injection, I.P., B.P.

Testosterone implants, B.P.

Testosterone esters injection, B.P.C.

Testosterone phenylpropionate injection, B.P.

Other important derivatives of testosterone in clinical use are 17-β-methyl testosterone, fluoxymesterone (9-β-fluoro and 11β, 17β-dihydroxy groups).

Nandrolone, which is without the methyl group at C-19, is another important derivative of testosterone. Among the other useful androgens are ethylestrenol (17-β-ethyl, no CH_3 at C-19, and no keto group at C-3) and methandienone.

Brand Names : Aquaviron® inj., Nuvir®, Testoviron® inj.

b) Nandrolone

3-Oxoestr-4-en-17β-ol.

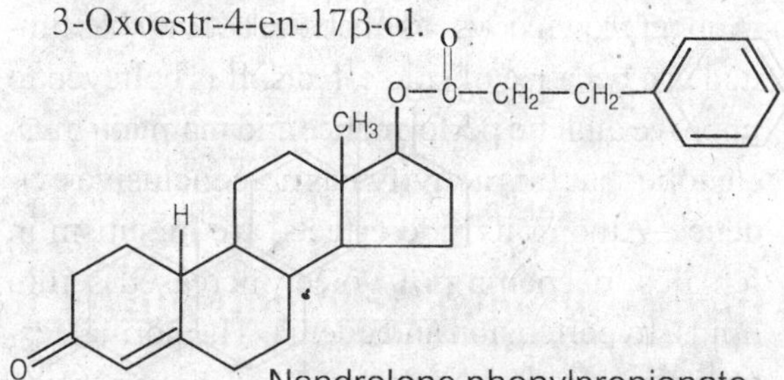

Nandrolone phenylpropionate

It is official in I.P. as the decanoate and phenylpropionate esters.

Properties : Nandrolone decanoate occurs as a white to creamy-white crystalline powder with a faint charactertistic odour. It is very slightly soluble in water; very soluble in alcohol; soluble in fixed oils and in esters. It is dextrorotatory.

Storage : It should be stored under nitrogen at a temperature between 2°C to 10°C, protected from light.

Actions and uses : Nandrolone has both anabolic and androgenic properties, similar to testosterone and methandienone. It causes nitrogen and calcium retention and promotes protein synthesis. It is used as an anabolic agent in the treatment of osteoporosis and during post operative recovery. It is also used in the treatment of breast cancer. It is not active when given by mouth.

Dose : IM injection 50 to 100 mg.

Preparations : Nandrolone decanoate injection I.P., B.P.

Nandrolone phenylpropionate injection B.P.

Brand Names : Growdeca®, Decaneurabol®, Neurabol®

II] Oestrogens (estrogens) and progestins

Source : Estrogens are produced in large quantities in ovaries and placenta. They are also produced in adrenals, in low quantities. About 50 to 350 mg per day are produced in ovaries during the menstrual cycle. During the first month of pregnancy, this amount goes up by 1000 times in blood. Progesterone, on the other hand is produced in ovaries, testes and adrenals. Most of the progesterone is immediately converted to other hormonal intermediates.

The main therapeutic use of estradiol and estrogens is for replacement therapy in deficiency states and for the treatment of conditions such as primary amenorrhoea and delayed onset of puberty and post menstrual problems. Progestins are used in progesterone deficiency. Besides this, progestins are used in the treatment of uterine bleeding to prevent habitual abortion and also as a pregnancy test. Both estrogens and progesterone and their chemical derivatives are used as ovulation inhibitors as oral contraceptives (see section on 'chemical contraceptive agents' below).

Progesterone, impregnated on intra-uterine devices (like copper T) are being used lately as contraceptive devices and it has been claimed that such devices give protection for a longer period of time.

However, there are many side effects of these two steroids. Large doses especially in post menstrual periods of women may lead to cancer, thromboembolism and myocardial infarction, edema and masculinisation of female fetus.

Estradiol (oestradiol) is the main estrogenic hormone in the ovaries. It is related to the nucleus of 5α-estrane (C18 steroid), in which ring A is benzenoid and, therefore hydroxyl group (-OH) at 3 position is phenolic, but -OH group at 17 position is alcoholic.

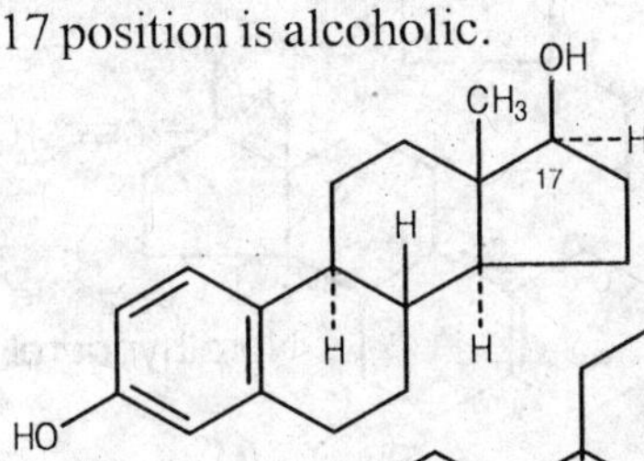

17-β-Estradiol

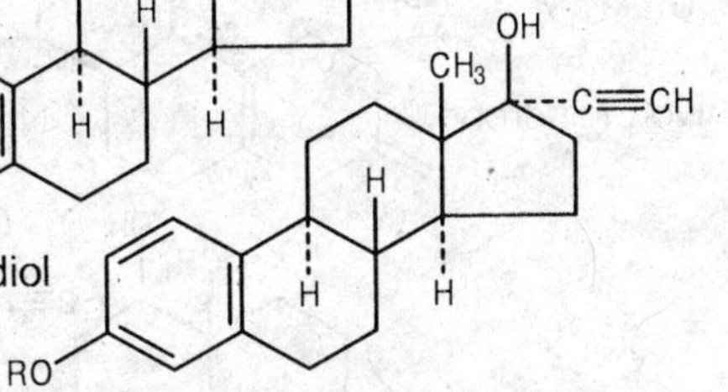

Ethinyl estradiol (R=H), Mestranol (R=CH_3)

a) Estradiol : (Oestradiol)

Estra-1,3,5 (10) trien-3-, 17β diol.

It is official in I.P. as benzoate and dipropionate esters.

Properties : Estradiol benzoate occurs as odourless, colourless crystals or white crystalline powder. It is practically insoluble in water, slightly soluble in alcohol, in arachis oil and in ethyl oleate. It is dextrorotatory.

Storage : It should be protected from light.

Actions and uses : Estradiol is the most active of the naturally occurring estrogens. It is used in therapeutics for replacement therapy in cases of its deficiency, for the treatment of primary amenorrhoea and delayed onset of puberty. It is also used to treat menopausal syndrome and some disturbances of menstruation. The estrogens can be given by the oral route.

Dose : IM injection 1 to 5 mg at intervals of 1 to 14 days.

Preparations : Estradiol injection, I.P., B.P.

Brand Names : Estraderm MX 50® patches, E-2® gel, Systen-50® patches

Introduction of 17-α ethynyl group at C-17, gives a very valuable derivative which is an oral contraceptive agent called ethinyl estradiol. Similarly its methoxy derivative, with-OCH_3 at C-3, gives another oral contraceptive agent, mestranol.

Simple non-steroidal synthetic compounds have been found to have potent estrogenic activity. A good example of such a compound is stilbestrol or diethylstilbestrol and some of its derivatives like dienestrol, methallenstrill. All these agents have actions and uses similar to those of estradiol.

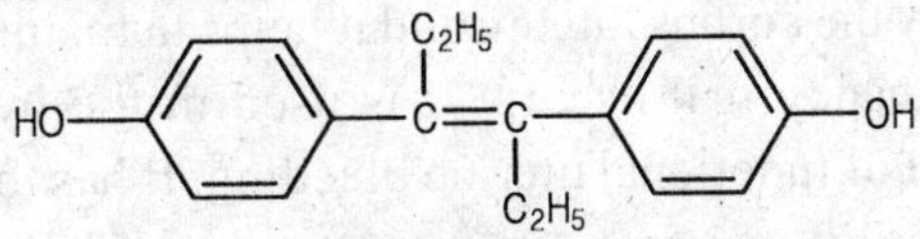

Diethylstilbestrol

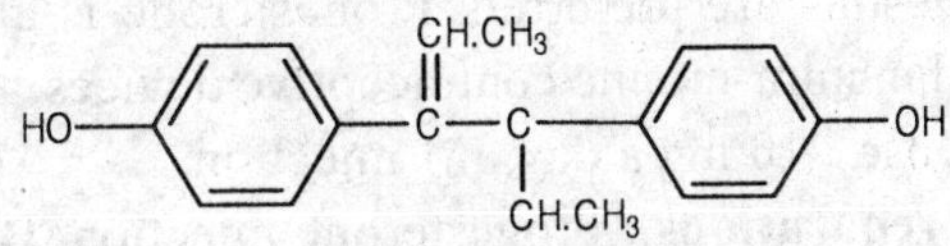

Dienestrol

Among the progestins groups, the main compound is progesterone. They are used in the treatment of functional uterine bleeding, and are often used in combination that estrogens in menstrual disorders and the treatment of neoplasms of breast.

b) Progesterone

4-Pregnene-3,20-dione.

Progesterone is related chemically to 5-α

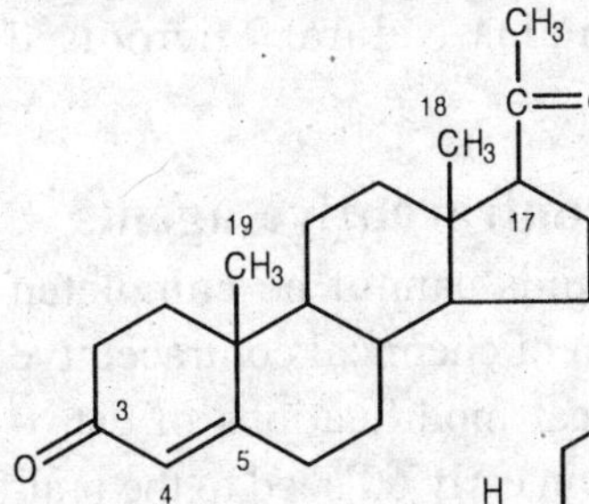

Progesterone

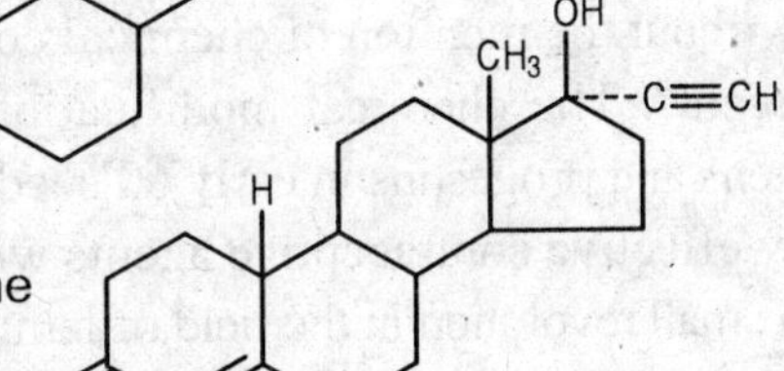

Norethindrone

pregnane nucleus and is a steroid with 21 C-atoms. It has two keto groups at C-3 and C-20, a double bond between C-4 and C-5 and three methyl groups at C-18, C-19 and C-21 respectively.

Properties : Progesterone occurs as odourless, colourless crystals or white or slightly yellowish-white crystalline powder. It is practically insoluble in water, freely soluble in alcohol, sparingly soluble in arachis oil and in ethyl oleate. It is dextrorotatory.

Actions and uses : Progesterone is secreted by the corpus luteum and it helps to maintain pregnancy if it occurs. It is used in the treatment of functional uterine bleeding. It has to be given by intramuscular injection and the oral progestins are preferred. Progesterone is also used in intra-uterine contraceptive devices.

Dose : 10 mg a day, IM injection.

Preparations : Progesterone injection, B.P.

Some of the derivatives of progesterone, like ethisterone (17-β hydroxy and 17-α ethynyl group) and lynestrenol (with a similar structure, but no keto group at C-3) are also as active as the parent compound, progesterone. Other steroids of clinical importance are norethindrone (oral contraceptive agent), medroxyprogesterone acetate, and megastrol acetate all are related to progesterone.

Brand Names : Dubagest®, Naturogest®, Puregest® (all contains Natural Micronised Progesterone)

III] Chemical contraceptive agents

Chapter on steroids cannot be completed without the mention of chemical contraceptive agents. The chemical modifications of estrogens and progestins in early 60's led to the orally effective contraceptive agents which caused a small revolution in the field of family planning. Some of these agents have been mentioned in the early parts of this chapter, but once again their structures can be given as below. Some of the major orally effective chemical contraceptive agents are,

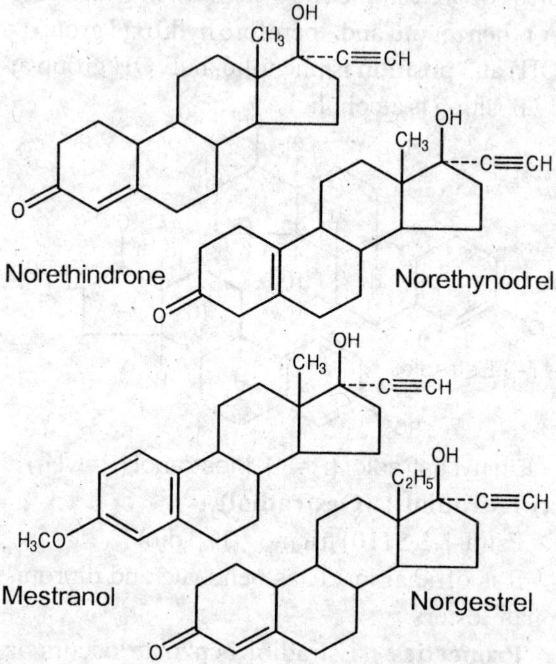

Norethindrone

Norethynodrel

Mestranol

Norgestrel

All these agents are ovulation inhibitors, and thereby bring about the contraceptive action.

Very often combination tablets are used wherein two of these agents are formulated together in different doses to bring about more effectiveness. Some of the commonly used combinations are,

1) Norethindrone (1 mg) + Ethinylestradiol (20 mcg)

2) Norgestrol (0.5 mg) + Ethinylestradiol (50 mcg)

3) Norethindrone (1 mg) + Mestranol (60 mcg)

4) Norethynodrel (1 mg) + Mestranol (60 mcg)

Sometimes sequential tablets, like estrogen followed by a progestin are also used. Thus mestranol (80 mcg) is used from 5th to 18th day of the mensural cycle followed by norethindrone from 18th to 25th day of the cycle. Progestin only, or sometimes called as 'mini-pill', is nor-ethindrone (0.35 mg) or norgestrel (0.075 mg) to be taken daily throughout the year to get proper protection. Injectable depots of medroxyprogesterone have been tried, so also 'once-a-month' or 'once-a-week' pill of ethinyl estradiol and nor-ethindrone acetate have been tried. Intrauterine implants coated with low doses of progestin have also been tried with high promise.

Synthetic non-steroidal compounds like diethylstilbsterol have been advocated as post-coital contraceptive agents.

All these agents have varying degrees of success, but combination oral pills have the highest rate of success, so far. Yet none of the agents is hundred per cent safe.

IV] Adrenocortical Hormones (ACTH) and Related Compounds

The adrenal glands (adrenal cortex) which are just above the kidneys, secrete over 50 different steroids, including precursors to many steroids. These steroids of adrenocortical origin fall into two main groups namely (i) Glucocorticoids causing primary effect on intermediary metabolism like gluconeogenesis, glycogen deposition, protein metabolism etc. eg. cortisone, hydrocortisone. (ii) Mineralocorticoids having their main action on electrolyte and water metabolism causing salt and fluid retention eg. aldosterone.

Therapeutically, glucocorticoids are more important because of their anti-inflammatory, immuno-suppressive effect and anti-allergic activity. Glucocorticoids are also used in the treatment of collagen vascular diseases and in rheumatoid arthritis. They are also used typically to treat various inflammatory and allergic conditions.

Mineralocorticoids are used primarily for the treatment of Addison's disease which is due to deficiency of adrenocorticoids due to either failure of adrenal or anterior pituitary gland.

The glucocorticoids and mineralocorticoids have related structures and are derivatives of 5-α-pregnane. They have 21 carbon atoms, with a side chain at C-17 (-CO-CH_2OR). At 11th position, there is an -OH or a ketone group (especially in glucocorticoids). A methyl group is usually present at C-10 and C-13 position, a ketone group at C-3 and a double bond between C-4 and C-5, are the other features of these steroids. Some of the important drugs are as follows,

Glucocorticoids

Among the glucocorticoids; hydrocortisone and cortisone are the main agents. Other agents of therapeutic importance are prednisolone, betamethasone and dexamethasone. The structures of these agents are as follows,

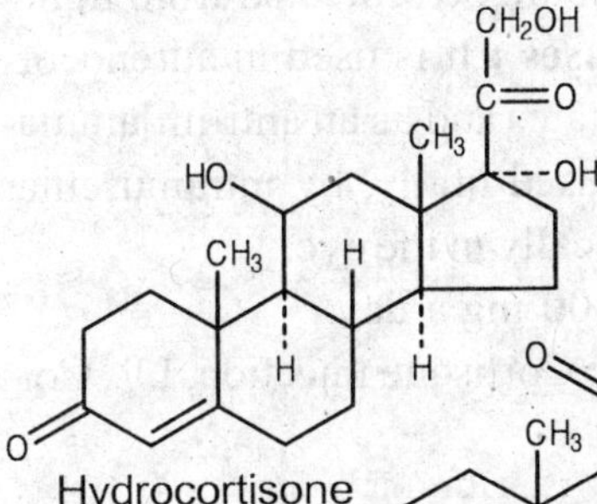

Hydrocortisone

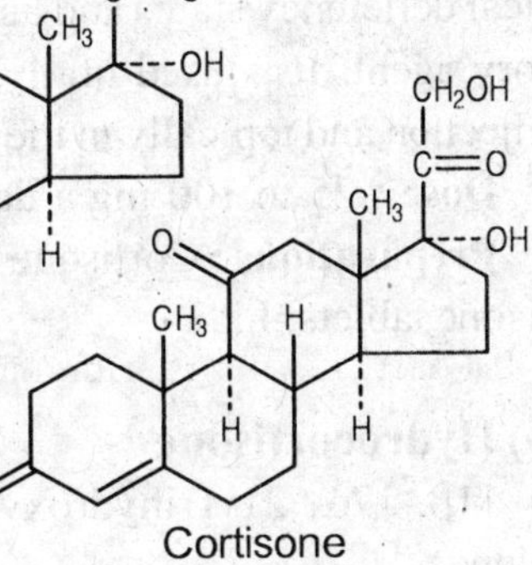

Cortisone

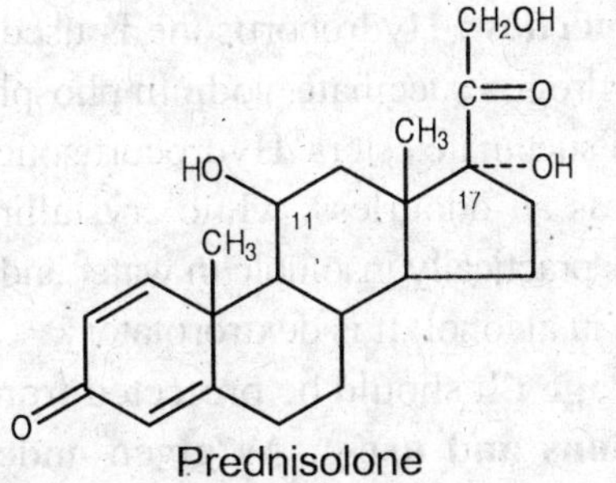

Prednisolone

(Double bonds at C-1-2 and C-4-5 positions, -OH group at C-11 and C-17)

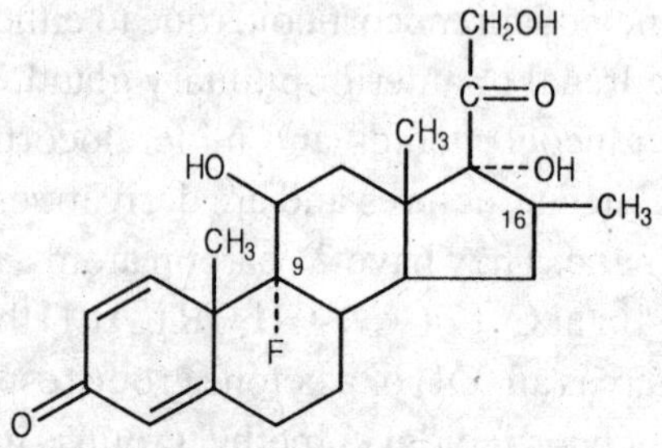

Betamethasone
(Double bonds at C-1-2 and C-4-5 positions, -OH at C-11 and C-17, a fluoro group at C-9 and additional $-CH_3$ group at C-16)

a) Cortisone

17α, 21-Dihydroxypregn-4-ene-3,11,20 trione

Properties : Cortisone acetate occurs as a white crystalline odourless powder. It is very slightly soluble in water and slightly soluble in alcohol. It is dextrorotatory. It exists in several polymorphic forms.

Storage : It should be protected from light.

Actions and uses : It is used in adrenocortical deficiency states and as an anti-inflammatory agent. It is used orally, by intramuscular injection and topically in the eye.

Dose : 25 to 100 mg a day.

Preparations : Cortisone injection, I.P., Cortisone tablets, I.P.

b) Hydrocortisone

11β, 17α, 21-Trihydroxypregn-4-ene-3,20-dione.

Properties : Hydrocortisone is used as acetate, hydrogen succinate, sodium phosphate and sodium succinate esters. Hydrocortisone acetate occurs as an odourless, white crystalline powder. It is practically insoluble in water and slightly soluble in alcohol. It is dextrorotatory.

Storage : It should be protected from light.

Actions and uses : As given under cortisone. It is also given by intra-articular injection into inflammed joints. It is also applied on the skin for anti-inflammatory action.

Dose : 10 to 40 mg a day.

Preparations : Hydrocortisone acetate injection I.P., B.P.

Hydrocortisone eye ointment, I.P., B.P.C.

Hydrocortisone sodium succinate injection, I.P., B.P.C.

Hydrocortisone cream, B.P.C.

Hydrocortisone lotion, B.P.C.

Hydrocortisone tablets, B.P.C.

Hydrocortisone suppositories, B.P.C.

Hydrocortisone eye-drops, B.P.C.

Hydrocortisone ointment, B.P.

Brand Names : Hycoson® inj., Wycort® inj., Lycortin®-SS

c) Prednisolone

11β, 17α, 21-Trihydroxypregna-1,4-diene-3,20-dione.

Properties : Prednisolone occurs as an odourless, hygroscopic, white, crystalline powder. It is very slightly soluble in water and soluble in alcohol. It is dextrorotatory. It is also used as acetate, pivalate and phosphate esters.

Storage : It should be stored in airtight container, protected from light.

Actions and uses : Prednisolone has actions similar to cortisone. Compared to cortisone, it causes less sodium retention and is, therefore, preferred as an antirheumatic agent. It is useful in the treatment of nephrotic oedema, as it produces diuresis.

Dose : 5 mg a day.

Preparations : Prednisolone tablets, I.P., B.P.

Prednisolone pivalate injection, B.P.

Prednisolone sodium phosphate injection, B.P.

Prednisolone enema, B.P.C.

Prednisolone eye-drops, B.P.C.

Brand Names : Deltacortil®, Hostacortin H®, Wysolone®

d) Betamethasone

9α-Fluoro-11β, 17α, 21-trihydroxy- 16β-methylpregna-1,4,-diene-3,20-dione.

Properties : It occurs as a white to creamy-white odourless powder. It is very slightly soluble in water; sparingly soluble in alcohol. It is dextrorotatory. It is also official as valerate and sodium phosphate esters.

Storage : It should be protected from light.

Actions and uses : It is widely used as an antirheumatic. Its glucocorticoid activity is 5 times that of prednisolone.

Dose : 0.5 to 2 mg a day.

Preparations : Betamethasone tablets, I.P., B.P.

Betamethasone sodium phosphate tablets, I.P., B.P.

Betamethasone sodium phosphate injection, I.P., B.P.

Betamethasone eye-drops, B.P.C.

Betamethasone valerate cream, B.P.C.

Brand Names : Betacortil®, Betnelan®, Betnesol®

Drugs For Further Study

Oestrogens

1) Tibolone - Livial®, Tibofem®, Tibomax®
2) Ethinylestradiol - Evalon®

Progestins

3) Dydrogesterone -Duphaston®
4) Medroxyprogesterone - Deviry®, Medarin®, Medtet®,Orgamed®
5) Hydroxyprogesterone - Gestimax®, Gravidin®, Hyprogres®
6) Norethisterone - Norgest®, Noristerat®, Noritis®
7) Allylestrenol (to prevent abortion) - Fetugard®, Fulterm®, Gestin®, Maintane®
8) Levonorgestrel (emergency contraceptive) - Ecee 2®, Norlevo®, Pill 72®

Oral contraceptives (Progestin + Oestrogen combination)

9) Levonorgestrel + Ethinyl estradiol - Duoluton-L®, Femilon®, Loette®, Ovral®, Triquilar®
10) Desogestrol + Ethinyl estradiol - Novelon®

Exercise

Q1. What do you know about sex hormones? Give properties, stability and storage and uses of progesterone. (Winter 04)

Q2. What are sex hormones? Give their examples and describe in detail uses of each hormone. (Summer 03)

Q3. Draw structures of - i) 5-α-androstane & ii) 5-α-pregnane. (Summer 06)

Q4. In what dosage form is the following drug administered - testosterone. (Summer 06, May-June 04)

Q5. Give uses of prednisolone. (Summer 06, May 07)

Q7. Write note on - steroids. (May-June 04)

Q8. Write note on oral contraceptives. (May 07, Nov 06)

28 Anti-neoplastic Drugs (Anti-cancer Drugs)

Cancer

Cancer still remains an unconquered disease. Inspite of voluminous research work, on all fronts, the disease still claims nearly 2.5 million victims per year all over the world. As compared with the success achieved by chemotherapy in the area of microbial infections, success of these agents against cancer remains limited. However, combination of surgery, radiations and chemotherapy has worked well in many cases and in many others brought some relief for a few years. Hence, the anti-cancer compounds currently available are mainly palliative in action, except in a few types of cancer.

Classification of Anti-Neoplastic Drugs

The drugs commonly employed in the treatment of malignant diseases are classified according to their mode of action as follows,

I) Alkylating agents

i) Nitrogen mustards eg. cyclophosphamide, chlorambucil.

ii) Ethyleneimines eg. Thiotepa

iii) Alkyl sulphonates eg. Busulphan.

II) Antimetabolites

i) Folic acid antagonists eg. Methotrexate.

ii) Purine antagonists eg. 6-mercaptopurine and Azathioprine.

III) Antibiotics

eg. Actinomycin-D, Mitomycin-C.

IV) Radioactive isotopes

eg. Radio-iodine, Radiophosphorus.

V) Miscellaneous agents

eg. Vinca alkaloids (eg. Vinblastin, vincristine), procarbazine, 1-aspargenase, cisplatin and hormones like androgens, estrogens, progestins, corticosteroids, etc.

Some of these agents are discussed briefly here.

I] Alkylating agents

Nitrogen mustards are called 'alkylating agents', because these compounds can transfer an alkyl radical to a suitable receptor site. Alkylating agents being nucleophilic, react with the nucleic acid bases and inhibit DNA synthesis. They also bring about the cross linkages of DNA strands and thus interfere with cell replication process.

Some of the important agents of this class are

i) Nitrogen Mustards

1) Cyclophosphamide

Properties : It occurs as a fine, white, crystalline powder. It is odourless and has a slightly bitter taste. It is soluble in water and freely soluble in alcohol.

Stability : It discolours on exposure to light. In aqueous solutions, stored above 30°C, hydrolysis occurs with the removal of chlorine atoms.

Storage : It should be stored in airtight

containers, protected from light.

Actions and uses : Cyclophosphamide is a typical nitrogen mustard with a phosphoramide moiety incorporated in it. It has similar actions like its parent compound mechlorethamine (Mustine). It is widely used, generally in combination with other agents, in the treatment of a variety of malignant diseases like Burkitts' lymphomas, Hodgkin's disease and other lymphomas. This drug is given orally (50 mg) or through intravenous injection (2-3 mg/kg). It is not a tissue irritant or vesicant.

Dose : Oral 50 mg. IV 100 mg a day.

Preparations : Cyclophosphamide injection, I.P., B.P.

Cyclophosphamide tablets I.P., B.P.

Brand Names : Cycloxan®, Endoxan-Asta®, Eldamide®

2) Chlorambucil

4-[4-Bis(2-chloroethyl)aminophenyl] butyric acid.

Chlorambucil is a new addition in I.P. 1996.

Properties : It occurs as a white crystalline powder with a slight odour. It is practically insoluble in water; freely soluble in alcohol. Its contact with skin should be avoided.

Storage : It should be stored in airtight containers.

Actions and uses : This is another drug of the class of Alkylating agents and is chemically related to the parent drug of this class, i.e., mustine. This drug is especially useful with proliferation of white blood cells, particularly lymphocytes. It is used in the treatment of chronic lymphocytic leukaemia, lymphomas and Hodgkin's disease. It is also used in carcinoma of breast, ovary and testis. It also has immunosuppressive properties.

Dose : Orally 5 to 12 mg and IV 0.1 to 0.2 mg/kg.

Preparations : Chlorambucil tablets, I.P., B.P.

Brand Names : Leukeran®

3) Mechlorethamine (Mustine)

This is the main agent of this class of nitrogen mustards, often known as mustine hydrochloride.

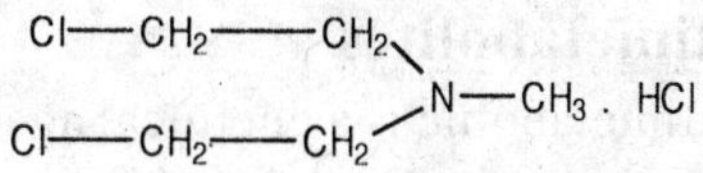

Mustine hydrochloride

Mustine is used in the treatment of Hodgkins disease, usually in conjunction with vinca alkaloids, prednisolone, followed by chlorambucil. Usual dose is 0.4 mg/kg of body weight given in 2 to 4 divided doses for 4 to 6 weeks.

Ethyleneimines also act like nitrogen mustards. Chemically these compounds are called aziridines. Thiotepa is the official compound in this class. Thiotepa is chemically named as phosphorothioic acid tri(ethyleneamide). It has a phosphorous, a sulphur and 3 aziridine rings all linked through phosphorus atom. The drug has actions similar to mustine, and is useful in the treatment of carcinoma of breast, ovary and various lymphomas.

Among the alkyl sulphonates, busulphan is the main compound.

iii) Alkyl Sulphonates

1) Busulphan

Tetramethylene bis (methane sulphonate)

$CH_3\text{-}SO_2\text{-}O\text{-}(CH_2)_4\text{-}O\text{-}SO_2\text{-}CH_3$

Properties : It occurs as a white crystalline odourless powder. It is slightly soluble in water, very slightly soluble in alcohol. It is irritant and its contact with skin should be avoided.

Storage : It should be stored in airtight containers, protected from light.

Actions and uses : Busulphan is a cytotoxic agent. Its effects are caused by inhibition of cell division. It has a selective depressant action on the bone marrow, especially on the production of granulocytes. It is given orally in the palliative treatment of chronic myeloid leukaemia.

Dose : 2 to 4 mg a day.

Preparations : Busulphan tablets I.P., B.P.

Brand Names : Mylefan®, Busuphan®

II) Antimetabolites

An antimetabolite is a chemical agent which has a very closely related structure to a normal metabolite and which can take part in the biochemical processes of a cell. However, at a vital step of cell metabolism, it blocks the metabolic transformation. This it does either by preventing the normal metabolite with a specific enzyme or by itself combining with the specific enzyme and thus getting transformed into a compound which is either metabolically inactive or harmful to the cell. Thus antimetabolites, in a way, 'fool' the cancerous cell.

Clinically useful antimetabolites are structural analogues of (a) substances essential for the synthesis of nucleic acid bases eg. folic acid antagonists like methotrexate (b) substances which get incorporated in the nucleic acid chains and ultimately affect the DNA synthesis eg. 6-mercaptopurine, 5-fluorouracil, azathioprine.

i) Folic acid Antagonists

1) Methotrexate (Amethopterin)

Methotrexate is a 4-amino substituted analogue of folic acid, which acts as an antagonist of folic acid.

Properties : Methotrexate occurs as a yellow to orange crystalline powder. It is very slightly soluble in water and in alcohol. It is soluble in dilute solutions of alkali hydroxides and carbonates.

Storage : It should be stored in airtight containers, protected from light.

Mode of action : In cellular metabolism, folic acid gets reduced to dihydrofolic acid and then to tetrahydrofolic acid (THFA). Methotrexate competitively inhibits the enzyme dihydrofolate reductase and thus prevents the formation of THFA which is further needed for the formation of purine and pyrimidine in the nucleic acid chain. Consequently the formation of DNA and RNA are impaired and further cell replication is stopped.

Uses : This drug is used in acute lymphoblastic leukaemia in children. It is especially useful in choriocarcinoma and in some cases it is reported to have produced complete cure. It is somewhat useful in the treatment of soft tissue sarcoma, breast cancer, acute myeloid leukaemia and in skin conditions called psoriasis.

Dose : It is given orally in 2.5 to 5 mg doses for children and 2.5 to 10 mg for adults and also intrathecally 0.1 to 0.5 mg/kg of body weight.

Preparations : Methotrexate tablets, I.P., B.P.

Methotrexate injection, I.P., B.P.

Brand Names : Biotrexate®, Neotrexate®, Imutrex®

ii) Purine Antagonists

1) 6-Mercaptopurine and Thioguanine

Purine-6-thiol

These two compounds are analogues of

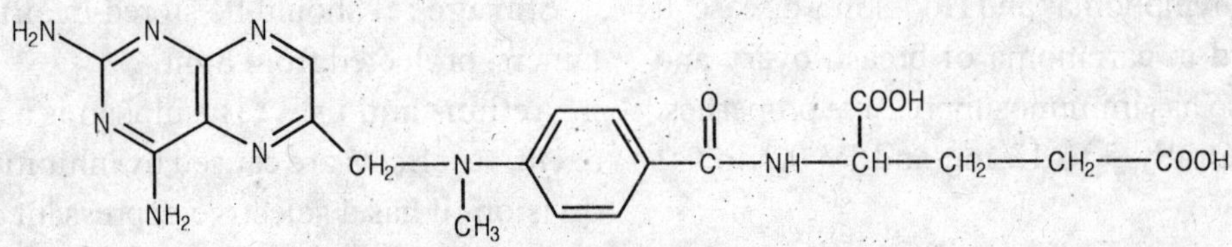

Methotrexate

naturally occuring purines and are structurally related to the naturally occuring adenine and guanine.

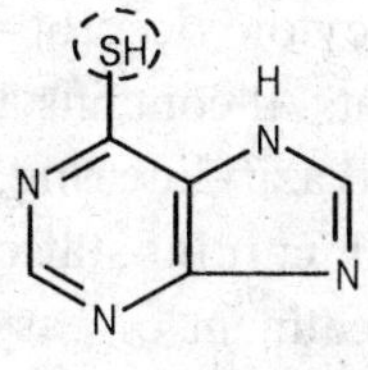

6-Mercaptopurine

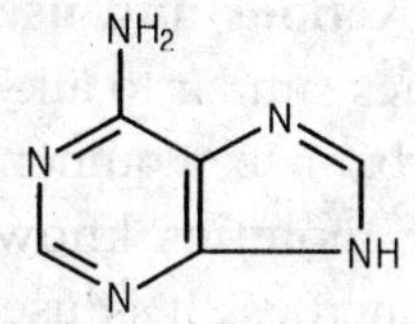

Adenine

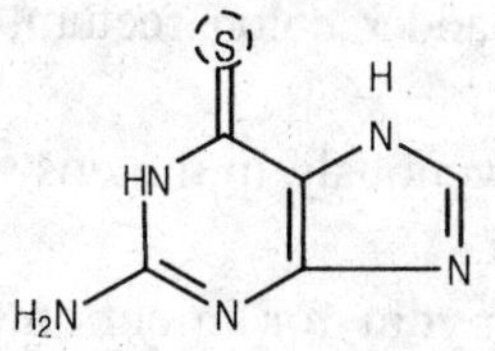

Thioguanine

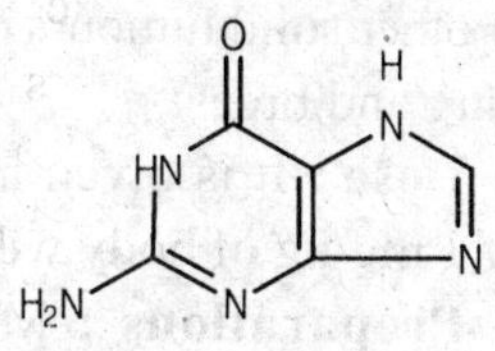

Guanine

Properties : Mercaptopurine occurs as an odourless yellow crystalline powder. It is very slightly soluble in water; slightly soluble in solutions of alkali hydroxides.

Storage : It should be stored in airtight containers, protected from light.

Actions and uses : Both these compounds interfere with the nucleic acid biosynthesis, being analogues of adenine and guanine. Mercaptopurine is used in acute leukaemia of children. It is also effective in choriocarcinoma. The drug acts slower than methotrexate, but there is no cross resistance to other antileukaemic drugs, and this is a great clinical advantage.

Dose : 2.5 mg per kg of body weight a day, in divided doses.

Preparations : Mercaptopurine tablets, I.P., B.P.

Brand Names : Mesna® inj., Mercapthol®

Other purine antagonists like thioguanine and azathioprine also possess cytotoxic actions. Azathioprine is especially an immunosuppressive agent useful in organ transplants.

There are also other drugs in this class like azaserine, duasomycin, though not exactly purine analogues, but they also interfere in purine metabolism. However, clinically they are not so effective.

2) 5-Fluorouracil

5-Fluoropyrimidine-2,4-dione

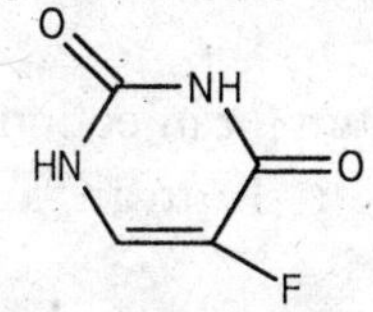

Properties : It occurs as a white, almost odourless powder. It is soluble in water; very slightly soluble in alcohol.

Storage : It should be stored in airtight container, protected from light.

Actions and uses : Fluorouracil is a pyrimidine analogue and acts as an antimetabolite of uracil. It interferes with the synthesis of DNA and RNA. It also possesses immunosuppressive properties. It is used in the treatment of carcinoma of stomach, colon, rectum, breast and ovaries. Recommended dose is 15 mg/kg of body weight daily for 3-5 days. It is also administered intravenously and as intra-arterial infusion.

Dose : 15 mg per kg of body weight a day, by IV infusion.

Preparations : Fluorouracil injection I.P., B.P.C.

Brand Names : Fludin® inj., Fluracil® inj., Oncourcil® inj.

3) Azathioprine

6-(1-Methyl-4-nitroimidazol-5-yl thio) purine

Properties : It occurs as a pale yellow odourless powder. It is practically insoluble in water; very slightly soluble in alcohol. It is soluble in dilute solutions of alkali hydroxides.

Storage : It should be stored in airtight containers, protected from light.

Uses : Azathioprine is an immunosuppressant and antineoplastic with actions similar to mercaptopurine. It is slowly converted to mercaptopurine in the body. It is used as immunosuppressant to facilitate survival of organ and tissue transplants.

Dose : 1 to 5 mg per kg body weight a day.

Preparations : Azathioprine tablets, B.P., U.S.P.

Azathioprine sodium for injection, U.S.P.

Brand Names : Imuran®, Azoran®, Azimune®

III) Antibiotics

Many antibiotics have been shown to be active against neoplasms. Some of them have found clinical use also. Three groups of antibiotics have been found to be therapeutically useful. They are actinomycins, mitomycins and anthracyclines. Actinomycin C has properties similar to actinomycin D.

1) Actinomycin-D (Dactinomycin)

It is an antibiotic produced by the growth of *Streptomyces chrysomallus* and *S. antibioticus.*

Properties : It is a bright red, crystalline powder. It is somewhat hygroscopic. It is soluble in water and freely soluble in alcohol.

Storage : It should be stored in airtight containers, protected from light.

Uses : Due to its high toxicity, its use is very limited. It inhibits the synthesis of DNA and RNA. It is used in the treatment of Wilm's tumour, uterus and testes tumours.

Dose : IV 15 mcg/kg body weight a day, for five days.

Preparations : Dactinomycin for injection, U.S.P.

2) Mitomycin-C (Mitomycin, Mitomycin X)

It is an antibiotic produced by the growth of *Streptomyces caespitosus.*

Properties : It occurs as a blue violet crystalline powder. It is soluble in water. Aqueous solutions are most stable at pH 6 to 9.

Storage : It should be stored in airtight containers, protected from light.

Actions and uses : It has cytotoxic properties similar to alkylating agents. It contains a carbamate, a quinone group and aziridine ring, the moieties known for their carcinostatic properties. It is used in the treatment of gastric and pancreatic carcinoma. It is also useful in other solid tumours of bladder, colon, rectum, lung and breast.

Dose : It is given intravenously in the dose of 1 mg/kg of body weight.

Preparations : Mitomycin for injection, U.S.P.

Brand Names : Mitomycin-C® inj., Mitocin® inj., Mitodus® inj.

3) Daunorubicin (Rubidomycin)

This antibiotic belongs to the anthracycline group. It is a glycoside and the aglycone portion contains anthraquinone structure, somewhat similar to the one in tetracycline antibiotics. The sugar part is daunosamine (an amino group containing sugar). This antibiotic is also produced by a species of *Streptomyces.*

Properties : Daunorubicin hydrochloride occurs as an orange-red hygroscopic microcrystalline powder. It is soluble in water and in methanol.

Storage : It should be stored in airtight containers, protected from light.

Uses : Daunorubicin is useful in the treatment of acute leukaemias and is used along with other antineoplastic agents like vincristine and prednisolone.

Dose : IV 45 to 60 mg per sq.m. of body surface,a day.

Preparations : Daunorubicin hydrochloride for injection, U.S.P.

Brand Names : Daunotec® inj.

IV) Radioactive isotopes

Various radioactive isotopes capable of emitting radiations have been used, like radio-iodine I^{131}, radio-phosphorous P^{35}, radio-gold Au^{198}. They have specific use, since they get deposited only in certain organs. Thus radioiodine is useful only in certain cases of thyroid carcinoma, radiophosphorus is useful in bone marrow and spleen neoplasms and radiogold is used as a palliative measure in malignant pleural and peritoneal infusions. All these radioisotopes give only symptomatic relief and other therapies have to be given along with them.

V) Miscellaneous agents

1) Vinca alkaloids

Various alkaloids isolated from periwinkle plant, Vinca rosea (*Catharanthus roseus*). Two compounds namely, vinblastine and vincristine (as sulphate salts), are therapeutically useful.

Uses : Vinblastine is mainly useful in Hodgkin's disease, choriocarcinoma and lymphosarcoma resistant to methotrexate. Vincristine is useful in the treatment of acute lymphatic leukaemia in children.

Dose : The weekly IV dose is 0.03 to 0.15 mg/kg of body weight and for adults it is 0.02 and 0.0075 mg/kg of body weight.

Brand Names :

Vincristine - Biocristin® inj., Cytocristin® inj., Oncocristin - AQ® inj.

Vinblastine - Cytoblastin® inj.

2) Hormones and related agents

Hormones act differently than cytotoxic agents and hence can be usefully combined with other antineoplastic agents. They act in several ways like inhibition of cell growth, stimulation of differentiation of cells, inhibition of circulatory concentration of substances that stimulate malignant cells and extension of their normal physiological functions. Thus adrenocorticosteroids (ACTH) are able to suppress mitosis of lymphocytes, glucocorticoids are of value for acute leukaemia in children and often are used to reduce immune responses to organ transplantation. Sex hormones like androgens and estrogens are also useful in women with advanced neoplasms of breast. Estrogens are used to control inoperable and metastatic neoplasms of prostate. Diethyl stilbestrol is generally preferred. Progestins are used in the treatment of inoperable neoplasms of endometrium. They have also been tried for neoplasms of kidney and prostate, medroxyprogesterone has also been found useful for this purpose.

3) Other agents

a) Hydroxyurea

Hydroxyurea is an antineoplastic agent. It also inhibits the synthesis of DNA and is useful for chronic myeloid leukaemia, malignant melanoma and inoperable tumours of ovary.

b) Cisplatin

Cis-diammine dichloroplatinum.

Cisplatin is another new addition in I.P. 1996.

Properties : Cisplatin occurs as white powder. It is slightly soluble in water. It is incompatible with aluminium and sodium bisulphite.

Storage : It should be stored at 2-8°C.

Uses : Cisplatin is a platinum containing complex and acts like alkylating agents. Cisplatin is of value in the treatment of metastatic tumours of testes, and is usually a component of combination chemotherapy.

Dose : IV - 20 mg per sq.m. of body surface every month.

Preparations : Cisplatin injection, I.P.

Brand Names : Blastolem® inj., Cisplat® inj., Plantinex® inj.

Summary of Drug Therapy of Neoplasms

The advent of chemotherapy has definitely helped improve this otherwise hopeless area of disease. And yet, chemotherapy of cancer, is still palliative in nature. Only in few conditions, long term remissions can be obtained by appropriate use of drugs (discussed in this chapter). These are acute lymphatic leukaemia in children, Hodgkin's disease, choriocarcinoma in females, Wilm's tumour in children, and testicular cancer (see table 28.1). In majority of other cases, anticancer drugs are only suppressive and help the patient to return to near normal mode of life.

Since all anticancer drugs are potentially very toxic and give rise to a number of adverse reactions such as secondary infections, depression of bone marrow, megaloblastic anemia, GI upset, ulceration etc., the diagnosis of the disease must be firmly established before the use of these drugs. Obviously, management of malignancies with various drugs needs considerable experience, as the choice is empirical rather than rational. A judicious combination of palliative surgery, radiation therapy and use of these drugs help a lot to fight this deadly disease. Also of importance is the overall care of the cancer patient, maintenance of nutrition, treatment of anemia, protection against infection, relieving pain and anxiety, occupational therapy and above all, adequate emotional support to the patient and the family. Good results are generally obtained in patients with adequate hepatic, renal and bone marrow functions, in good nutritional state and without severe metabolic disturbances, infections or other complications.

The following table gives some of the better managed malignancies with the use of drugs.

Table 28.1 : Treatment of different types of cancer

No.	Type of Cancer	Drug of Choice	Other supportive Drugs
1	Acute lymphatic leukaemia	Vincristine with prednisolone	Methotrexate, mercaptopurine, cyclophosphamide
2	Chronic lymphatic Leukaemia	Chlorambucil	Cyclophosphamide, prednisolone
3	Chronic myeloid leukemia	Busulphan	Hydroxyurea, mercaptopurine, radiations
4	Hodgkin's disease	Methotrexate, vincristine, prednisolone	Cyclophosphamide, chlorambucil
5	Choriocarcinoma	Methotrexate	Mercaptopurine, Actinomycin-D
6	Carcinoma of breast, ovary	Cyclophosphamide	Fluorouracil, methotrexate

Drugs For Further Study

Alkylating agents

1) Ifosfamide - Ifex-M®, Ipamide®, Isoxan®
2) Melphalan - Alkeran®
3) Lomustine - Lomustine®

Cytotoxic antibiotics

4) Doxorubicin - Adriamycin®, Adrim®, Doxobin®
5) Idarubicin - Zavedos®
6) Epirubicin - Alrubicin®, Farmorubicin®
7) Bleomycin - Bleochem®, Bleocin®, Oncobleo®

Antimetabolites

8) Cytarabine - Arasid®, Cytabin®, Cytarine®
9) Fludarabine - Fludara®

Miscellaneous

10) Vinorelbine - Vinbine®, Vinelbine®
11) Etoposide - Beposid®, Etoside®, Fytosid®
12) Paclitaxel - Altaxel®, Paxtal®, Petaxel®
13) Docetaxel - Daxotel®, Docet®
14) Irinotecan - Irinotel®
15) Topotecan - Topotel®
16) Carboplatin - Carbopa®, Carbotinal®, Karplat®
17) Dacarbazine - Dabaz®, Dacarex®, Dacarzine®
18) Procarbazine - Indicarb®, Neozine®, P-carzine®
19) Dactinomycin - Cosmegen®, Dacmozen®

Exercise

Q1. Define anti-neoplastic agents. Classify them with examples from each class. (Winter 04, Summer 03, Summer 06)

Q2. Give uses of - i) Flurouracil & ii) Busulphan. (Summer 03)

Q3. Explain interferone with suitable example. (May-June 04)

Q4. Write a note on cytotoxic agents. (Nov 06)

■

29 Anticonvulsant Drugs

Introduction

The primary use of anticonvulsant drugs is in the prevention and control of epileptic seizures. In most cases, the treatment is symptomatic. Majority of anticonvulsant drugs are non-specific depressants of central nervous system. However, converse is not true. Thus, some of the classical CNS depressant drugs like morphine, reserpine or tranquilisers do not abolish epileptic convulsions. The disease affects approximately 0.5 to 1 per cent of the population. In India, every one person in 200 is affected by this disorder. Although the disease is not fatal, consequences of the seizures can be disastrous. For example, if an epileptic attack takes place while driving a car, it can be very dangerous.

Each type of epilepsy may be distinguished by clinical and electroencephalographic patterns (EEG) and each responds differently to the various classes of anticonvulsant drugs. The major types of epileptic seizures are,

a) Grand Mal

Sudden loss of consciousness followed by general muscle spasms, lasting for 2 to 5 minutes.

b) Petit Mal

Sudden, brief loss of consciousness with minor movement of head, eyes and limbs, lasting for only about 5 to 30 seconds. The person becomes immediately alert. This type is more common in children.

c) Psychomotor Seizures

Automatic, patterned movements lasting for 2 to 3 minutes. Often, no memory of incident remains.

Classification of Anticonvulsant Drugs

I] Barbiturates
II] Hydantoins
III] Oxazolidinediones
IV] Succinimides and
V] Miscellaneous agents

The anticonvulsant drugs have a common structural feature as shown below

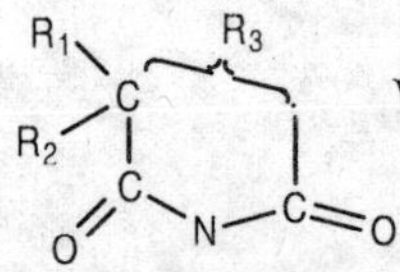

When R_3 is

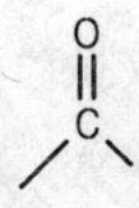

NH = Barbiturates

—NH = Hydantoins

—O = Oxazolidinediones

—CH_2 = Succinimides

—NH_2 = Phenacemide

I] Barbiturates

The most commonly used barbiturates are phenobarbital, mephobarbital and metharbital. The anticonvulsant activity of the barbiturates is not related to the sedation they produce. Actually, they offer protection from convulsions at a nonsedating dose. The barbiturates are especially useful in grand mal seizures, but not effective in petit mal or psychomotor seizures. The barbiturates are also discussed in the chapter on hypnotics and sedatives.

Brand Names :

Phenobarbital - Beetal®, Gardenal®, Phenobarb®

Primidone (Deoxybarbiturate) - Mysoline®

II] Hydantoins

The hydantoins have a cyclic structure related to barbiturates, and most of the substitutions are at 5 and 3 positions as follows,

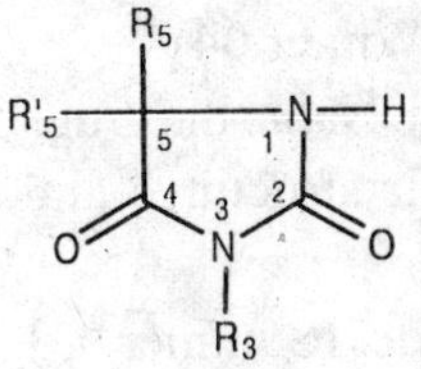

Phenytoin (Dilantin), R_5 and R'_5 = phenyl, R_3 = H,
Mephenytoin (Mesantion), R_5 = phenyl, R'_5 = Ethyl and R_3 = Methyl Ethotoin (peganon), R_5 = phenyl, R'_5 = H and R_3 = Ethyl

Phenytoin, mephenytoin and ethotoin are all used for grand mal epilepsy and they are not of much use for other types. They also have the same side effects like blood dyscrasias, skin rash, ataxia and gum hypertrophy.

Dose : Phenytoin, 200 to 600 mg a day.

Mephenytoin, 200 to 600 mg a day

Ethotoin, 1 gm a day

Brand Names : Phenytoin - Dilantin®, Epilan®, Eptoin®

III] Oxazolidinediones

The oxazolidine-2,4-diones, are related to hydantoins by substitutions of an oxygen for nitrogen. Oxazolidinediones are effective in the treatment of petit mal, but are not effective against grand mal. Trimethadione (Tridione) and paramethadione (Paradione) are the two effective drugs in this class having the following structure.

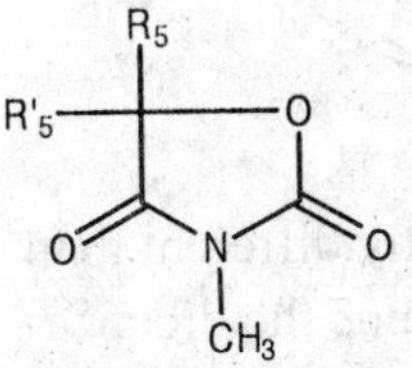

Trimethadione, $R_5 = R'_5 = CH_3$
Paramethadione, $R_5 = CH_3$, $R'_5 = C_2H_5$

Dose : Trimethadione, initial 300 mg, three times a day.

Paramethadione, initial 300 mg, three times a day.

IV] Succinimides

In succinimides, $-CH_2$ group is substituted for nitrogen in hydantoins. Ethosuximide, Phensuximide and Methsuximide are three major drugs in this class and have the structure as follows,

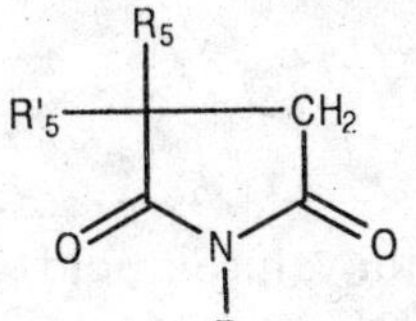

Phensuximide, R_5 = phenyl, R'_5 = H & $R_3 = CH_3$
Methsuximide, R_5 = phenyl, $R_5 = CH_3$ & $R_3 = CH_3$
Ethosuximide, $R = C_2H_5$, $R_5 = CH_3$ & R_3 = H

V] Miscellaneous agents

1) Phenacemide

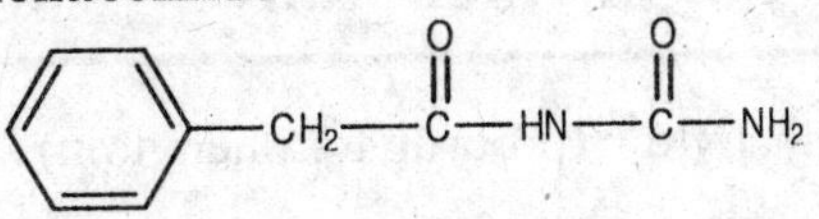

(Phenurone), Phenyl acetylurea is an open chain compound and a derivative of urea.

The drug was used for the treatment of psychometer seizures, grand mal and petit mal. But it had serious side effects like personality changes, suicidal tendencies, liver damage and bone marrow depression, due to which it is no longer used.

2) Carbamazepine

5H-dibenz (b,f) azepin-5-carboxamide

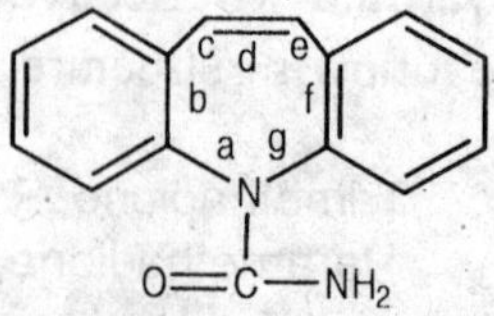

Carbamazepine is structurally different than the drugs in this class. It contains the dibenzazepine ring and is closer in its structure to imipramine (see chapter no. 10 on transquilisers). Carbamazepine is an effective agent for the control of major motor and psychomotor epilepsy. Its efficacy in grand mal seizures is approximately equal to phenobarbital. However, it is ineffective for the treatment of petit mal and minor motor epilepsy. Side effects include, dizziness, drowsiness, ataxia and dermatological reactions.

Dose : 300 mg to 2 gm per day.

Brand Names : Tegretol®, Mazetol®, Carmaz®

3) Other agents

Include primidone, diazepam, valproic acid, and some diuretics, have also been found marginally useful in the treatment of epilepsy.

Drugs For Further Study

1) Fosphenytoin (prodrug for phenytoin) - Fosolin®
2) Oxcarbazepine - Carbox®, Oxcarb®, Oxetol®, Oxrate®
3) Sodium valproate - Epival®, Valate®, Valcontin®
4) Clonazepam - Clonotril®, Clozep®, Epitril®, Lonazep®
5) Clobazam - Clodus®, Clozam®, Lobazam®
6) Gabapentin - Gabantin®, Gabapin®, Gabatin®
7) Lamotrigine - Lamepil®, Lametec®, Lamidus-DT®
8) Topiramate - Epitop®, Topamate®, Topex®
9) Divalproex - Diproex®, Dilvapro®, Valance®

Exercise

Q1. Classify anticonvulsants and write the structure of phenytoin and ethosuximide. (Karnataka Univ.)

Q2. Define anticonvulsants. (Winter 04)

Q3. Explain the term hydantoin. Name the drugs from the class, give their structures and uses (Winter 04)

Q4. Give uses of ethosuccimide. (Summer 03)

Q5. Define the following term with examples of drugs - anticonvulsants. (Summer 03)

Q6. What is epilepsy? Explain use of hydantoins as antiepileptics. (Summer 06)

Q7. Name one anticonvulsant drug possessing a pyrimidine derivative. (Nov 06)

30 Vitamins

Role of Vitamins

Vitamins are organic substances present in food and other natural products, but are not indigenous to the human body. They are required in small quantities by the body and are important constituents of many enzyme systems, metabolic processes and body constituents. Some of the vitamins are synthesised inside the body through some chemicals naturally found in foods, like vitamin A and vitamin D, which are synthesised *in vivo* through their precursors found in food stuffs. Vitamins also are important for the biochemical metabolism of carbohydrates, proteins and lipids, that human body consumes through the foods. Thus, in short, vitamins are required for the proper utilisation of these three vital components of our food. Vitamin deficiency can cause certain diseases and shortage of vitamins to the body may impair some of its vital processes. For example, deficiency of vitamin D can weaken the bones, while deficiency of vitamin B_{12} can cause anaemia. Deficiency of vitamins can occur due to various reasons like poor dietary intake, improper intake of food, unbalanced diet, etc. Vitamin deficiency can also take place due to certain physiological and pathological conditions like chronic diarrhoea, jaundice or during pregnancy, lactation or other stress conditions. Sometimes, vitamin deficiency (although temporarily) may be caused by certain drugs taken during an illness, like antibiotics which affect intestinal flora, drugs which affect absorption, or drugs which interfere with utilisation, for example diphenylhydantoin interferes with folic acid and INH with pyridoxine. Clinical manifestations of deficiency of vitamins are often not specific or clear cut. Although some of the diseases and deficiency symptoms are well established as indicated in the Table 30.1.

It is beyond the scope of this chapter to discuss in detail the various biochemical pathways in which vitamins and their coenzymes take part, hence the discussion here will be limited to chemistry, sources, physiological aspects and therapeutic uses.

Fat Soluble Vitamins

1) Vitamin A

Source : Vitamin A is present in the diet as the pre-formed vitamin, retinol, or as esters of retinol or in the form of carotenoids, especially β-carotene, which is considered to be a provitamin A. Carotenes are present in green leafy vegetables and fruits, carrots, papaya, mango etc. Retinol is present in eggs, milk, and meat products. Rich source of retinol is fish livers such as cod liver, shark liver and halibut liver.

Chemistry : Different forms of naturally occuring vitamin A are either geometrical isomers of vitamin A_1 (Retinol), or simple derivatives of vitamin A_1 which also exists in several stereochemical forms.

Table 30.1 : Deficiency diseases of vitamins

No.	Vitamin	Deficiency disease and/or deficiency symptom
1	Vitamin A	Nightblindness, xerophthalmia
2	Vitamin D	Rickets, bone weakness, osteomalacia
3	Vitamin E	Sterility, impairment in reproductive functions.
4	Vitamin K	Impairment in blood clotting process.
5	Thiamine or Vitamin B_1	Beriberi, polyneuritis
6	Riboflavin or Vitamin B_2	Syndrome called angular stomatitis, glossitis, magenta coloured toungue (ariboflavinosis)
7	Nicotinic acid or Nicotinamide	Pellagra
8	Pyridoxine or Vitamin B_6	Lesions of the skin, in children
9	Pantothenic acid	No specific deficiency disease, but causes fatigue, dermatitis
10	Biotin	No clinical deficiency symptoms
11	Ascorbic acid or Vitamin C	Scurvy
12	Folic acid	No specific deficiency disease
13	Vitamin B_{12}	Malabsorption of vitamin B_{12} from GI tract due to lack of intrinsic factor, is the cause of pernicious anaemia

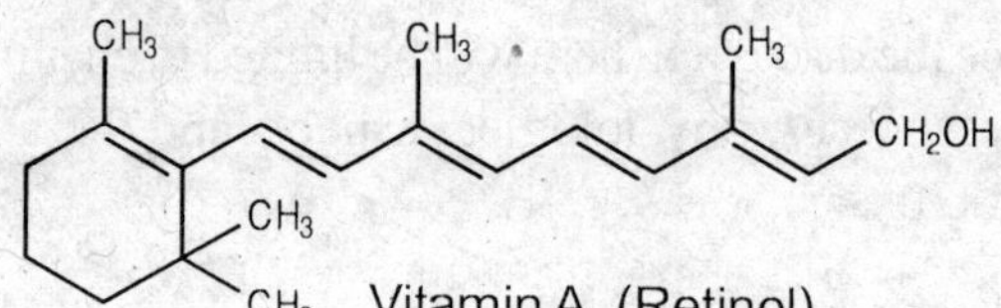

Vitamin A_1 (Retinol)

Commercially available vitamin A is almost exclusively synthetic, starting from the natural source, β-ionone which is obtained from lemon grass oil. Vitamin A is stabilised by converting it to its esters, acetate or palmitate, or by addition of antioxidants like vitamin E. Vitamin A occurs as pale yellow crystals, insoluble in water, but freely soluble in alcohol or oils.

Storage : It has to be stored in tightly closed, light resistant containers.

Physiological, biochemical functions and therapeutic uses : Vitamin A plays a vital role in the phenomenon of dark adaptations where it is essential for the synthesis of rhodopsin a photosensitive pigment of rods. Clinical deficiency of vitamin A is characterised by night-blindness, which, if untreated, aggravates in xerophthalmia. In the treatment of night-blindness or xerophthalamia, vitamin A is administered in the dose of 1,00,000 units by IM injection. Prophylactic use of vitamin A from 50,000 units to 2,00,000 units orally are recommended.

Dose : Daily requirement of vitamin A is about 5000 units for adults and 3000 units for children. Enough vitamin A, about 1500 units, should be given during the first six months of infancy. About 35 gm of green vegetables, 100 gm of mango, fish, glass of milk provide enough vitamin A for a day.

Brand Names : Advit-A®, Beetrion®, Vistamina®

2) Vitamin D

Source : Vitamin D (cholecalciferol) occurs in many fish liver oils, notably in tuna liver oil, halibut liver oil and cod liver oil. Milk and eggs are also good sources. Commercially, vitamin D is obtained by irradiation of ergosterol, a yeast sterol, which gives vitamin D_2 or calciferol which is also known as ergocalciferol. It appears as colourless crystals or white crystalline powder, practically insoluble in water and slightly soluble in fixed oils.

Storage : It has to be stored in tightly closed, light-resistant containers at about 15°C. The solutions cannot be heat sterilised and, therefore, have to be sterilised by filtration.

Chemistry : Vitamin D is a group of closely related substances which are derivatives of sterols having antirachitic activity. Ergosterol, a yeast sterol, on ultraviolet irradiation yields vitamin D_2, called calciferol or ergocalciferol. It is closely related to vitamin D_3, called cholecalciferol. Chemically cholecalciferol is named as 9,10-secocholesta- 5,7,10(19)-trien-3β-01. There is breaking of bonds between 9, 10 positions of the steroid nucleus, and hence the prefix 'seco'. The structure of cholecalciferol (vitamin D_3) is similar to ergocalfiferol except that the double bond between 22-23 is saturated and there is no methyl group at position 24.

Physiology, biochemistry and therapeutic uses : Vitamin D group is closely associated with antirachitic properties. Severe deficiency of this vitamin is known to cause rickets, especially in children. There is no definite biochemical role of vitamin D, but it is believed that vitamin D plays an important role in the mobilisation of calcium and phosphorus and their build up in bones. Vitamin D is used in deficiency conditions and in pregnancy and lactation periods as supplement to the diet.

Dose : Prophylactic - 400 to 1000 I.U. a day.

Therapeutic - 5000 to 50,000 I.U.

For prevention of rickets - not more than 20 mcg.

One international unit of vitamin D is equivalent to 0.025 mcg of crystalline vitamin D_2.

Brand Names : Shelcal®, Macalvit®, Calcimax®

3) Vitamin E

Source : Vitamin E is present in soyabean oil, wheat germ and rice germ oil. Green leafy vegetables and lettuce are also good sources. Synthetically, vitamin E is made from trimethyl hydroquinone and phytylhalides, which yields after several steps α-tocopherol.

Chemistry : There are at least four compounds of vitamin E group, known as tocopherols (α, β, γ and δ) and they are derivatives of chromanol. Tocopheryl acetate (α-tocopheryl acetate) is official.

Physiological and biochemical functions and uses : Vitamin E deficiency in lower animals may lead to sterility in males and abortion in females. However, deficiency syndromes are not established in humans. Vitamin E has been found to be important in maintaining the integrity and stability of membranes. Thus, it is essential for normal structure and functions of nervous system. Vitamin E has been used empirically in a variety of disorders, like sterility, myopathies and in chronic fat malabsorption. But there is no clear cut physiological or biochemical function associated with vitamin E.

Dose : Prophylactic 5 to 30 mg a day.

Brand Names : Evion®, E-Toplex®

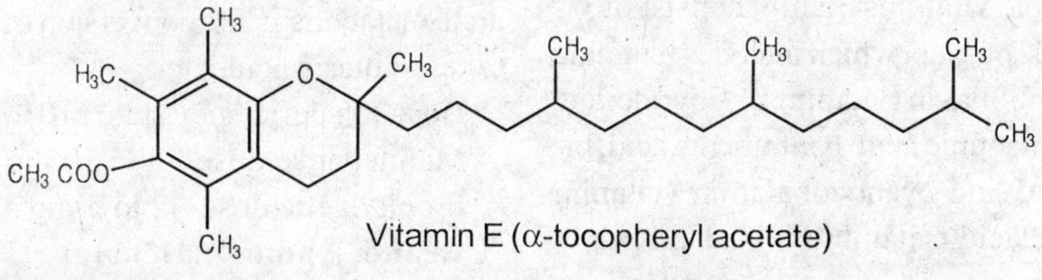

Vitamin E (α-tocopheryl acetate)

4) Vitamin K

Sources : Vitamin K is present as vitamin K_1, in fresh green vegetables, fruits and egg yolk. Synthetically, it is made as menadione which is a synthetic analog of vitamin K.

Chemistry : Natural vitamin K is phytomenadione, which is chemically, 2 - methyl, 3-phytyl-1,4,naphthoquinone. Synthetic menadione is 2-methyl-1, 4, naphthoquinone (without the phytyl side chain).

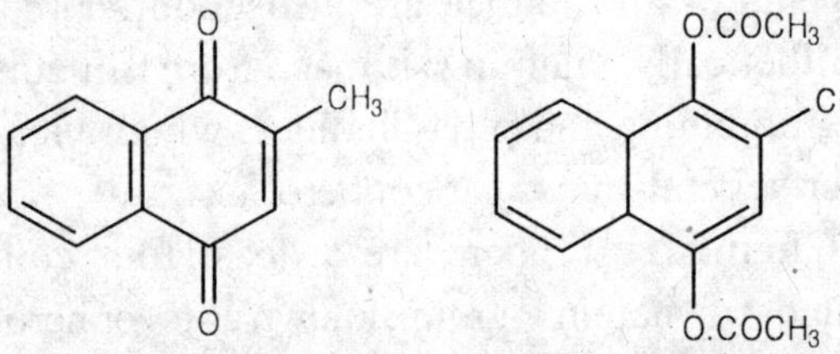

Menadione Acetomenadione

Physiological functions and therapeutic uses : Vitamin K is essential for the formation of prothrombin and other clotting factors and for the maintenance of normal prothrombin level in plasma. Menadione is used in the treatment of hypothrombinaemia and haemorrhage, especially caused by prolonged anticoagulant therapy. There is not specific biochemical coenzyme function; but vitamin K is involved in all steps of the process of the formation of blood clots.

Dose : As antidote to anticoagulants (except heparin) 5-20 mg. For haemorrhagic diseases of new born, by IM or IV 0.5 to 1 mg.

Water Soluble Vitamins

Water soluble vitamins mainly consist of vitamin B complex group, which includes thiamine (vitamin B_1), riboflavin (vitamin B_2), pyridoxine (vitamin B_6), nicotinic acid, pantothenic acid, biotin, folic acid and cyanocobalamin (vitamin B_{12}). Ascorbic acid (vitamin C) is also a water soluble vitamin.

1) Thiamine (Vitamin B_1, Aneurine)

Source : Peas, beans, germinated cereals, oatmeal, peanuts, mammalian organ meat are rich sources of this vitamin. Vegetables and fruits are also good sources of vitamin B_1. It is also made synthetically.

Chemistry : Thiamine molecule contains a pyrimidine and a thiazole ring linked by a methylene bridge. The nitrogen of thiazole ring is charged (+ve) and forms salt with chloride ion. Thiamine has a basic character and therefore almost white, freely soluble in water. Thiamine decomposes rapidly in alkaline pH, and is incompatible with oxidising and reducing substances.

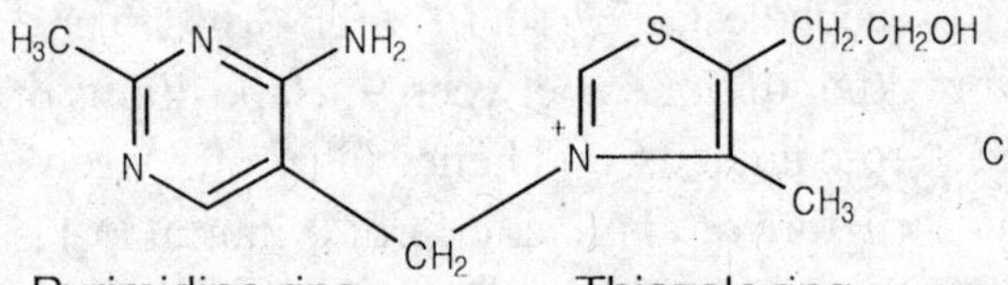

Pyrimidine ring Thiazole ring

Physiological, Biochemical functions and therapeutic uses : Thiamine deficiency causes a deficiency disease called beriberi. Besides beriberi, the deficiency of this vitamin also causes confusion, blurred vision and tremors. Other symptoms include epigastric pain, anorexia, constipation, easy fatigue etc. Thiamine deficiency can be prevented by improvement in the dietary intake and by preventing overpolishing of rice and other cereals. Acute beriberi responds dramatically to oral or parenteral administration of thiamine.

Biochemically active form of thiamine is called thiamine pyrophosphate and it constitutes the prosthetic group of enzyme, decarboxylase. This enzyme takes part in many steps of carbohydrate metabolism like conversion of pyruvic acid, α ketoglutaric acid, etc.

Dose : In deficiency state : 10 to 30 mg orally
Maintenance dose - 5 to 10 mg
Prophylactic dose - 2 to 5 mg a day

Brand Names : Benalgis®, Becosules®,

Beceflor®

2) Riboflavin (Vitamin B_2)

Source : Liver, Kidney, meat, eggs, milk, yeast and green vegetables.

Chemistry : Riboflavin molecule consists of a complex heterocyclic ring (isoalloxazine), a D-ribityl group (derived from pentose sugar D-ribose), attached to the central nitrogen of the isoalloxazine ring. When made into a solution it gives a greenish-yellow fluorescence. It is soluble in water 1:20. In presence of alkali or heavy metals, it is not stable.

Storage : It has to be stored in airtight, light-resistant container.

Physiological, Biochemical functions and therapeutic uses : Riboflavin deficiency in man gives a peculiar syndrome characterised by a magenta coloured tongue, glossitis and angular stomatitis. Other minor symptoms of riboflavin deficiency are dermatitis, 'burning feet' sensation, lacrimation and photophobia. The biochemically active form of riboflavin is formed by phosphorylation. The two coenzymes, flavin adenine dinucleotide (FAD) and flavin mononucleotide (FMN) are the active forms of riboflavin. These two coenzymes play an important role in electron transfer in cytochrome system, which is involved in oxygen transfer. They also play important roles in carbohydrate and amino acid metabolism.

Riboflavin is used therapeutically for the treatment of ariboflavinosis, in the dose of 2 to 10 mg a day, besides, it forms a component of multivitamin tablets or other preparations.

Dose : Prophylactic - 1 to 4 mg a day (as riboflavin phosphate)

Therapeutic dose - 5 to 10 mg a day.

Brand Names : Beplex®, Bexoplex®, Cordiet®

3) Nicotinic acid and nicotinamide

Sources : Nicotinic acid is present in large quantities in rice polishing, liver, milk, eggs and in lesser quantities in potatoes and vegetables. Nicotinic acid and nicotinamide are synthesised in fairly easy manner by oxidation and amidation of β-picoline.

Chemistry : Nicotinic acid or niacin is chemically pyridine 3-carboxylic acid. The amide-nicotinamide or niacinamide differs from the acid in being freely soluble in water. Niacin occurs as white or off-white crystals, sparingly soluble in water, but heat resistant. The amide is also a

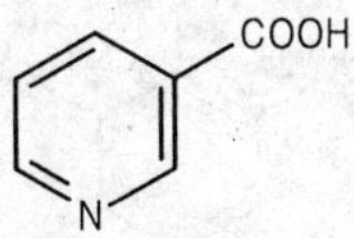

Nicotinic acid

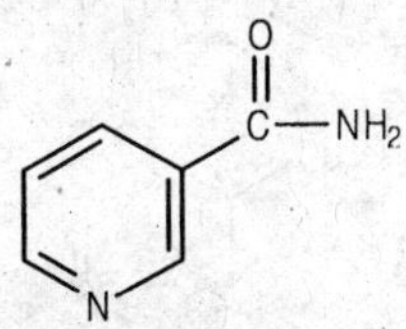

Nicotinamide

white crystalline powder.

Physiological, Biochemical functions and therapeutic uses : Deficiency of niacin causes the deficiency disease called pellagra. The characteristic features of pellagra are dermatitis, pigmentation of skin, anorexia, lethargy, mental confusion and in extreme cases degeneration of spinal cord and spastic paraplegia. Nicotinic acid causes peripheral vasodilation by direct relaxation of the vascular smooth muscle and causes flushing. Large doses of nicotinic acid are known to lower serum cholesterol levels.

Biochemically active forms of nicotinic acid are nicotinamide adenine dinucleotide (NAD) and its phosphate (NADP). These two coenzymes are involved in many biochemical pathways of protein and amino acid metabolism and in electron transfer reactions in the respiratory chain.

Therapeutically, niacin is used to treat pellagra in the dose of 50 to 500 mg. Usually, nicotinamide is preferred. It is also used in the treatment of peripheral vascular disorders.

Dose : Daily requirement - 15 to 20 mg

In pellagra - 50 to 500 mg

Therapeutic dose - 50 to 250 mg

4) Pyridoxine (Vitamin B_6)

Source : Pyridoxine is present in yeast, cereals, legumes, milk and meat. All the three forms of pyridoxine are converted to pyridoxal phosphate in the body, which is considered to be the active form.

Chemistry : Pyridoxine, pyridoxal and pyridoxamine are together known as vitamin B_6. These are the derivatives of pyridine and have the following structures.

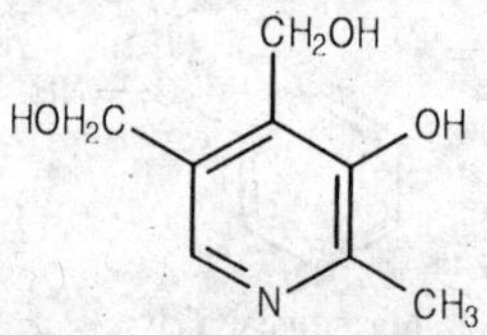

Pyridoxine

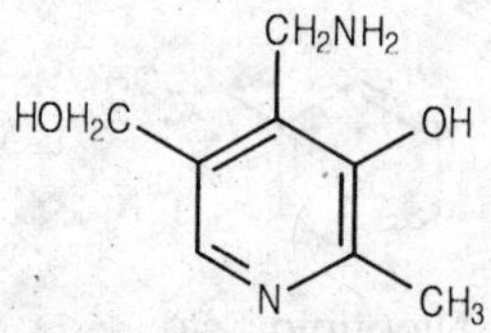

Pyridoxamine

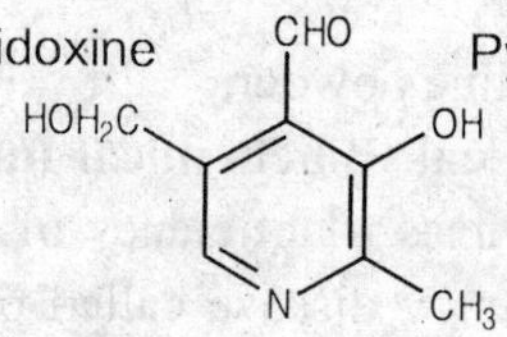

Pyridoxal

All the three forms are converted to pyridoxal phosphate in the body.

Physiological, biochemical functions and therapeutic uses : There are no clear cut symptoms of pyridoxal deficiency in man. But deficiency may cause lesions of skin and mouth, peripheral neuritis, convulsions. Macrocytic anaemia may result due to inadequate utilisation of iron for erythropoiesis. Deficiency syndromes in infants result in indigestion of milk, irritability, twitching and failure to gain weight.

Biochemically active form of pyridoxine is pyridoxal phosphate which is a coenzyme for amino acid decarboxylases and transaminases. It is, thus, intimately involved in the synthesis and degradation of biogenic amines like catecholamine, 5-HT and other biologically important agents like GABA.

Pyridoxine is used to treat convulsions due to its deficiency. Anaemia, secondary to its deficiency, usually responds to 50 to 150 mg daily dose of the vitamin. Pyridoxine is also found to be useful in controlling vomiting during pregnancy and in radiation sickness. It is somewhat useful in muscular dystrophies but without conclusive benefits.

Dose : Prophylactic 2 mg a day.

Therapeutic 10 to 150 mg daily in divided doses.

Brand Names : B-long®, Pyricontin®, Vitriv-B®

5) Pantothenic acid

Source : Pantothenic acid is found in yeast, wheat, peanuts, cereals and milk. Liver contains large amount of this vitamin. It is also made synthetically.

Chemistry : Pantothenic acid chemically is a derivative of aminopropionic acid and is a straight chain compound. β-alanine (an amino acid) is one of its degradation products. It occurs as an odourless, white microcrystalline powder. It is very soluble in water and is unstable in acid and alkali.

Physiological, Biochemical functions and therapeutic uses : Pantothenic acid forms an integral part of the coenzyme A (CoA) molecule which takes part in several biochemical pathways such as transfer of acetyl group, through Acetyl CoA, in fatty acid metabolism, carbohydrate metabolism, etc. In drug metabolism also, CoA takes part through benzoyl - CoA, succinyl-CoA as its 'active' forms.

Although pantothenic acid deficiency in man is not known, in animals, its deficiency causes dermatitis, retardation of growth, loss and depigmentation of hair.

However, pantothenic acid as calcium salt is employed in variety of conditions, such as streptomycin toxicity, in some post-operative conditions and in rheumatoid arthritis. It is used as a member of vitamin B complex formulations.

Dose : Calcium pantothenate - 10 to 50 mg

Dexpanthenol - IM or IV 250 to 500 mg.

6) Biotin

Biotin is an organic acid, containing an imidazolidone, a thiophene ring (joined together) and a valeric acid side chain.

Biotin takes part as a coenzyme in numerous carboxylation reactions. Although biotin deficiency in man is not known, it can be artificially created by feeding large amounts of raw egg white which contains avidin. Therefore biotin was called 'egg-white-injury' curative factor.

Daily requirements of this vitamin are not well established and since deficiency syndromes are not established, this vitamin finds little therapeutic applications.

Brand Names : Essvit®, Essvit-M®

7) Folic acid (Pteroylglutamic acid)

Source : Folic acid is found in both animal and vegetable sources. Liver, yeast, leafy vegetables are good sources of this vitamin. It is also prepared synthetically.

Chemistry : Folic acid molecule contains three main parts namely pteridine, p-amino benzoic acid and L-glutamic acid. (Fig. 30.1)

It is a yellow or yellowish orange coloured, tasteless, crystalline compound. It is practically insoluble in water, but soluble in alkaline solutions. Sodium salt of folic acid is freely soluble in water and injections can be made by cold sterilisation process.

Physiological, Biochemical functions and therapeutic uses : Folic acid and vitamin B_{12} are intimately involved in the treatment of macrocytic and megaloblastic anaemias. In both these conditions, folic acid duplicates the effects of liver therapy and increases the reticulocytes, red and white blood cells, platelets and haemoglobin. Folic acid performs a specific function in the maturation of the various cells of bone marrow.

Folic acid, through its active forms such as folinic acid, tetrahydrofolic acid (THFA), N_5-N_{10}-methylene THFA, N_5-methyl-THFA and formimino THFA (-CH=NH) takes part in the introduction of single carbon unit into purines, pyrimidines, nucleotides and hence in the synthesis of DNA. It is also involved in some amino acid conversions, like histidine. Therefore, a large number of structural modifications of folic acid have been synthesised as antimetabolites of folic acid, with the hope to find a chemotherapeutic agent against cancer.

Dose : Prophylactic dose : 0.2 to 0.5 mg a day

Therapeutic dose in anaemias : 5 to 20 mg a day

Brand Names : Folvit®, Fol-5®, Sysfol®

8) Vitamin B_{12} (Cyanocobalamin)

Source : Vitamin B_{12} is found only in animal sources. Liver and kidney are the richest sources of this vitamin. It is also present in milk and eggs. Commercially vitamin B_{12} is made by fermentation.

Chemistry : Vitamin B_{12} is a cobalt and cy-

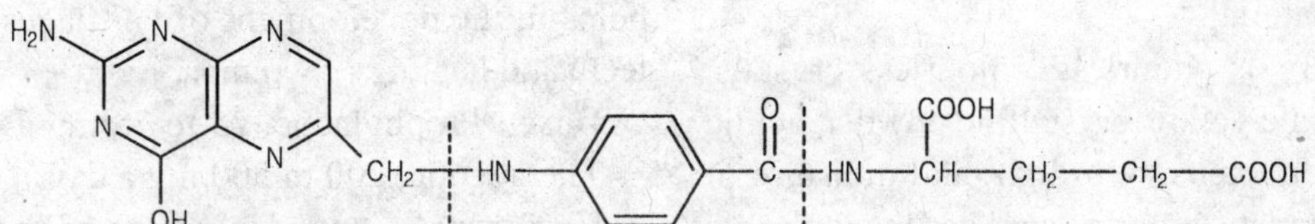

Fig. 30.1

ano containing compound having a complex structure containing porphyrins; 5,6 dimethylbenzimidazole, 1-aminopropanol and α-ribazole moieties.

It occurs as a dark bright red, odourless, hygroscopic crystalline powder. It is sparingly soluble in water (1:80). The solutions can be sterilised by autoclaving. It is not stable with oxidising and reducing agents.

Physiological and Biochemical function and uses : Vitamin B_{12} is most effective in the treatment of pernicious anaemia and its resulting neurological complications. In pernicious anaemias, it is believed that it is the failure to absorb vitamin B_{12} from the GI tract, due to lack of "intrinsic factor". Before vitamin B_{12} could be made by fermentation, purified animal liver extracts, were widely used as "anti- pernicious principle", to treat anaemias.

Dose : In anaemias : 1 to 2 mg, in divided doses by IM injection. For maintenance : 250 mcg every three to four weeks.

Brand Names : Cobadex forte®

9) Ascorbic acid (Vitamin C)

Source : Rich sources of vitamin C are abundant in vegetables and fruits. Citrus fruits of all kinds like lemons, oranges, tomatoes, mangoes are rich in vitamin C. Green vegetables, germinated cereals, potatoes also have good amount of vitamin C. 1 ml of lemon juice contains as much as 0.5 mg of this vitamin.

Chemistry : Ascorbic acid is chemically related to the carbohydrate 2-keto-1-gulonic acid and it is actually synthesised from D-glucose as starting material.

It occurs as odourless, colourless crystals, white or pale yellow crystalline powder, acidic in taste. On exposure to light and moisture, it turns brownish. Ascorbic acid has the ionisable hydrogens, and in presence of oxidising agents,

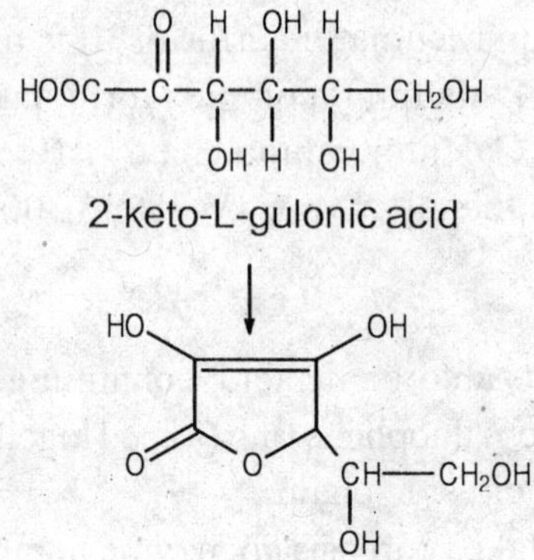

2-keto-L-gulonic acid

Ascorbic acid

quickly gets converted to dehydroascorbic acid.

Physiological and Biochemical functions and uses : Since very early times of Columbus and other voyagers of the 16th century, outbreak of scurvy due to vitamin C deficiency is known. Sailors after long voyages on sea would get this disease, which would get dramatically cured, after landing and eating fresh fruits.

Ascorbic acid deficiency leads to the development of scurvy, which is characterised by perifollicular hemorrhage, particularly in saddle areas and posterior thigh. Other symptoms are swollen or inflamed joints, spongy gums and loss of appetite, etc.

Ascorbic acid and its oxidation product dehydroascorbic acid are intimately involved in many oxidation-reduction reactions of biological importance such as respiration. It is involved in carbohydrate metabolism and in the oxidation of aminoacids phenylalanine and tyrosine. It is required for the functional integrity of -SH group of enzymes and therefore takes part in the collagen and intracellular matrix formation. It thus helps in the development of cartilages, bones, teeth and healing of wounds.

Dose : Prophylactic, 25 to 75 mg a day

Therapeutic, 200 to 500 mg a day

However, prolonged ingestion of large quantities of vitamin C in the belief of cure for cancer or prevention of common cold may lead to the formation of oxalates in urine and ultimately to the formation of kidney stones.

Brand Names : Celin®, Chewcee®, Limcee®

Multivitamin Combinations

Multivitamin formulations in the form of tablets, capsules and liquid-orals are now aggressively marketed by companies and widely prescribed by the physicians. Prophylactic multivitamin preparations should contain about 1 to 1.5 times the recommended dietary allowance (except vitamin D which should not exceed recommended dietary allowance). The recommended daily allowance for various vitamins for adults per day are given in Table 30.2.

Multivitamin preparations for therapeutic use may contain 4 to 5 times the recommended daily allowance. Selective deficiency of one single vitamin occurs rarely in a population which takes fairly nutritious food regularly. Hence, multivitamin therapy is commonly employed prophylactically and also therapeutically for the management of generalised avitaminosis. Multivitamin therapy should be used only for deficiency states and during periods of increased vitamin requirements such as pregnancy or during convalescence period. Its indiscriminate use as dietary supplements to "keep energy and vigour" is wasteful and may be even harmful. Moreover, some of these preparations are very expensive as they contain massive doses of water soluble vitamins, which get washed out and excreted in urine within 24 hours.

Megavitamin therapy or 'Forte' multivitamin preparations contain several times the amounts of vitamins required for normal body metabolism. Such therapy has been advocated only in selective disorders or in selective situations like convalescence period after a massive antibiotic therapy. But in normal population such megavitamin or forte vitamin preparations are not at all needed. It is a misguided attempt by many a people to take such preparations regularly with the hope for better "vitality and vigour" which may actually result in adverse effects of some of the vitamins like vitamin D, vitamin C, folic acid or pyridoxine.

Marketed products containing vitamins B_1, B_2, B_6, nicotinamide, folic acid and calcium pantothenate include - Becosules®, Beneuron® Forte, Beplex®, Cebexin®, Cobadex® Forte,

Table 30.2 : Recommended dietary allowance (dose) of vitamins for adults/day

Vitamin	Recommended Dose	
	For Indian population by ICMR	For World population by WHO/FAO
Vitamin A	750 mcg	750 mcg
Vitamin D	5 mcg (200 IU)	2.5 mcg (100 IU)
Thiamine	1.2 to 2.0 mg	1.0 To 1.5 mg
Riboflavin	1.3 to 2.2 mg	1.3 to 2.1 mg
Pyridoxine	–	1.5 to 2.0 mg
Niacin	16 to 26 mg	–
Vitamin C	50 mg	30 mg
Folic acid	100 mcg	200 mcg
Vitamin B_{12}	1 mcg	2 mcg

Polybion®.

Exercise

Q1. Define and classify Vitamins with examples. Write properties and uses of Ascorbic acid (vitamin C). (Winter 04, Karnataka Univ., Summer 03)

Q2. Name the vitamin, deficiency of which leads to : i) Beri-beri, ii) Pellagra, iii) Scurvy & iv) Xerophthalmia. (Summer 06)

Q3. Define and classify vitamins. Give names of vitamins and their sources, that are useful in treating : i) Dental carrie ii) Anemia iii) Scurvy iv) Poor blood clotting v) Xerophthalmia. (May-June 04)

Q4. Define Vitamins. Classify them and write a note on fat-soluble vitamins. (Nov 06)

Index

Bibliography

1) Block J. H. & Beale J. M. (Ed.): Wilson & Gisvold's Textbook of Organic Medicinal and Pharmaceutical Chemistry; Lippincott Williams & Wilkins, Philadelphia, 2004.

2) Brunton L. L., Lazo J. S. & Parker K. L. (Ed.): Goodman & Gilman's. The Pharmacological Basis of Therapeutics, McGraw Hill, New York, USA, 2006.

3) Finar I. L.: Organic Chemistry Vol. 1 & 2; Pearson Education Ltd., Essex, UK, 1975 (Indian Reprint 2006).

4) Moffat A. C. (Ed.): Clarke's Analysis of Drugs & Poisons, Pharmaceutical Press, London, UK, 2004.

5) Morrison R. T. & Boyd R. N.: Organic Chemistry; Pearson Education, Inc., Essex, UK, 1992 (Indian Reprint 2006).

6) Shargel L., Mutnick A. H., Souney P. F. & Swanson L. N. (Ed.): Comprehensive Pharmacy Review, Lippincott Williams & Wilkins, Philadelphia, 2004.

7) Williams D. A. & Lemke T. L. (Ed.): Foye's Principles of Medicinal Chemistry; Lippincott Williams & Wilkins, Philadelphia, 2002.

8) British Pharmacopoeia 2005, Vol. I – IV: The Stationary Office on behalf of MHRA, London, 2005.

9) European Pharmacopoeia: Directorate for Quality of Medicines, Council of Europe (EDQM), Strasbourg, France, 2004

10) Indian Pharmacopoeia: Minister of Health & Family Welfare, Government of India, New Delhi, 2007..

11) The Merck Index: Merck & Co., Inc., Whitehouse Station, NJ, 2001.

12) United States Pharmacopoeia. (USP 25& NF 20): U. S. P. Convention Inc., Rockville, USA, 2002.